McGraw-Hill Series in Nursing

LUCILE PETRY, *Consulting Editor*

Careers for Nurses

McGraw-Hill Series in Nursing

LUCILE PETRY, *Consulting Editor*

CAREERS FOR NURSES

Dorothy Deming, R.N.

Consultant, Public Health Nursing
Professional Examination Service
American Public Health Association
Formerly General Director
National Organization for Public Health Nursing

SECOND EDITION

New York   Toronto   London
McGRAW-HILL BOOK COMPANY, INC.
1952

CAREERS FOR NURSES

Library of Congress Catalog Card Number: 51-12598

*The names of doctors, patients, and nurses used
by the nurse-writers of the job descriptions in
this book and by the author are purely fictitious;
they are not intended to belong to any living
person or persons. Any resemblance to actual
individuals is purely a matter of coincidence.*

THE MAPLE PRESS COMPANY, YORK, PA.

FOREWORD

You have read a great many books in whole or in part as you studied nursing. There were texts on sciences and nutrition; there were references on psychology and new therapies, reports on medical research, manuals on nursing care, bulletins on vital statistics, studies of patients' problems, and even novels about community and interpersonal relationships. All these you read to understand patients and the nursing of patients.

Here is a book written about and for *you*. When you entered a nursing school, you chose nursing as a career. Actually, nursing is a great variety of careers. Now, about to graduate or to seek a new position, you are choosing that one career in nursing in which you can serve most effectively and in which you can find greatest personal satisfaction. "Careers for Nurses" is presented to you as a guide in making a wise choice.

Dorothy Deming, the author of this book, has had wide experience herself. She has traveled extensively and knows nurses and nursing everywhere. This book is a series of delightful conversations with her. She may tell you of opportunities you haven't thought of. She will help you to line up the advantages and disadvantages so that you may make an intelligent decision. She will help you to make a long-term plan as well as an immediate plan. She will guide you in that decision about continued study and answer questions about details of applying for a position in person or by mail. She will tell you how to use professional placement services.

To participate in these conversations with you, Miss Deming has invited successful young nurses to tell you what they like about the work they are now doing. Perhaps these informal, friendly chats will lead you not only to analyze the advantages and the disadvantages of various types of positions, but also to analyze yourself as to your talents, interests, and preparation. The conversations set a pattern that you can follow if you wish to discuss your problems and your decisions with still other nurses and interested persons.

With the sound advice so charmingly given here and with your own intelligent analysis of your plans, you can move forward into a rewarding way of life, both professionally and personally.

LUCILE PETRY

PREFACE TO THE SECOND EDITION

The first edition of this book was written at the close of the Second World War. It was written especially for the thousands of cadet nurses just graduating from schools of nursing and for the nurses being discharged from the armed forces who were returning to civilian service with fresh perspective on the career opportunities in nursing. Since then the years of peace in the United States have moved nursing forward and outward, new fields have opened, higher salaries have been established, and more opportunities for postgraduate education have been developed. About forty-five thousand students now graduate from our schools of nursing each year and still search eagerly for the branch of nursing in which they can serve best.

This second edition has been almost entirely rewritten, with the necessary changes to bring it up to date. It has been prepared without the sense of postwar pressures, but with the ever-present awareness that a third world war may disrupt the most carefully planned career. The aims of the book, however, remain the same: to assist professional nurses to select the specialty best suited to their interests and abilities, to prepare for it, to apply for a position in it, and to grow in it.

The arrangement of each chapter is planned to facilitate quick reference to sources of employment, and lists of additional reading materials appear at the end of each chapter. A bibliography on counseling and guidance forms Appendix B, and at the request of many nurses, brief suggestions for making a recruiting speech are offered in Appendix C. Practical nursing, together with its opportunities, has been added as a last chapter in the book.

All the descriptions of on-the-job experiences—the heart of each chapter —have been reviewed, rewritten, or newly prepared. The authors are successful nurses, qualified for their positions and actively at work in the field they describe. The writer is very much indebted to them for interrupting their own busy programs long enough to put down the informal account of "what goes on" day by day and how they feel about it all.

The list of those who have contributed suggestions for this revised edition is even longer than in 1946. It seems particularly appropriate to mention with grateful appreciation the nurse consultants in the specialties in the national and Federal agencies who actually wrote whole paragraphs for me to incorporate in the book. I have also had the advice of those who interview and place nurses as well as of employers in large and small agencies. I have talked with student nurses about to select their first jobs and with young graduates in the act of changing their jobs. In short, the book is a cooperative enterprise, almost a team activity, of more than a hundred people, and I could not, even if I would, say who has contributed most to its pages. From 2 hours of conference granted by the president of a national agency to 1 hour of play foregone by my little Scottie dog so that I could finish typing a chapter, time has been generously given by all involved, not forgetting a very patient publisher. My appreciation for such help is deep and lasting.

DOROTHY DEMING, R.N.

New York, N.Y.
January, 1952

HOW THIS BOOK CAME
TO BE WRITTEN

Sarah Brinton, R.N., M.A., stood at her office window in Harrison Hospital and watched the swirling snowstorm usher in an early twilight. From where she stood she could see the lighted windows of the west wing of the hospital and on the other side, partly veiled by the drifting snow, the gaunt steel girders of the new east wing under construction. Ten years, she reflected, ten years today as superintendent of this hospital and never a moment of peace! She had dragged the institution out of the debts left by the depression only to see it plunge into the war shortages of personnel and matériel. Shortly, now, there would be another hundred beds in the new wing. Growth, change, challenge—always more to do, more to learn, wider horizons to reach! How she loved it!

A knock sounded on her door, which opened at once, and Dr. Forsythe, president of the board of trustees, stepped in. He carried a rosy cyclamen plant in full bloom.

"A small recognition of the anniversary, Miss Brinton." He beamed at the superintendent and placed the plant on the window-sill. "Congratulations!".

"Thank you! How *do* you remember the date so accurately, Dr. Forsythe?"

"Because your arrival was a momentous day for Harrison Hospital, and tonight you have come to another milestone. How would you like to take six student nurses from Memorial Hospital for general ward experience? Seems that hospital hasn't enough clinical material to meet state requirements and—"

"Of course! With our new wing we shall have more than enough patients, and we can develop a school of nursing as soon as Mrs. Green and I can find qualified instructors."

Dr. Forsythe chuckled. "I offer you six students and you found a school of nursing! Excellent. The endowment fund was established with that purpose in mind. Now we shall prepare the best student nurses in the country and our patients will get the best care!"

Miss Brinton spoke quickly, "Ah, but those are not our only goals, Doctor. Our school must turn out the best *graduate* nurses in the country. I want to prepare every student for the professional specialty for which she is best fitted. From the day she enters here, each girl will be observed, tested, and guided toward the professional field for which she is suited *after* graduation. I want to send out successful graduate nurses, not just provide skilled students for our own patients here."

"I'm with you there!"

"There ought to be a book—a book for young graduates as well as students—that would describe all the wonderful opportunities open to nurses. Something to help them select a satisfying career and build wisely toward it. We need that kind of guidebook very much."

"Good. Let's find someone to write it so we can use it in building careers for nurses."

Well, here it is, Dr. Forsythe: "Careers for Nurses." I hope you and Miss Brinton like it, and all the students and graduates everywhere for whom it is written.

My warm appreciation goes to those many professional nurses whose accounts of their work in the following chapters brighten and make factual the descriptions of the various nursing specialties. Also to the many others, including student nurses, who have shared information with me, made suggestions as to the content of the book, and offered ideas, I should like to express my formal thanks.

DOROTHY DEMING, R.N.

New York, N.Y.
October, 1946

TO DIRECTORS, SUPERVISORS, INSTRUCTORS AND OTHER COUNSELORS OF NURSES

The material in this book is intended to give you a bird's-eye view of the various fields of work open to student nurses and graduates seeking new positions. Many chapters will merely supplement your own knowledge of requirements for the special fields. There will be other chapters in which the writer hopes you will find fresh information pertinent to the problems of employment that nurses bring to you. The last part of Chap. I has suggestions useful for interviewing applicants.

This is an age of specialization in nursing as well as in many other professions. We owe it to our students to acquaint them as early as possible in their nursing experience with the various fields of specialized service for which they may prepare. The information should not be saved until they are ready to graduate but should be available to them currently as they study the subjects in which a high degree of specialization has been achieved. Thus, by the time they reach the course in professional adjustments, they should be ready to prepare a list of careers which appeal to them and for which they have already learned the prerequisites. They should have discussed the opportunities with their advisers and made plans for the first steps toward their goals. Good counseling never seeks a final answer for the young nurse looking for her first job. It merely attempts to lay the appropriate opportunities before her and suggest a direction in which to start.

It is suggested that this book be placed where it can be picked up and read by the students and graduates at any time and that assigned reading be given to students when a specialty is being studied or previous to an affiliation in a specialty. If observation of formal advanced clinical nursing programs is not possible in the parent hospital, or if there is no opportunity for observing a specialty, such as industrial nursing, in the community, the related chapter and suggested reading will partially fill the gap and open the way to class discussions. A perusal of the pertinent chapters might well be a preliminary to lectures by the representatives of the various national, Federal, or state nursing organizations who are so frequently invited to speak to student bodies.

Special attention has been given to the personal qualities desirable in each field of work, to help counselors guide students and graduates to an appropriate choice of occupation. For the most part, these are valid discriminations. For example, the nurse who dislikes teaching or is very self-conscious, shy, and retiring is not a likely candidate for public health nursing, but she would do a good job in research; the nurse who is imaginative, creative, and enjoys change and a constant contact with new situations and people will not be happy as supervisor of an operating room but would be satisfied in the out-patient service. If a young nurse has her heart set on a certain position, it is well to let her try it, the authorities believe, the counselor having done her duty by pointing out the demands of the chosen field and the applicant's shortcomings, if she has them. It does no harm for the newly graduated nurse to explore the possibilities of several specialties, provided the experience is under good supervision. Nurses do not automatically fall into particular niches, like oranges screened for size. Most people, including nurses, can do more than one job well, but a maximum of ability without interest and liking brings less satisfaction than keen interest plus a second or even third degree of ability.

This book makes no attempt to touch upon the principles of counseling and guidance, which constitute a specialized field. It merely offers information regarding the fields into which students and graduates may be guided. When, how, by whom, or where guidance and counseling are given depends on the organization of the school or employment agency. The plan should be formulated and directed by a person *qualified in this specialty* and, for students, integrated throughout their curriculum and practice. All too few schools of nursing have sought the advice of trained counselors.

It has been suggested that part-time consultant service from trained vocational counselors may guide faculty and students in developing an effective program in a school of nursing. Small schools do not always take advantage of as much part-time service from colleges, universities, and other recognized sources as they might. There are also advantages to an elective experience as an aid to senior nurses in vocational choice. Such electives may offer a wide and desirable variation from the home hospital experiences.[1]

In this specialized field of guidance and placement, tests of various types are used as tools in guiding and placing individuals. A word regarding their function is necessary here. Tests of any kind, to be relied upon, must be in competent hands. The type used in testing for job placement should be compiled and administered by people trained to give tests. It is essential that the results be interpreted by an experienced staff who understand the limitations and advantages of various types of tests and their proper application to the individual's case. Those who take this responsibility should be members of the American Psychological Association. Advice and assistance in arranging tests can usually be secured from the department of psychology in colleges and universities, or from the American Psychological Association. Aptitude and guidance tests are "skilled procedures," as we nurses would say. Like a nursing treatment, they can do more harm than good in untrained hands.

Student nurses are familiar with tests of all sorts. They have had aptitude tests preceding acceptance in their schools and examinations, quizzes, ratings, and term papers along the way. They anticipate "finals," "comprehensives," "orals," and "state boards" before they can secure graduate and registered nurse status. It is well to accustom them to the idea of additional tests when they apply for future positions or attempt to qualify for university matriculation or for job promotion. Colleges and universities will almost surely give entering or qualifying tests in a more or less formal way, as well as course examinations. Civil Service (merit system) appointments frequently are made only from those satisfactorily completing a written examination. Increasingly, other employment agencies are giving preemployment and promotional tests, and employers are using tests as in-service guidance and training tools.

The point to emphasize with prospective job applicants is that tests are but one part of the appointing or placement procedure and that any well-qualified nurse has nothing to fear from them. They can be, as a matter of fact, of great service to the candidate in helping her strengthen her weak points, in placing her in congenial work, and in saving her from the bitter experience of finding a job too difficult for her.

[1] For example, see BIXLER, ELIZABETH S.: Elective Experience for Seniors, *American Journal of Nursing*, p. 673, October, 1950; also Career Studies for Senior Nurses, *American Journal of Nursing*, p. 101, February. 1951.

Another special type of test of inestimable value to nurses, when in proper hands, is that offered by vocational and guidance services to candidates who are trying to discover their special aptitudes or "bent." Sometimes these assist an unsuccessful, discouraged nurse to find her proper sphere and "make good." The battery of tests may include interest tests; reading time and comprehension test; scholastic aptitude, manipulation, and vocabulary tests.

Nor must counselors overlook the nurse who needs more than guidance, advice, encouragement, and information. There will always be some students and graduate nurses who need both psychological and psychiatric guidance service before they will be able to succeed or be happy in any job. These services should be on tap and should be consulted freely by all those assuming the very grave responsibility of influencing the future lifework of human beings.

A reading list of interest to those who counsel appears in Appendix B under Guidance. Familiarity with the contents of the books in the list and with this book will not be a substitute for professional guidance and counseling service in schools of nursing and in employment agencies. Such a service should be directed by a full- or part-time specialist familiar with the tools and techniques of guidance and the principles of counseling, working through all those in contact with students or applicants, wherever they are. It is especially important for the counselor to be familiar with the changing trends in employment and the shifts in the demand for nurses and the supply of them.

CONTENTS

CHAPTER I

Choosing a Career

To you who have taken the important step of becoming a nurse, the world is beckoning. A wide field of useful service which should return personal satisfactions and professional success awaits your choice. What shall it be? Nursing in hospitals, homes, clinics, schools, industries, on transportation lines, in the country, in the city, here, or abroad? Do you like to be your own boss and work alone, or do you prefer to be one of a staff of 20, or 100, or 1,000 nurses? Do you want to seek out the unusual job like missionary work in Africa or industrial nursing on a rubber plantation in Brazil, or would you like to be in charge of a 10-bed hospital in Alaska or teach nursing in Hawaii? Perhaps you cling to city life and would prefer to work in the office of a world-famous surgeon, in a hotel of 800 guests, or in the largest department store in the world. Or, if you have an artistic bent, would connections with an art museum, a theater, a library, or a Hollywood movie studio appeal to you? If a yen to be near writers, or to write, is yours, you may find a job as an industrial nurse in a large publishing house, a newspaper office, or a printing firm—or yourself be the editor of a professional journal.

Then there are the "specialties," the advanced clinical nursing fields that we know as medical, surgical, obstetric, pediatric, orthopedic, and psychiatric nursing, to say nothing of industrial nursing, public health, the fields of nursing education and administration in all types of agencies and institutions. The demand for nurse educators far exceeds supply.

If you enjoy travel, you might want to join the staff of one of the national or Federal agencies. Here you would travel all over the United States, quite possibly abroad. The United Nations and the World Health

1

Organization provide opportunities to travel to distant countries and quite literally to "see the world." However extraordinary your ambition, nursing offers something to match it, together with the reassurance that you are always prepared for emergencies—those of war when you can serve your country through the armed forces, that of disaster when you respond to the call of the American Red Cross,[1] or those in your own home town, when your family, friends, and neighbors turn to you in extremity. The demand for nurses, especially for those well qualified, has not been filled in the last 10 years, and even in time of general unemployment there has always been a place at the top for well-prepared nurses. You have chosen a profession that is always wanted, needed, and entering upon a great future. It is your responsibility now to pick the field of nursing in which you can serve best and be happiest.

DECIDING ON A CAREER
GENERAL CONSIDERATIONS

Most of us do well the work that interests us, and usually we grow interested in the work we find we can do well. This book is intended as a guide in choosing the branch or specialty of professional nursing that suits you best. It should save you both time and money by helping you to discover, without too many trials and errors, which job appeals to you and fits your abilities and qualifications. After a thoughtful reading of the description of the job of your choice, it should not be necessary for you to say, a few months after taking a job, "But I did not know special training was needed for this type of work," or "If I had only known I would have to teach in this position, I would never have taken it!"

This book presents information about employment in the major fields of nursing. It stresses the beginning or entering positions in each field, rather than the supervisory and administrative responsibilities, although in each specialty the future opportunities for advancement are indicated. Unless otherwise stated, the fields described in this book are open to registered nurses of either sex.

The second half of this chapter offers suggestions to guide a nurse (a) in making application for a position, (b) in attending a personal interview, and (c) in deciding whether or not to accept a job. The chapters in the rest of the book are divided into three parts:

[1] For the addresses of all organizations mentioned in this chapter, see Appendix A.

1. Information about the field as a whole, its scope, requirements (educational and personal), salary ranges, and future opportunities
2. A description of the work in each major field written by a successful nurse on active duty in that field, in her own words
3. A list of sources of employment and a reading list which offers more information about the field

HOW STUDENT NURSES MAY USE THIS BOOK

If you already know what you want to do after graduation from your school of nursing, turn to the description of that job (see Table of Contents) and find out what special requirements and personal qualifications are desirable among applicants in this field. Read the story of the nurse who has won professional success and personal satisfaction in work of this kind and then, if you are not already familiar with the books and articles on the subject, look up some of the reading references to give you further insight and information in your chosen field. Consult with your faculty advisers regarding your choice. Then consider carefully the special training (or additional general experience) you will need, where you can get it, what it will cost, and where you can apply for financial aid, should that be needed. If a job is to precede special study, note the sources of employment for work in your chosen field. In selecting your first job be sure to seek guidance from a qualified professional counselor.

If you are *not* sure which field of nursing interests you, even after consulting with your faculty advisers, read all the sketches written by nurses "on the job." Which one appeals to you most? Which ones do you feel you could do? Read the rest of the chapter in which each of them appears. Then list your choices in order and talk them over with your faculty adviser. She may suggest that you study the field more closely, talk with nurses already employed in it, or visit them at their work before making a decision. *It is never too early to be thinking about your future career.* You will be a jump ahead of your classmates if you can decide upon a specialty before you graduate and make your plans accordingly.

GRADUATE NURSES

If you are one of the many nurses still undecided as to your specialty, or if you are thinking of making a change from your present job to another field of nursing, then after reading this chapter, browse through the list of specialties in the Table of Contents and check those that interest you. Read all of each chapter carefully, thinking always of your own abilities, educational qualifications, likes and dislikes in relation to the job described and to its future opportunities and financial returns compared to those in your present position. Check the places at which you will apply for a job.

STUDENTS AND GRADUATES

Do not be afraid to think of yourself in the highest paid position described in this book, but be realistic about it and consider carefully what is said about prerequisites in relation to the following points:

1. Educational qualifications: What basic and advanced courses or special training are necessary?
2. Years of experience: How many years of experience (of what type and where) are called for? Must the experience have been under supervision?
3. Character of the responsibilities: What are the duties of the job?

Under this last heading there may be duties expected of you which you have never undertaken or which you would not want to undertake at any salary; for example, constant travel, a heavy assignment of public speaking, or a program of academic teaching entirely removed from contact with patients. Nearly every top-salaried position in nursing today carries with it considerable administrative responsibility, desk work, overtime, public appearances, addresses at conventions, and committee work. The positions paying more than $6,000 are reached mainly through successive and successful job experiences over a period of at least 7 or 8 years. One almost never jumps from staff nursing to a directorship. Nevertheless, if the top is where you want to go, the trail to the summit is blazed for you in this book, and the short cuts, if any, are indicated.

THE FIRST JOB

Advisers experienced in giving students help in selecting a first job, and vocational counselors redirecting graduate nurses to new fields of employment, stress two points:

1. For the beginner, the position that offers a *solid groundwork* of knowledge and practice is better in the long run than one that skips the

first grades, so to speak, and offers a higher salary with many advanced duties. The bright beginner will progress rapidly anyway, but she will have had the elementary background experience that is fundamental to a clear understanding of the superstructure and absolutely essential if she is ever to *teach* beginners.

For instance, here is a promising young graduate nurse who accepts as her first job the supervision of a new out-patient department in her home-town hospital. For 3 years she struggles along, never failing to meet the demands of the service, but never a growing leader in it. Then she applies for a supervising position in a large city health department and finds she must accept a temporary staff position because she lacks general public health nursing experience under supervision and has had no formal preparation for supervision. She has lost the greater part of 3 years by skipping grades.

A second nurse accepts a staff nurse position under qualified supervision at a moderate salary immediately after graduation. She enrolls in evening classes in her specialty and by her third year she is promoted to be an assistant supervisor. Then, with additional courses, she is appointed as a supervisor 4 years after graduation.

2. The selection of a position under qualified and adequate *supervision* may make the difference between success or failure in the first job. Not only does good supervision assure the inexperienced graduate nurse of a smoother introduction to her new duties, better teaching and skills, but also the development of her capacities and aptitudes for special phases of the work. Promotion—if it is deserved—is more rapid where there is good supervision. The qualified supervisor will put all sorts of unusual opportunities in the way of the promising employee and take time to help her conquer personal difficulties as well as professional inadequacies.

Most important of all, many supervisory and teaching positions state as a definite requirement for the position that the applicant must have had general nursing experience (in hospital, clinic, or homes, depending on the field) *under qualified supervision*. Most of the Civil Service specifications for positions in public health, in institutions and clinics, and many positions on the teaching staffs of schools of nursing and universities, make this a prerequisite for appointment. If you have the choice of beginning your work on a well-supervised staff at a low salary or of accepting a position at a far better salary working alone, be wise: You will get ahead faster, with surer ground under your feet if you start your work under supervision.

CHANGING JOBS

"When should I change jobs?" This is one of the frequent questions that both young and old nurses ask themselves and their advisers. It is easy to say "When you feel like it," but this is a risky rule to follow. Every job has its dark days and its difficulties. The nurse who changes too frequently acquires the reputation of being an unstable worker. She owes a certain loyalty to her employer if she has received an expensive period of training for her job on the job. But there is the opposite extreme: Clinging to a job because it is easy, congenial, and a friendly place to work. Almost before the nurse realizes it, the desire, ability, and capacity to change jobs are gone. She grows into her rut, she cannot see over its sides, and no one wants her anywhere else.

There are of course happy exceptions to this statement. We have nurses who remain in one job all their lives, making it a true life work, growing with it, contributing their best to it, so that one never thinks of B—— Hospital without thinking of Miss A——. But these nurses are usually dynamic leaders. They have never stood still in their jobs. The "followers" by nature will do well to weigh the advantages of change.

It is well to remember another fact regarding a change in job. Among the growing numbers of elderly workers in the population, we may expect to find more nurses actively at work after the age of fifty. A change in job—at least in the type of job—after this age might be unwise both from the standpoint of its demand on physical capacity and mental adjustment, and from the point of view of lively competition.

Between these two extremes, drifting from one job to another and remaining buried in just one, there is a happy medium. Counselors usually ask two questions:

1. Do you feel you are still growing in your present job, does it hold untried responsibilities, fresh developments, and a real future for your talents?
2. Have you reached the limit of what *you* have to give to your present job?

In the latter case, perhaps your need is merely to break away for a year of study or travel. A restocking of your mental furnishings is called for. Whatever may be the cause, and it may be fatigue or ill health, a lagging interest in your job is a warning signal. There is nothing so discouraging to a supervisor or employer as to see a conscientious nurse carrying out her daily duties without zest or love of the work. The end results are bad for all concerned. You should feel free to talk with your advisers or placement counselors about your attitude toward your job. If you do not like it, say so. Genuine interest in and liking for your job are indispensable to success.

The essential point to remember in pursuing a career is that your next step should be *forward*. Marking time or seeking a well-paid, easy job may be a backward step. In nursing, luckily it is almost never too late to change your direction, provided you are physically strong and mentally flexible.

WHAT DO I DO IN THIS JOB?

The job descriptions are the most valuable part of this book. They give you the report of a nurse at work, on the job, writing straight from her own day-by-day experience in her specialty. After you have read them for enjoyment, read them slowly, seeking to see what abilities and training are implied in what the nurse says she does. Picture yourself in her place. Think of the chances for your own growth in such a position. All the authors chosen to write the sketches are experienced nurses and, as you will note, they speak frequently of the value of supervision and of the special courses which have helped them "make good."

The reading lists at the end of each chapter have been selected to provide more information on the conditions under which a nurse serves in the specialized fields and to amplify the desirable qualifications for successful service. They are *not* intended as bibliographies covering the principles, practices, techniques, or policies of nursing service in the specialties. Some semipopular books are included to give you the "feel" of the specialty and an idea of its place in human welfare.

A general reference reading list relating to vocational problems and guidance aids for counselors will be found in Appendix B. Job descriptions appear currently in the *American Journal of Nursing* and in *Public Health Nursing*.

RESIGNATIONS

A word should probably be said regarding resignations from the job. It is customary for nurses holding salaried positions to give at least a month's notice of their withdrawal; if the position is an important one or difficult to fill, 3 to 6 months. A similar courtesy is expected of the employer when a resignation is requested, except when an employee is being dismissed for gross neglect of duty, falsification of records, infringement of rules, or unprofessional conduct, when the dismissal may take effect immediately. These rules are usually defined in the leaflet or outline of personnel policies provided by the employer at the time of appointment.

If, after a reasonable length of service with an agency, you request a leave of absence for study, and if you expect the position to be held for you, you should plan to return and remain with the agency following your leave of absence for at least a year.

THE EMPLOYMENT FIELD FOR SPECIAL GROUPS

MEN NURSES

In 1940, there were 8,169 men who were registered professional nurses or professional students.[2] A sampling of the occupations of 271 men nurses, prior to their entry into the armed forces, indicated that they were usually employed in institutional nursing as supervisors or general staff, in industrial nursing, and in private practice. Men nurses are especially well-fitted for the care of men in mental hospitals, in the heavy industries where employees are chiefly men and liable to serious injuries, and in hospitals with large surgical divisions caring for orthopedic conditions, as in the hospitals of the Veterans Administration. When possible, men nurses usually have the special care of men suffering from diseases of the genitourinary tract and find a need for their help among patients who require supervision in sports, corrective exercises, and the like, where active participation of the supervisor is necessary or desirable. Many elderly male invalids refuse care from women. Men are better suited also to the nursing jobs in labor camps and heavy construction projects, which call for service under very rough or out-of-door conditions. Among the latter are lumbering, exploration, and marine operations, in which the workers are exclusively men. Venereal disease programs in all their phases as they affect men—public health, clinic service, and hospital care and treatment—form a promising field for men nurses.

At present, the most pressing need for professional men nurses exists in the field of psychiatric nursing in the mental hospitals of our country (see Chap. VII); and as this is written, Congress has been asked to con-

[2] *Facts about Nursing*, p. 14, American Nurses Association, 1948. (This is an annual publication.)

sider a bill to "provide for the appointment of male citizens as nurses in the Army, Navy, Air Force and for other purposes."[3]

A comprehensive survey of the opportunities for men nurses in New York State (1948) indicated that

> The existing barriers to the employment of men nurses appear to be due more to sentiment and tradition than to any sound reason of their ineptitude because of sex. The survey shows that there are more positions for men nurses than there are applicants. . . . There are many strong arguments for recruiting men into the nursing profession and for expanding the opportunities for their service.

(The full report may be obtained from the New York State Nurses Association.) It was also found that general hospitals throughout the state were seeking the man nurse for many new positions, one of which was as supervisor of orderlies. Paraplegic and urological nursing, central control supply, admitting wards, treatment clinics, plaster and operating rooms, blood banks, anesthesia, physiotherapy, hydrotherapy, laboratory, pneumothorax therapy, and x-ray were all activities which offered employment to men nurses.

These conclusions concerning New York are probably true for many of the states, especially those with large population.

It is also well to point out that men nurses have found nursing an excellent preparation for collateral positions such as administration (hospital and welfare agencies), personnel work, clinical psychology, scientific research, physical education, first-aid instruction, and editorial work in professional subjects.

Information regarding the activities of men nurses may be secured from the Men Nurses Section of the American Nurses Association and from the American Psychiatric Association.

NEGRO NURSES

The first school for Negro nurses opened in 1891. There are now about ten thousand graduate Negro nurses in the United States. They are employed chiefly in public hospitals in the North and in official and private public health nursing agencies in areas with large numbers of

---

[3] For the progress of this effort, the reader is referred to an article by GREEN, WILLIAM: Men Nurses and the Armed Forces, *American Journal of Nursing*, p. 237, April, 1951.

Negro patients. Only 6 per cent are in private practice and 1 per cent in industry. At this writing only 3 per cent of the graduate nurses in the United States are Negro, while Negroes compose 10 per cent of the population.

Negro nurses are being employed in increasing numbers in Federal agencies and in a consultant capacity to national organizations. During the war the Army and Navy Nurse Corps included them for assignment for active duty. The growing awareness that the health of the Negro is important to the nation as a whole is a forceful argument in favor of recruiting more Negro doctors and nurses. There is no doubt that the war opened many doors heretofore closed to Negro nurses. It is anticipated that the demand for qualified Negro nurses will be greater in the South and continue to grow fairly steadily in Northern cities.

Educational opportunities for Negro nurses are also developing rapidly, both on the basic and advanced clinical levels. A course for Negro nurse-midwives, for example, is currently being offered at Tuskegee Institute, Alabama.[4]

Although salary differentials between white and Negro nurses still exist in the South, positions in the North usually pay equally. The Federal services pay the same to all, as do positions under state and local Civil Service and merit systems.

Opportunities for advancement for Negro nurses are greater in institutional work than in public health. There is pressing need for a larger body of Negro nurses prepared for supervisory, teaching, and administrative positions. A few scholarships are available.

Information regarding the development of new opportunities for Negro nurses may be secured from the American Nurses Association.

SPECIAL FACTORS IN CHOOSING YOUR
FIELD OF SERVICE

In selecting a field for your future career, there are several searching questions which you must answer for yourself or find answers for from outside sources—all of them quite aside from the problem of your capacity to do the job well. The order in which these considerations are listed here is not significant, as it makes no difference where your thoughts start with relation to your work—in the end you will need all the answers.

[4] For information, write to the Children's Bureau, Social Security Administration, Federal Security Agency, Washington, D.C.

Before deciding on a specialty, ask these questions:

1. Is there a fairly universal, constant demand for nursing services in this field? Or is it seasonal, geographically restricted,[5] or declining in frequency or intensity?

2. How fast is the need for nurses in this type of occupation being recognized by the public or, putting the question another way, how general is public support of this service? Is it a "pioneer" field? Is there great competition among nurses in this field, or is it relatively unexplored? What is its probable future?

3. Do I qualify for the beginning positions in this field? If not, how long will it take me to qualify? How much will it cost me? Can I earn while I study? Are the necessary courses easily available at recognized, nearby schools or colleges?

4. How much qualified supervision can I count on?

5. How does the salary compare with other fields for which I am qualified? How long will it take me to reach the maximum salary? Will additional qualifications assure me of higher salary? What is the rate of salary increases? What will be involved in the way of salary deductions for taxes, dues, pension, or insurance?[6]

6. What do the jobs in this field offer in old-age security?

7. Will qualification for this field prepare me for any other field, in case I have to switch? What side-line jobs might it lead to? Is it so highly specialized that I will grow away from the usual nursing services or lose my general skills?

8. Have I special skills or abilities that will put me ahead of others in this field, such as knowledge of a foreign language, stenography, or photography? Are there any drawbacks that would make the job unacceptable to me, such as constant travel (or no travel), absence of

---

[5] It is of interest to note that in 1940, 37.3 per cent of all employed professional nurses were in the Northwestern states, 13.3 per cent in the West. In the Northeastern states, however, there was 1 professional nurse to every 370 persons, and 1 to every 292 persons in the West, while the South, with 20.4 per cent of the nurses, had only 1 nurse to 574 persons! See "Professional Nurses, The Outlook for Women in Occupations in the Medical Services," Women's Bureau, Department of Labor, Washington, D.C., Bulletin 203, No. 3, p. 2, 1945.

[6] It must be pointed out that the salary scales quoted in this book are constantly shifting, that they vary with the area of the country, size of agency, cost of living, and national income level. At present (1951) nurses' salaries are at a high level, the highest in history. Therefore, all *the salary ranges cited must be checked from time to time with local rates.*

supervision (or too close supervision), rural rather than urban life (or vice versa), too much teaching, too little nursing?

9. Are there "leadership potentialities" in this field, or is it all routine?
10. How much chance will a job in this field give me to live my own life when off duty, develop hobbies, study, enjoy recreational activities, travel, or do creative work (such as music, painting, or writing)?

Assuming that you have answered these questions about the job to your satisfaction, the next considerations are about you.

HEALTH

It is eminently appropriate that first and serious consideration be given to your health—now, on the job, and in the future. Are you in good health and able to pass a fairly stiff medical examination for acceptance on a job? Will jobs in your chosen field be a hazard to your health? What will employers do for you if you are sick? What protection is offered you against service-connected illness or injury? It is just plain good sense to consider these points before starting any job in any field.

You have been nursing long enough to know how essential good health is to rendering satisfactory service. A sickly nurse, besides offering low resistance to infections, can seldom give efficient care, makes an unfortunate impression on the public, and is a cause of worry to her observant patients. You owe it to yourself and your job to keep well after graduation and to secure the yearly medical examination—including chest x-ray—to which you should have been accustomed during your school days. Routine visits to your doctor, dentist, and oculist pay dividends in unbroken periods of employment and confidence in yourself.

Some fields of nursing, it is true, demand more resistant physical and mental health than others. The public health nurse is exposed to all kinds of weather and meets more undiagnosed communicable conditions among her patients than does the nurse in the operating room. Yet she has more regular exercise and much more fresh air. The supervising nurse in a mental hospital must develop and foster a reserve of emotional composure to enable her to remain "calm, cool, and collected" under stress, a reserve that is not demanded to so great an extent of the nurse who is working in the private office of an eye specialist. The peculiar physical demands of each job described in this book are indicated at appropriate points.

It is well to remember that many jobs can be adjusted to a nurse's temporary or permanent handicap. The public health nurse who develops a cardiac condition, the operating-room nurse with a game knee, or the industrial nurse with a thoracoplasty may all benefit by rehabilitation, retraining, job placement, or adjustment, just as patients do. The door to the field of a nurse's choice should never be closed against her because of her handicap until it is ascertained that it bars her from any share in any part of the program. Almost every field offers a few opportunities to handicapped nurses, although imagination and initiative are needed in finding nontaxing, out-of-the-ordinary, yet lucrative jobs which can utilize the nursing background.

HEALTH EXAMINATIONS

Employing agencies which follow the best modern practice usually request the candidate for a position to conform to one of the following procedures:

1. Arrange for a complete medical examination by a physician of the employer's choice at the expense of the agency or at a very moderate charge. The examination usually includes all blood tests and a chest x-ray, and is followed, if the candidate is accepted, by any necessary immunizations. If serious defects are found, the applicant may be assisted to correct them before employment, or will be advised to seek more appropriate work.
2. Present a report, on a form supplied by the agency, of physical condition as found by the physician of the applicant's choice. This report is frequently followed by a second examination by the agency's physician before permanent appointment is made.
3. Present a report secured within the last year from a physician of the candidate's choosing. (This is the least satisfactory procedure for all concerned.)

Yearly examinations and x-rays are required by many employing agencies, usually without charge to the employee. The most rigid requirements are usually found in the examinations given by the Federal services, because compensation for disabilities is involved under Civil Service rulings.

HEALTH, HOSPITAL, SICKNESS, AND ACCIDENT INSURANCE

In nearly all institutional positions, a nurse employee is given necessary medical and nursing care without charge, unless extensive treatments or special nursing over a long period are needed. The same professional courtesy is often extended to any sick or injured professional nurse in the community. However, such service cannot always provide the extras that become essentials in critical illness, especially if a nurse is not in her own home town or hospital. It is therefore wise to take out hospital insurance and carry accident and sickness insurance as soon as you start to earn your living outside of your own hospital.[7]

Many agencies offer coverage for illness and hospitalization to their staffs under group insurance contracts. Workmen's compensation laws in nearly all states cover nurses injured while at work or suffering from service-connected compensable illness. These are all points to be checked when applying for a position in your chosen specialty.

SECURITY AND THE FUTURE

Most of us crave a sense of security in our jobs. That is natural and right. A job that is stable and permanent, that promises advancement in an interesting career and a dependable pension or annuity in old age, offers that kind of security. An example is found in the positions in the Veterans Administration. If a nurse is doing acceptable work, Civil Service regulations offer her permanency of position and an increasing salary, promotion, stated vacations, and leaves of absence for sickness, and a generous retirement pension (see Chap. XVI). At the opposite extreme of security is private duty nursing, or private practice, as it is called in this book (see Chap. X). It is uncertain in demand, in length of employment, in degree of difficulty, in amount of pay, and in a secure future. It carries with it no paid vacations, sick leave, or promotion. On the other hand a too-secure job tempts the ambitionless nurse to mark time, grow into fixed habits, and lower her nursing standards. There is much to be said for wholesome competition in an open market.

The degree of security and provisions for the future offered to nurses by the various nursing fields are described in the succeeding chapters. It is perhaps sufficient to point out here that all nurses should—and thousands do—look ahead from the very first day of their working lives to the proverbial rainy day and old age and embark upon a savings plan that will give them protection, as well as a fund to be spent for future fun and self-improvement.

Nurses self-employed in private practice or on salary in so-called

[7] Of the many hospitalization plans available to nurses, the most familiar is the Blue Cross plan.

covered employment may now take advantage of the pension plan offered at age sixty-five by the Old Age and Survivors Insurance program. Many more nurses are now eligible than formerly as a result of congressional extension of the Act in 1950. The current monthly deduction (2¼ per cent from self-employed earnings or 1½ per cent each from employer and employee salary payments) will yield at most to fully insured persons $80 monthly after age sixty-five. Full information as to definitions of covered employment, rate of payment, accumulated funds, anticipated returns, and benefits due survivors—all of which the individual earner will want to investigate carefully—may be secured from the Bureau of Old Age and Survivors Insurance, Social Security Administration, in your neighborhood.[8]

Since even $20 a month for life may be very welcome after you are sixty-five, this Federal insurance plan is well worth looking into. It is a backlog of security around which you should build your whole retirement program. The sooner you enter it, the better will be your monthly pension after age sixty-five.

Fine as is "OASI," it will not yield at most enough to provide a financially ample living after sixty-five, and many nurses must retire before then. It is well to show a wise foresight and plan for a supplementary pension in one of the following ways:

Regular monthly savings, personally made on a well-thought-out plan, or annuities, or both.

Monthly payroll deductions or saving plans offered by the employing agency. Such plans are voluntary. Hospitals as well as many public health nursing agencies take advantage of this plan to provide security for their employed staffs.

One of these plans in which voluntary social, health, and welfare agencies participate is that of the National Health and Welfare Retirement Association, Inc. This offers life insurance and retirement pensions. For information, write to the Association (see Sources of Information, Appendix A). The American Hospital Association is cooperating with this association in offering group plans to hospital staffs.

In the formal and group voluntary plans which may be coordinated with Social Security, the usual monthly payroll deduction is 5 per cent.

Relatively few nurses are now covered by unemployment insurance.

[8] See your telephone book. The main office is in Baltimore, Md.

If you have any question about your status, write to the Social Security Administration in Washington, D.C., or to the office of the U.S. Employment Service nearest you.[9]

MARRIAGE

Unless noted in the job descriptions, married nurses are eligible for most of the positions described in this book. Occasionally a hospital or agency will have vacancies open only to single nurses, or will have set a quota for employment of married nurses. If you are thinking of getting married, it is wise to ask the employer's policy with relation to married nurses. Attitudes toward this vexing problem are far more liberal than they were 10 years ago. Employers are agreed, however, that when married nurses are employed their first responsibility is to their job. Except in genuine emergencies, family illnesses and housekeeping complications must take second place, and the employed nurse is expected to secure other help to release her for her work. It is especially important for employed nurses with little children to have competent and reliable assistance at home, because worry over what is happening to Johnny or Louise in her absence can practically incapacitate the best of nurses. Some employers prefer not to take nurses with babies less than a year old, feeling that such separation is bad for both parties—to say nothing of Father! On the other hand, one director of nurses permitted a member of her staff to bring her two-months-old breast-fed baby to the hospital and provided a sunny room for him in the nurses' home. Both mother and baby flourished, while the student nurses had to be literally driven away from the nursery of their adopted mascot, who was supplying them with firsthand experience in the care of a *well* baby.

MATERNITY LEAVE

Nearly all employers are willing to give maternity leave without requesting a resignation. It is customary in many public agencies to require the employee to inform her supervisor when she becomes pregnant. Great variation exists in the amount of time allowed, or required, before and after the baby's birth. Most nurses prefer to leave work by the seventh or eighth month; some agencies prefer to have them leave as soon as the condition is noticeable.

Modern obstetric advice generally suggests a ruling suited to the conditions of each case. An early leave may be provided for the individual

[9] For retirement provisions for nurses employed by the Federal government, see Chap. XVI.

showing abnormalities, while another may be permitted to work up to the day of delivery. The work, of course, must always be adjusted to the nurse's condition. Heavy lifting, stairs, rough automobile travel (as over rural roads), long standing, or other unwise strains are removed if possible, and the nurse is shifted to easier work.

· After the baby is born, leave is generally continued for at least 3 months, much depending on home circumstances, on the health of mother and baby, and on arrangements for the infant's care.[10]

PERSONAL QUALIFICATIONS

There are certain universal personal qualities that all employers expect to find in a nurse, no matter what specialty or field she represents. (These will not be repeated when discussing the special nursing fields, unless the type of job emphasizes that quality as an outstanding requisite.)

The universally expected personal qualities are neatness, reliability, good judgment, tact, and poise. We often express these qualities in synonymous terms, as good grooming or pleasing personal appearance, accuracy, dependability, honesty, common sense, and emotional stability. An employer expects loyalty, cooperation, and conscientious performance of duties. He usually likes to find initiative, dignity, imagination, and a timely sense of humor. Most positions call for a degree of leadership and ability to act fast in emergencies.

You will notice that most of these qualities are the same that we expect in any good businessman or businesswoman. If, however, we were to pick out any one of them as a first and absolute necessity in a nurse we should have to bow to the popular conception of a professional nurse and stress *neatness*—that shining spotlessness which makes a glance at a nurse like a breath of fresh air. There is something profoundly reassuring about the presence of a perfectly groomed, tidy, clean nurse in a crisp white uniform, something decidedly disturbing in a sloppy, grimy, careless appearance. One feels that the first person is a reliable nurse, that the second is shiftless and may prove indifferent to her patient's needs.

Reliability and all that it implies in honesty, loyalty, and alertness would certainly be the outstanding quality that doctors and other nurses expect of a nurse.

[10] Regulations relating to maternity leave under Federal, state, and local Civil Service and merit systems show great variation in practice. Inquiry had best be made when applying for a position. Helpful information is also available from the Women's Bureau, Department of Labor, Washington, D.C. See especially "Standards for Maternity Care and Employment of Mothers in Industry," a four-page leaflet.

Patients look for something more in every nurse. "Miss Black and Miss White are both excellent nurses, but I prefer Miss White because she is interested in me as a person." Beyond technical skill, conscientious performance of duties, and pleasing appearance is that intangible something that makes the truly successful nurse. The quality is hard to define. It is the sort of devotion to duty which keeps the captain of a great ship on his bridge for 48 hours without sleep when danger threatens; it is the dogged determination to trace effect to cause that the laboratory worker displays in testing 1,000 formulas to find the right one; it is the absorption in creative work of the composer of music, the sculptor, or the painter for whom all sense of time, place, and self is lost as he seeks for the right expression of his skill. Yet it is still something more, for the nurse is not dealing with ships, test tubes, notes, or colors, but with the human body —the temple of the mind and of the spirit. Some call this quality "selflessness or self-sacrifice," some, "the true spirit of nursing," others know it as religion. By whatever name, it is a spiritual quality that patients recognize instantly, that employers long to find in every nurse, and that can be most simply and unsentimentally called *interest plus*. When a nurse has this quality, it pervades all she does for patients and lights the way of those who must perform their executive and supervisory tasks far from the beds of sick people.

BASIC EDUCATIONAL QUALIFICATIONS

Nearly all salaried positions in professional nursing are for nurses who have completed high school and are graduates of state-accredited schools of nursing connected with registered hospitals having a minimum daily average of 50 patients. The basic nursing course must have included experience in medical, surgical, pediatric, and obstetric nursing. Experience in communicable disease, including tuberculosis, and psychiatric nursing is now considered essential, and these services are frequently provided through affiliations in other hospitals.

These standards are *minimum* for nearly all jobs and are often—and increasingly—higher, the usual requirement now reading that nurses must be graduates of schools of nursing connected with general hospitals having a daily average of 100 patients or be able to pass a standard written objective test of nursing ability. High school seniors are now being advised to select schools of nursing connected with collegiate (degree) programs and there is no doubt but that the better jobs will go to college graduates in the future.

If you have been unwise in your selection of a school of nursing—perhaps one connected with a very small hospital offering limited clinical experience—what can you do about it? There are cases on record of undaunted nurses who have chosen one of the better schools of nursing and repeated the entire course. Many other nurses consult the state board of nurse examiners in the state where they plan to practice and find out how and where they can make up their deficiencies. It has taken some unfortunate nurses 18 months to repair the omissions of the poor school they attended. Usually the deficiencies have been in one of the specialties —pediatric or obstetric nursing, for example—and enrollment in a recognized course giving theory and practice will be advised. Or you may obtain the advice of the director of nurses who has rejected your application for employment, or the department of nursing education in a college or university, or the National League of Nursing Education. If there are deficiencies in your basic nursing preparation, the sooner you discover them the better. It is easier to correct the mistakes when you are young.

In some ways it is easier to make up for the lack of a high school diploma than it is to fill the gaps in nursing experience, as evening schools permit a nurse to complete the course while working. Again, the advice of your supervisor, vocational counselor, or future employer should be sought before enrolling for high school study. Older nurses are not always benefited by working for a high school diploma and would gain more from intensive work in the branch of nursing for which they have shown proficiency. It must always be remembered that some nurses are fitted for general duty and staff work, enjoy it, are successful in it, and have no desire or potential aptitude for executive positions. There must always be followers, or the leaders will have no one to lead. Staff nursing is an art in itself. Its successful practitioners should not be made to feel that their performance cannot reach an acceptable level or that it will necessarily be greatly improved by adding an academic degree to the R.N.

A word of warning should be offered regarding home study and correspondence courses which promise to "put you through high school" or give you the "equivalent" of a high school diploma. Check with the principal of the local high school or with the state board of education (state university) before purchasing such help with a view to obtaining credit for high school courses or a diploma. If you are interested merely in "brushing up" on a high school subject, such as algebra or English, the home study courses offer a way to do so. This is a second choice, however, to joining a class in your own neighborhood, such as an evening extension course, in which you will be under the direct guidance of a qualified teacher and have the fun of studying with others. But beware of the quick and easy promises on paper.

OTHER BASIC QUALIFICATIONS

Citizenship in the United States is a usual requirement expected of professional nurses. It is an absolute necessity for employment in many tax-supported agencies and for the positions in the Federal government.

Registration in the state in which you are practicing is a requirement under state law, unless reciprocal recognition is permitted, and it is expected by most employers of out-of-state nurses within a reasonable time after permanent appointment. Nurses who are students are considered exempt from the regulation during their practice periods, the employing agency or the university taking the responsibility for seeing that the spirit of the law is complied with and that, on completing the course, nurses who plan to remain in the state obtain registration. Until the day when we have national registration through a national board of nurse examiners, professional nurses will find it necessary to secure a license to practice when transferring from one state to another, unless the second state accepts their original registration. *If there is any doubt* about the legality of your practicing professional nursing in the state where you do not hold a license, write to the state board of nurse examiners for complete and up-to-date information regarding the law.[11] Nurses have had the bitter and expensive experience of accepting a position in a distant state only to find that they could practice there for a limited period only or not at all without taking the state examination for a license. Look before you leap!

Age limits vary with the field of nursing and type of work in it. Few positions have a minimum age limit, because most nurses are twenty-one when they graduate. Since a year or two of experience and study is required for any position above staff level, an applicant for such a position is seldom less than twenty-two. There are *upper* age limits, especially for entering positions. For example, nurses over forty are not advised to enter public health nursing. The entering age limit is noted in subsequent chapters wherever it is pertinent. The armed forces usually set a very definite age limit; other branches of nursing sometimes waive restrictions in emergencies.

Residence requirements (state or city) are frequently found in positions

[11] Addresses are in the official directory of the *American Journal of Nursing*.

under Civil Service. They may be for 1, 2, or 3 years. Privately supported (voluntary) hospitals, visiting nurse associations, and private schools are unlikely to require previous residence in the town or state. One way, therefore, of acquiring resident status in a community is to secure a position with a voluntary agency for the time required to qualify for Civil Service examinations.

Preparation for Advanced or Specialized Positions in Nursing

There is much to be gained from advanced study, whether or not it is required for a position and quite aside from the preparation for a specialty in which a higher salary may be anticipated along with letters after one's name. The interchange of experiences, ideas, methods, and opinions among fellow students from all parts of the country, and frequently the world, a new perspective on the job, the stimulation of discussing the latest developments in nursing, and the inspiration of meeting and hearing leaders in the medical and nursing professions are worth many hours of study, while the friendships formed stand one in good stead for all the years to come. Nothing can equal the sense of satisfaction, security, and self-confidence that comes from mastering a subject or a skill.

Advanced study is compulsory for the nurse who wants to grow with her profession and increase her earning capacity. Among the many reasons for the increased need of advanced clinical study by professional nurses is that more and more procedures formerly performed by physicians only have now been transferred to them. Also, with the multiplication of medical and nursing specialities, it is obviously impossible to give advanced preparation during the years of basic nursing education. Not the least of the reasons is the appreciation on the part of the profession itself that the fields of education, counseling, and administration call for highly prepared nurses. Opportunities for graduate study at all levels are increasing yearly, and the content of the courses is becoming more clearly defined. Nurses are urged to make inquiries as to the best places for special preparation. The least expensive are not always the best—or the worst!

Full-time study as against part-time study accompanying employment is a matter of personal choice, usually decided by financial circumstances. No nurse in frail health should ever undertake to combine the activities. Most educators agree that full-time study is preferable when working toward a degree. The proposition might be stated even more strongly: Justice to two demanding programs, work and study, cannot be done by a tired nurse. It is wiser to work and save to study full time, than to attempt to combine these activities.

Just as there is a saturation point of experience in one job, at which the worker may fail to improve and may regress, so there comes a time when additional education, the gathering of degrees and credits, does not add any more competency to one's service. It may, indeed, demonstrate a reluctance on the part of the student to face the realities and struggles of a full-time job. The confirmed degree collector and bookworm may not be a good employment risk. A placement agency or an employer will look with as much skepticism on the degree-saturated job seeker who has failed to balance theory with practice as on the nurse who is unable to hold a job for more than 2 or 3 months at a time or who has had *no* advanced preparation for a difficult job.

Remember that the employer looks at your records of education and experience not as of value in themselves, but as evidence that you possess the knowledge and abilities upon which she, or he, may *judge and predict* your success in the job for which you are applying. Actual experience among other professions in rating training and experience has proved that this prediction is very difficult without additional tests. Help your prospective employer all you can by giving your complete history and accepting any tests suggested in your case. A familiar parallel to this situation is that of the doctor who cannot make a satisfactory diagnosis when the patient fails to locate his pain, describe his symptoms, or give dates or duration of previous attacks. The doctor, too, must resort to additional tests to verify his conclusions.

When enrolling in a postgraduate course for advanced study, certain precautions are advisable:

1. Assure yourself that the course is approved by the National League of Nursing Education or other appropriate national professional group.
2. If you are aiming to acquire a degree, inquire carefully as to whether the course offered will be recognized for credit toward the degree in the university you have in mind.
3. Find out how much of the time must be spent in residence and whether there is a limit of time within which you must complete the requirements for an advanced degree.

4. Estimate as far as possible the cost of the program and the living costs, with a generous allowance for the inevitable extras.
5. If the course is offered in a hospital as a "refresher" or "special" course, be sure that the hospital is not planning to benefit unduly from your service as a student. The course should be an educational experience for you under qualified supervision and instruction, not a means of securing cheap labor for the hospital in exchange for maintenance and a little teaching.

Institutions usually request a medical report on the applicant's physical ability to carry the academic program, and many offer a scholastic-aptitude test as a means of guiding the student to the most needed courses, as well as achievement tests.

Questions regarding the standing of an institutional program of study may be referred to the National League of Nursing Education, questions related to public health preparation to the National Organization for Public Health Nursing, and those in industrial nursing to the American Association of Industrial Nurses (see Appendix A).

SCHOLARSHIPS AND LOANS

Preparation for advanced positions in nursing and in specialized fields costs money. Such courses are usually given in colleges and universities, occasionally as postgraduate refresher courses in hospitals. Nearly all require a period of supervised experience in actual practice in hospitals, clinics, or public health agencies.

A limited number of scholarships are available to meet the costs of study and practice in advanced nursing. A few of these are exclusively for Negro nurses.[12] Scholarships are awarded to the best qualified applicants. They may be outright gifts, loans (with or without interest), part payment on expenses, or free maintenance. They always cover tuition costs.

When funds come from a national source, the applicant must meet the requirements of the school, college, or hospital where she wishes to enroll. Veteran preference sometimes operates in connection with choice of applicants, as does residence. For information regarding allowances for veterans, inquire at the college of your choice or at the nearest office of the Veterans Administration.

As the number, amount, requirements, and sources of scholarship aid

[12] Inquiry should be made at the American Nurses Association. Federal aid to nursing education should also be investigated.

change constantly, it is well to ask for a current list from the American Nurses Association.

In applying for a scholarship, loan, or fellowship, besides submitting your credentials, a recent photograph, professional and social references, and job history to date, it is a good idea to state how you plan to use the knowledge and skill to be secured through further study and when you expect to be available, and—when it is feasible—to ask your supervisor to write a letter to the scholarship committee, sponsoring your application.

It is not unusual to find that there is an age limit for those granted scholarships, and a medical examination is a frequent prerequisite for obvious reasons. There is less likely to be restriction of any kind on loans.

MEMBERSHIP IN PROFESSIONAL ASSOCIATIONS

A word should be said about the importance of keeping in touch with professional nursing organizations—local, state, and national—after graduation. The point is mentioned here only to stress its relation to successful job finding and holding. Membership in professional associations benefits the individual nurse by

1. Increasing her prestige and standing among other nurses and other professions
2. Enlarging her outside interests and bringing her new friends, especially if she is in a strange city
3. Giving her desirable contacts, which may stand her in good stead when seeking a new job
4. Supplying up-to-date information on employment trends, including the development of new job opportunities and changes affecting her security (for example, her status under the revisions of the Social Security Act)
5. Offering inspiration and education through special programs, conventions, and institutes
6. Enabling the nurse to answer the questions on job application blanks which frequently request affirmation of professional membership connections, because membership in itself is evidence of having met basic qualifications (for example, membership in the National League of Nursing Education)
7. Offering congenial social and recreational activities

Subscriptions to professional journals serve much the same purpose as items 4 and 5 in the preceding paragraph. The journals carry lists of employment opportunities and professionally approved placement services and will publish "want ads" from nurses seeking positions. The current official directories printing the names of nurses in executive positions in Federal, national, and state organizations should be used when writing to individuals in these agencies regarding employment. The directories appear at least once a year in the journals, and quarterly in the *American Journal of Nursing*. It is much more courteous, as well as more intelligent and diplomatic, to address the director or superintendent of an organization by name rather than to say, "Dear Madam" or "Sir." (See following section, Applying for a Job, for letters of application.) It also saves clerical time in routing mail.

From time to time colorful descriptions of specialized nursing jobs appear in the pages of professional journals. There are also notices regarding new courses, scholarships, current salary surveys, and statements of recommended personnel policies.

APPLYING FOR A JOB

Your application for a position in the field of your choice is, of course, the first step in your career and—like marriage—not to be entered upon lightly. There is an advantage in seeing the place of work and the kind of service with which you are planning to connect yourself before applying for the job, but this is not always possible. If you know anyone engaged in similar work elsewhere, you might ask her about it, but if she is unhappy or not well suited to the position, you might be unwarrantedly prejudiced against a position that might be ideal for you. After all, the proof of the pudding is only in the eating and you are the diner, not your friend. If you cannot see the work but wish to give it a trial, be careful not to commit yourself to stay after a certain period if you have any misgivings about the position.

Increasingly, employers are listing their vacancies and job needs with recognized professional employment agencies and receiving the names of qualified candidates from these sources. This procedure is timesaving, efficient, and more satisfactory to all concerned. Through the careful investigation of the candidate's abilities and detailed knowledge of the job requirements, the professional placement secretary is more apt to

find the right nurse for the right job than is the employer who interviews a long list of unknown applicants, or the job seeker who responds
to a list of haphazard references. It is to your advantage, therefore, to
make connections upon graduation with a recognized professional placement agency and to benefit from its qualified counseling service and
wide familiarity with a variety of job opportunities. The listing of your
name with such an agency gives you greater assurance of satisfying employment, in a field with a future, than would your own chance selection
of an employer. The use of placement agency services is essential for
your own protection if you are seeking a job in an area of the country
entirely strange to you. You will also find that the professional counselor
can give you a very fair picture of employment conditions in the area
and the salary scales in force. Such a counselor can also help you by
evaluating the personnel policies effective in the position you are
contemplating.

Vocational guidance is a term that may desirably include a complete
review and analysis of the candidate's aptitudes, records, and job experience, with vocational tests of various types to assist the counselor
in predicting successful adjustment to a particular field of work. Reports from schools, employers, and supervisors are gathered and a vocational record opened and maintained for the applicant. Regrettably,
the term "vocational guidance" may mean in nonprofessional agencies
the mere listing of the applicant's name and address and her job
preference.[13]

Under the term "vocational placement" is included the best that is
meant by vocational guidance, plus a choice of positions selected to
suit the applicant's aptitudes and preferences. The placement bureau
should be able to give a description of the job being offered, the duties
involved, its opportunities for advancement, and its appropriateness for
you, as well as the salary scale and conditions of employment. Again,
nonprofessional placement may mean merely notifying you of a vacancy
and suggesting that you apply for the job, or simply notifying you that
your name has been sent to a prospective employer. If you have indicated your willingness to take any type of job within a specified compensation range, you may simply be told where and when to report for
duty. From these comments, you, as a job seeker, will understand why

[13] In some states, there are state vocational associations (general) with advisory committees from which one may obtain information on standards of guidance and
counseling and the names of accepted counseling agencies.

it is desirable to know how much and what kind of service you will receive from a placement agency and just what registering for a job implies.

Occasionally a job applicant resents the search into her past employment experiences. When you consult a vocational counselor, you may expect her to ask in some detail how you yourself felt about your previous jobs—what you liked about them and what you didn't like or found hard. It is also to be expected that the counselor will secure the impressions of your ability from your previous employers. The employer will be asked to say what your work showed with relation to your personality, interest, initiative, appearance, and dependability, as well as her rating of your nursing skills. She will surely report on your ability to get along with other people—patients, doctors, coworkers and how you handled yourself in various types of situations. Two of the significant questions asked on nearly all reference forms are: Did this nurse show promise of professional growth and did she possess leadership capacities? Such questions are evidence of the ever-constant search for the "nurse with a future" and should be welcomed by job candidates. If, incidentally, facts are revealed that will be helpful in guiding you into positions that will strengthen your weak points and bring you more satisfaction, that too should justify the bothersome red tape of filling in the necessary registration forms.

EMPLOYMENT THROUGH PLACEMENT AGENCIES

The American Nurses Association has sponsored a vocational placement and guidance service for all registered nurses. Its official name is American Nurses Association Professional Counseling and Placement Service, Inc., and it has two offices, one at the Association's New York headquarters and one (a branch) in Chicago (see Appendix A). Also, many state nurses associations, at the suggestion of the ANA, have established professional counseling and placement services within the state, with qualified counselors appointed to conduct the bureaus. Nurses wishing to consult a state service of this type should write to the state nurses association (the names of executive secretaries will be found in the official directory of the *American Journal of Nursing*) or to the national office.

Through these professional services you may secure "placement in your state or elsewhere, according to your wishes and qualifications, and the location of desirable positions. Because the service is nationwide in scope, you may have your professional record compiled and kept permanently in a central place, ready for use or transfer whenever you want it. Your records are kept confidential." This is a desirable connection for you because "Professional nurses—many of whom have special preparation or experience in counseling—are in charge of the national and state programs."[14] The service has the approval of the ANA and the cooperation of other national professional nursing organizations. Local centers will be developed as needed. *All service is free.*

The U.S. Employment Service or the state employment service in your state may be a desirable point of contact, if its professional division is conducted or sponsored by professional nurses or has their advice. As these services are tax-supported, there is no charge to the registrant or employer for placement. These bureaus are more apt to have positions available under Civil Service and in official agencies than in private homes and voluntary associations. Their coverage is wide, however, and experienced vocational counselors are usually available in the professional divisions.

The New York State Employment Service, because centrally located and professionally directed, has a wide placement service for professional as well as practical nurses. It aims to assist interested nurses in making suitable vocational plans and is thus a true counseling service as well as a placement agency. It has as assistants trained vocational counselors and committee advisers who are nurses. It accepts openings for all types of nursing jobs all over the country and abroad. Any nurse may register.

Nationwide placement service is also obtainable from commercial registries for a fee. The advertisements of commercial registries and commercial employment agencies are not accepted by the professional nursing journals.

LOCAL REGISTRIES

There are hospitals, professional nursing, and commercial registries or employment bureaus functioning on a local or regional basis.

The professional or officially approved registries (the current list may be found in the *American Journal of Nursing*) give varying amounts of counsel and vocational guidance and carry on placement in a variety of fields, with emphasis on private practice. A few registries—less than 50 per cent in 1951—enroll practical nurses and occasionally obtain visiting housekeeper services. For the most part, however, they are maintained

[14] Quoted from "Plan Your Own Career in Nursing" (ANA leaflet), 1946.

for professional nurses. They list positions in hospitals, homes, doctors' offices, and occasionally in the field of industry and public health. A few registries have attained the status of true community nursing bureaus, sponsored by representative lay and professional groups and receiving support from community chests. They make placements in every field of nursing. The professional registries are few in number compared to the commercial registries.

Professional registries attempt to cover their costs. They are not run for profit. If there is a deficit at the end of the year, the district or state nurses association sponsoring the registry decides on how it is to be met. In 1950, professional registry charges to registrants ranged from $15 to $50, annually.

The registries are concerned with keeping their registrants busy and satisfied. They try to offer opportunities for professional growth. Many make available educational information, sponsor institutes and refresher courses, provide a loan library, and offer friendly advice. The young nurse seeking private practice will find professional assistance from these registries. She is expected to conform to their rules and carry out their policies with regard to responding to calls, hours of work, and charges for service. Occasionally, complete vocational service is offered. Hourly service may now be obtained through most of the professional registries.

Locally, many hospitals maintain registries, especially in small communities and in cities where there is no professional registry. In large cities, the hospital registries confine their placements to graduates of their own schools of nursing and largely to service within their own walls or for their medical staffs. Small community and rural hospitals may register and place many types of nurses, including nurses' aides, both within the city and in the surrounding area.

Charges in hospital registries vary greatly. In some, the service is free; in others a small yearly fee is asked to cover expenses. Formal vocational guidance is not given.

If the field of counseling, guidance, and vocational placement interests you, the most recent requirements for nurses qualifying for the directorship of registries or professional placement agencies should be sought from the ANA. It is obvious that only the very well prepared nurse—professionally and personally speaking—should undertake to guide applicants into employment. A wide acquaintance with all types of nursing work and familiarity with the local situations and agencies are vital to wise counseling.

COMMERCIAL EMPLOYMENT BUREAUS

There is a limitless variety of these. Large cities may have as many as 30 to 40. (New York City alone has over 80.) Commercial registries are in business for profit. The registrant cannot be too careful about having a perfectly clear understanding of the fees and method of collection of the registry and its employment policies. The service expected of her must be clearly described and nothing signed until the printed rules and regulations are read and understood. Employment agencies that take fees for placement service are usually restricted by law in the amount of their charges. In many localities they must be licensed to operate. Information regarding the standing of placement agencies may be secured from local chambers of commerce, license bureaus, or better business bureaus.

It is evident that a commercial placement bureau that specializes in placing professional nurses and employs a registered nurse to handle these placements will probably render more understanding service than one dealing mainly with business and unskilled workers. Many commercial agencies advertise "nurses" among their available workers, but the placement service may be run by an ill-equipped clerk and place only practical nurses or nursemaids. There are a few well-organized, highly ethical commercial registries, run by well-qualified professional nurses, which give discerning service to registrant and employer alike, take a personal interest in finding the right nurse for the right job, and actually render a more far-reaching community service than some of the professional registries that function in a limited field, placing only one type of nurse.

PERSONAL APPLICATION FOR A JOB

Your application for a position, whether the job has been referred to you through a placement agency or discovered on your own initiative, may be by letter or through a personal interview with your prospective employer or both. Possibly the job has been offered you directly, without reference to a placement agency, registry, or at your own request. Personal applications and interviews are always more satisfactory than written applications. The former may not be possible, however, and therefore your letter should contain enough information, if it has not been supplied by a placement agency, to permit the prospective employer to decide whether she wants to send you a formal application blank, ask for additional information, or invite you for an interview.

Application by Letter. If you are applying for a position by letter, put yourself in the place of your prospective employer and think about the facts that you would like to know about a new member of your staff. As this letter is, in a sense, your first appearance in your employer's office, you will want to make a good impression. Employers draw quite a few conclusions from a letter of application. They have every right to assume that, if the applicant's letter is scrawled on scented, highly decorated note paper, misspelled, untidy, and poorly expressed, then the nurse's work may be superficial and careless, with little regard for the fitness of things and her charts and records are likely to be untidy, even illegible, like her note. On the other hand, a well-spaced, well-planned, correctly spelled letter on plain writing paper, giving clear but brief information about the candidate's qualifications and interest in the position, will go far toward favorable consideration among a number of candidates.

Two letters of application, in acceptable form, are offered here. They are strictly formal, but there would be no objection to including a sentence expressing your own interest in the field of work for which you are applying, or referring to the source of your information about the position. An employer likes to know how you heard about the position and will naturally feel gratified if you express enthusiasm at the prospect of working on her staff. Don't make the mistake of thinking only in terms of what *you* will get *from* the job; remember the job should be enriched by what you take to it. Enthusiasm is a good start.

A letter of application from a newly graduated nurse applying for a public health nursing position might read somewhat like this:

St. Timothy Hospital
Chicago, 10, Ill.
March 21, 1952

Miss Jessie Leighton, Director
Visiting Nurse Association
Middlefield, Ill.

Dear Miss Leighton:

I wish to apply for a position as staff nurse in your Association. I have just graduated from the St. Timothy General Hospital School of Nursing in the February 1952 class, and am now doing floor duty in the medical wards of the same hospital. I had six weeks in the out-patient service. I am registered in Illinois (#383111), am twenty-one years old and a Protestant. I would be interested in taking college work in public health nursing later if my work on your staff proved to be satisfactory.

The director of my school of nursing, Mrs. Mary Dale, will be glad to give you a report of my work. I am enclosing a picture of myself in uniform.

If there is a vacancy on your staff, may I be considered for it? I will be available after June 1. I could go to Middlefield for an interview on any Thursday afternoon of this month.

Very truly yours,
Elizabeth Bower, R.N.

A letter of application in response to an advertisement, from a graduate nurse (who has not been in military service[15]) might read like this:

914 East 54th Street
New York, N.Y.
June 20, 1952

Dr. Walter Smith
1005 X Street
New York City

Dear Mr. Smith:

I am very much interested in securing a position as office nurse with you. I was born in Albany, N. Y., in 1925 and am a graduate of Columbia Hospital School of Nursing, Albany, 1946. I am unmarried and a Catholic.

Since graduation I have held the following positions:

Columbia Hospital, Albany, N.Y., staff nurse, Orthopedic Service, 1946–1947, salary $175 a month.

American Red Cross, Pittsburgh, Pa., special instructor working with poliomyelitis patients, 1948, $200.

Johnson Hospital for Contagious Diseases, New York City, private duty nursing, 1949 to present time, at $10 a day.

[Any additional education or special courses would be listed here]

[15] If this application is from a veteran, the date of official discharge from the armed forces should be stated.

Since my major specialty has been in pediatrics and my work has been almost entirely with children, I feel that I am especially well equipped to be an office nurse for a pediatrician.

I should like the opportunity of a personal interview with you and could arrange an appointment at your convenience. I am enclosing a small recent photograph.

For references, may I suggest Miss Mary Jones, Director of Nurses at the hospital where I am now employed, and Miss Sallie Black, 2006 Cross Road, Albany, N.Y.

My home address is 914 East 54th Street, New York City, telephone Central 5-4218.

Sincerely yours,

Alice McDermott, R.N.

My New York State registration number is . . . .

Application in Person. If your application for a position is made in person, it is customary to write or telephone in advance for an appointment. This saves everyone's time. Keep the appointment promptly. If delayed for any reason or unable to keep the appointment, make every effort to let your interviewer know. It is neither polite nor businesslike to keep her waiting and uncertain of your intentions.

The following suggestions may strike you as childish and unnecessary, but the experience of many employment agencies, administrators, and directors of nursing service testify otherwise. Many nurses do not seem to realize that their personal appearance and behavior during this first interview with a prospective employer may determine their acceptance or rejection for the position. Here are a few do's and don't's to save you bitter and embarrassing experiences:

Wear simple tailored clothes, appropriate to the season and to a business call, moderate heels, and simple jewelry if any. Wear a plain hat. Tone down your makeup, especially nail polish and lipstick. Leave off mascara.

Be sure your grooming is as nearly perfect as possible. This means hair simply dressed, lifted well off the shoulders and collar, spotless accessories, clean hands with unpointed nails, straight stocking seams, well-polished shoes, even heels, and well-pressed suit, coat, or dress. Good posture suggests self-reliance.

Do not use strong scent, no matter how expensive. Do not chew gum or smoke.

During the interview, speak quietly, sit still, and look directly at your interviewer. Remember it is for her to direct the conversation and ask the questions; save yours until the end of the interview. Poise is not demonstrated by loud, assured voice and manner, nor knowledge of the job by a know-it-all attitude and questions that show off your ability to use technical terms.

Of course, the sizing-up is not all on one side. You too, as an applicant for the job, should be observant of factors that may be indicative of the conditions under which you will work.

Are the surroundings where you are interviewed attractive, clean, businesslike, and quiet? Does your interviewer conduct the conference in a friendly yet dignified manner? Is her (or his) appearance prepossessing? Are you given a fairly full description of your duties and are your questions answered frankly and satisfactorily? Do the general atmosphere of the place and the spirit toward its service attract you?

"I always look at an executive's bookcase, if I get the chance," a counselor of college students told her class. "Do the books look used, are there a few recent 'best sellers' in the professional field and any examples of recreational reading outside the professional field? A general reader is usually a leader."

The young nurse applying for a position for the first time may feel a bit overawed or timid about asking questions. It is especially hard to insist on perfectly definite answers; yet these are important. Remember that you have as much right to know all the conditions under which you are going to work as the employer has to know the details of your educational and personal qualifications for the job. Mutual frankness and a free exchange of information will do much to prevent misunderstandings and later disappointments. Too frequently, in the past, a disillusioned employee has resigned in a huff, saying, "You didn't tell me I would have to work evenings," or the irritated employer has dismissed a misfit saying, "You did not tell me you disliked working with children!" To which either speaker could have answered, "But you didn't *ask* me!" Something quite evidently was lacking in that preliminary interview. Don't hesitate to ask questions politely and tactfully. The trustworthy employer has nothing to hide.

If you are given an application blank, fill it out neatly and with care to see that every question is answered. If you do not understand a question, ask about it. Usually you will be asked to give references—

one professional, one social. If these can be local names, so much the better. It is customary and polite to let the persons to whom you have referred an employer for a social reference know of your action. Sometimes you will wish to ask their permission in advance.

A courteous step following a personal interview is a brief note of thanks for the privilege of the interview, with a renewed expression of your interest in the position. Such a note also serves to remind the employer of your application.

INFORMATION ABOUT THE POSITION

The information that you will surely want to secure during your correspondence or interview with your future employer, if the placement agency has not supplied it to you, will relate to the duties involved, supervision, opportunities for special training or study, promotion, salary, hours of work, vacation, sick leave, retirement benefits, if any, general rules and regulations for the staff, and the date when you are expected to report for work. If it concerns you, the agency's policy with regard to married nurses and/or maternity leave must be ascertained.

Nearly all large agencies have their "personnel policies" printed in leaflet form to be read at the applicant's leisure, while Civil Service positions state the regulations in their posted advertisements of specifications for the position.

Retirement, saving, sickness, and accident plans open to employees may also be discussed at the preliminary interview or described in the leaflet, as will the requirements for medical examination, immunizations, aptitude tests, or other prerequisites to appointment.

Nurses are well-advised to find out whether there is a quick turnover of the professional staff. A high rate of turnover would be more than 25 per cent of the staff leaving within a year—always assuming no outside factors, such as war, influenced the resignations. This situation usually indicates unsatisfactory or misrepresented working conditions. The trouble with ascertaining this fact is that, when the turnover is rapid, the employer will prefer not to reveal the situation. It is well to secure the information indirectly or from an outside source, if possible. This is another excellent reason for securing a job through a placement agency.

Before accepting the job, you will want to find out in more detail, quite possibly from outside sources, these facts about the salary offered:

1. Whether it compares well with the current rates paid by other employing agencies in the vicinity[16]
2. Whether it will be increased upon evidence of your good work, your further theoretical preparation, or the development of special skills; what the rate of increase is and how soon the maximum can be reached
3. Whether it is the policy of the employer to make salary adjustments in accordance with changes in the cost of living
4. Whether there are special privileges or opportunities offered to offset a low salary. Occasionally, the excellence of the supervision, the unusual opportunity to develop a specialty or take certain academic courses concurrently with the job make a low salary quite acceptable.
5. What deductions will be made on monthly salary checks, especially with relation to retirement funds, insurance, taxes, and dues (if any)

All positions classified under Civil Service may be secured for state positions from the state Civil Service (or merit system) Commission at your state capital; for Federal positions, write to the U.S. Civil Service Commission, Washington, D.C. In cities and counties offering positions under Civil Service, see the listing in the local telephone book under city or county Civil Service (or merit system).

CONTRACTS

A formal printed business contract, which both employer and employee sign, with witnesses, is not usual in a professional field and is rare in nursing. Generally, the agreement as to employment (date of starting work, rate of pay, and conditions of work) appears in a letter or official memorandum to the prospective employee from the employer, usually following a personal interview. Whether it appears in a letter, a memorandum on official letterhead, or in the form of a signed employment card, the employee *should secure the statement in writing in an official form*. This is important and a good business procedure. "A friendly understanding" or "a tacit agreement" as to the conditions of employment may prove worthless at a later date. Competent administrators invariably say, "I will confirm this appointment in writing." If not, the applicant should say, "May I please have these arrangements in writing?"

[16] The national nursing associations (see Appendix A) are always glad to share on request their information on current salaries paid in various fields all over the country. Placement agencies also have this information. For costs of living, see "Labor Review," the monthly report of the Department of Labor, Washington, D.C.

Written agreements concerning conditions of employment are not necessary for positions classified under the Civil Service, since these conditions are public property, unchangeable and regulated by law. The date of starting work, however, and any special promise with relation to place or type of assignment should be in writing, if for no other reason than that the appointing officer might be incapacitated and the employee have no proof that she was promised anything verbally.

In nonsalaried positions in which pay is by the hour or day, in part-time, hourly, or private duty service, formal contracts are not usual.

Should a nurse in private practice be working "free lance" and not making use of a placement bureau, she may be engaged on a long-time case and agree to work on a salary or reduced rate basis. She will be wise to have this understanding in writing from her employer with the date of employment and rate of pay clearly stated. Nurses attempting to collect overdue back wages under the law, following the demise of the patient or employer, have found such action difficult and expensive without substantiating data, properly signed, witnessed, and dated.

APPLYING FOR A CIVIL SERVICE POSITION

The number of positions for nurses in public agencies where Civil Service regulations apply is increasing. *General* information is given here on how to secure a Civil Service position, what entrance requirements are usually expected, and where to secure further information. Professional placement services are also prepared to assist their registrants in applying for such positions.

The applicant for a Civil Service position in a public agency must recognize three factors which differ from those involved in employment by a private agency:

1. All appointing processes under Civil Service are controlled by the rules and regulations of the personnel board, merit system council, or commission (whatever its name may be). The selection of a candidate is subject to these restrictions and, in order to make the appointment on an impartial, nonpartisan basis, the candidates are examined or rated on the basis of their training and experience by some form of objective test or rating scale. An oral (personal) interview, sometimes before an interviewing board, is usually a part of the selective process. It is a candidate's privilege to appeal or protest any step involved in the selective process which she considers unfair in

the light of the "specifications" (conditions) described in the advertised announcement of the job.

2. The information supplied on the application sheet by the candidate is given under oath and is, in a sense, a legal record. The candidate will be disqualified for the job for misrepresentation of facts.

3. After a candidate has qualified for a position and been rated, her name is placed on a register (list) of eligible nurses in the rank to which she is entitled by the grade she received in the rating process. Appointments of nurses are now made from registers established as a result of unassembled examinations (the office rating process); no written tests are required in the Federal Civil Service. It is usual to "certify" or refer to the appointing agency only the nurses at the top of the register. The top three or five names are usually certified first for appointment. Of course, if six or ten nurses are needed, the whole register might be used by the appointing authority. The setting up of a new register is, in some cases, required by law after a stated interval.

It can be seen from this statement that the Civil Service commission, board, or merit system council is the collector of eligible applicants, who, in turn, are referred for *appointment* to the appointing authority (future employer). The commission must follow the rules of the system in making the selection of nurses for the register, and the appointing authority must abide by the rules of the system in making appointments. Thus, there is much less flexibility and freedom of choice of candidates under a Civil Service system than in private agency practice. If properly administered, however, the system is much fairer to all applicants than the personal, often subjective, picking of an employee carried out in the private agency by one person only who may be partial, easily impressed by a good talker, or under outside pressure to make the appointment. Favoritism and "pull" do not enter into Civil Service appointments.

Although the rating of a candidate's training and experience and the personal interview may be the only formal steps in ranking and appointing a nurse, many Civil Service systems—notably state merit systems—are requiring written (objective) examinations. Most of the recent public health nursing appointments on a state level have been made from those who have given satisfactory evidence of their knowledge through written examinations.

The announcement or advertisement of a position for nurses in an agency under Civil Service regulations provides the following information:

1. The name of the position, its duties, location, and salary
2. The entrance or qualifying requirements, covering such points as age, professional education, experience, state registration, citizenship, residence, and physical condition
3. Information concerning the examination for the position—where and when held, where to obtain application blanks, what kind of examination it is—the fields of knowledge expected of a candidate, and the relative weights given to (a) the written test (if any), (b) rating of training and experience, and (c) the oral interview
4. An explanation as to the handling of veterans' preference accompanies these statements. For Federal Civil Service positions, photographs are not necessary.

Candidates are fingerprinted before employment and receive a thorough medical examination.

These regulations apply not only to nurses but to all applicants to Civil Service positions. Frequently an "additional data" sheet is sent to nurses who qualify under the general specifications for a position.

It is extremely important to fill out the application blank and any supplementary form completely and accurately. *Every question must be answered.*

Although these steps may sound complicated and the written tests formidable, actually the process runs smoothly. Qualified nurses will find the tests fair—often extremely interesting. The ultimate result of this method of selection should produce a staff definitely qualified to render superior public service. The benefits to the jobholder are

1. Assurance of appointment on the basis of merit and fitness, without regard to political considerations, personal favoritism, or "pull"
2. A definite promotion plan
3. A position with career possibilities and tenure

The nurse appointed to a Civil Service position is usually on probation for the first 3, 6, or 12 months.[17] (This is also the familiar practice in

[17] The probationary period should not be confused with a temporary, emergency, or provisional appointment.

private agencies.) At the end of that period, if the nurse's work is satis-factory, she receives a permanent appointment with full "Civil Service status." This latter phrase means, in most Civil Service systems, that she is entitled to the privileges of paid vacation, sick leave, holidays, pay-ment for overtime (time and a half), and disability and (usually) re-tirement benefits.[18] Dismissal (or "separation") from the job after this period is unlikely, except for very unsatisfactory service, misdemeanors, or serious neglect of duty.

The working day is 8 hours, the week 40 or 44 hours, vacation at the rate of 2¼ days per month, sick leave 1¼ days per month.

Efficiency or service ratings (reports of a nurse's work) are filed at regular intervals by the appointing agency. Unless these are "unsatis-factory," a nurse can plan on an increasing salary up to the maximum for the class of position she occupies. Promotion to higher positions usually is—and always should be—on the basis of higher qualifications, more study, and experience; not on years of service alone. Promotional examinations are given in some agencies.

Administrators of public service agencies are especially interested at this time in making nursing a "career service"; that is, making it possible for well-qualified staff members to reach the top positions in an agency by adding higher qualifications, advanced study, and specialized skills to their minimum qualifications for the job. In this way, an ambitious, energetic young nurse, if she throws in her lot with an agency under Civil Service, may feel that she is starting on a career with a promising, interesting future and assured old-age security.

The steps in securing a *Federal* Civil Service position are charted here:

1. The nurse reads the announcement of position and asks for an ap-plication blank.
2. She fills out the application and sends it to U.S. Civil Service Com-mission, Washington, D.C.
3. She receives a supplementary information blank and returns it.
4. She may be required to take a written examination—this is not cur-rently the practice (1951).
5. The C.S.C. rates the nurse and places her on a register, if she is qualified.

[18] Federal Civil Service positions for nurses all carry retirement benefits (see Chap. XVI). Unfortunately, state and local Civil Service systems have not all been so astute. This is a point to check when reading the announcements of positions.

6. The C.S.C. certifies (refers) the candidate to an employing agency.
7. The nurse is notified and given an appointment for a personal interview.
8. She receives an appointment for a probationary period, if accepted, and is given a medical examination by the employing agency.
9. She receives a permanent appointment at end of 12 months, if service ratings are satisfactory.
10. She receives promotion based on service ratings, qualifications, additional experience.
11. She receives retirement annuity upon resignation from service after specified length of service.

In local, county, state, and Federal Civil Service positions at the present time, salaries equal those in private agencies and frequently exceed them; for example, overtime pay is offered. At the same time, the employee is offered greater security (including retirement annuities) than is found in many private agencies.

Information regarding all Federal Civil Service positions open to nurses, their requirements, and the forms on which to apply may be secured from the U.S. Civil Service Commission, Washington, D.C., or from one of the U.S. Civil Service regional offices. Assuming, however, that you are interested in a special service, such as floor duty in a large hospital of the U.S. Public Health Service, the following letter would bring you the necessary forms and information.

380 Greene Avenue
Louisville, Ky.
March 1, 1951

Miss Elsie Berdan, Chief Nurse,
Division of Hospitals
U.S. Public Health Service
Washington, D.C.

Dear Miss Berdan:

I am interested in a position as general duty nurse in one of the large hospitals, preferably on the East Coast. I am twenty-seven years old, registered in Michigan and New York, and a graduate of the Harper Hospital School of Nursing in Detroit, Mich., class of 1945.

Since graduation my major specialty has been surgical nursing at Harper Hospital and at Mt. Sinai Hospital in New York. I have had one course in ward administration at Teachers College, Columbia University, in 1946.

Will you please send me information regarding the opportunities for me in the service and the necessary application forms? I am free to report for duty immediately.

Sincerely yours,

Helen Carpenter, R.N.

State registration numbers ....

THE BEST AVENUE TO A JOB—GOOD WORK

Although all these avenues to employment are open to nurses—direct application, advertisements, Civil Service, and employment agencies (national, state, regional, and local; professional and commercial; with and without charge)—the fact remains that most nurses find their jobs through friends and through rendering good service. A satisfied patient, pleased doctor, observant supervisor, or interested friend will suggest your name when another patient needs care, a job falls vacant, or a new position develops. This is not always the best way to secure a job. A good placement agency takes pains to match the applicant's qualifications with those the employer seeks, but a record of work well done, a series of positions adequately filled, of responsibilities shouldered and carried on without complaint, are good recommendations for a worker and will bring offers of better jobs. It is good sense to do one's best in the simplest job and in every job in order to build a successful job record. Only occasionally do circumstances excuse poor work. The alibi of "bad luck on that job" almost never holds. The exceptions are the worker's own ill health, for which she should take remedial steps, the employer's ill health or lack of ability, which are generally recognized by all, or the infrequent "impossible situation," from which the nurse should resign promptly, if, on seeking the advice of others more experienced than herself, she is convinced that there is no other way out. It must not be forgotten, however, that what appears as an "impossible situation" may be the best challenge in the world to a nurse who, if she succeeds in the job, will have gained infinitely in the experience and perhaps qualified herself for a position of far greater responsibility. The biblical declaration "Thou hast been faithful over a few things; I will make thee ruler over many things . . . " defines the policy most supervisors follow in promoting young nurses and, although discontented employees often complain that their companions are promoted through "pull" or favoritism while they are overlooked, there are not many places where a permanent appointment can be secured through "pull" *and* poor work.

Professional counselors are fair and impartial judges of employment situations and are in a position to distinguish between the genuinely impossible setup and that which only appears to be so to the young or discouraged nurse. They also know what constitutes fair employment practice. Their advice should be sought when the going gets tough and before a drastic step such as resignation is taken.

The Future Outlook for Employment

Nursing is not unique in giving back to you in proportion to what you put in it of yourself and of your energy. You have seen girls flit casually through their training, studying just as lightly as possible, doing as little as they can for each patient, and working hard only when a situation becomes critical. There will not be much of a career waiting for them. Nursing will never give them much material reward. You must always put more into a job than you expect to get out of it, indeed to get anything worth while out of it. Those who can offer the "big-time" jobs pay no attention to clock watchers or to those who are always trying to get by with doing as little work as possible. These nurses usually drop out of the profession soon after graduation or take an easy job and remain in it forever. If that is what you want out of nursing, you do not need this book.

After all, nursing is a profession. It is not a secretarial job or a behind-the-counter selling job. As Earl S. Johnson has so well stated:

A profession is based on intellectual as well as technical operations, and that involves a large degree of individual responsibility. . . . A profession is based on science, and this is refreshed through seminars and work in the laboratory. . . . This requires that a profession police itself and keep open the channels of communications and new knowledge, both social and professional. . . . A profession is, furthermore, in command of a technic capable of being passed on at a level higher than a simple apprenticeship. . . . A profession is also a self-governing body. . . . Finally, a profession is a group which is responsible to public interest and welfare and has an abiding sense of its obligation to society. On this score I challenge any profession to match the devotion of the profession of nursing.[19]

One more point before you select your future career. There are exceptions to every rule. The war emphasized that lesson for all of us. We forgot to say, "It can't be done," or "It has never been done." We did it. The most rigid requirements, the wisest counsel, the most time-honored tradition and unbroken precedent, all have gone down at times before the enthusiasm of a sincere, eager, conscientious worker. If you believe you are personally qualified for a job, have set your heart on it, and are *willing to work to get it*, apply for it whether you meet all the stated conditions or not. Possibly, just a few months of additional study and training will qualify you, or an interested employer will find a way to help you. Even among the jobs under Civil Service, with their rigid requirements, there may be found one which will serve as a steppingstone to the Civil Service job of your choice. Nursing is full of surprises. Administrators are human —often, luckily, inconsistent! Do not hesitate to ask for what you want. You may be the great exception, the genius who is a "natural" in the specialty, the long-awaited answer to a supervisor's prayer—in other words, the right nurse in the right job. It can do no harm to apply for a job if you really want it, but don't be discouraged if it is not for you. Nursing is a very broad field. Somewhere, someone is waiting to help you find the place in which you can serve best with the deepest personal satisfaction in return. Don't give up the search. "A horizon is nothing save the limit of our sight."[20]

"The opportunities for nursing in the next decade transcend anything we have ever known. The extent to which they are realized will depend, in large measure, on the nursing profession itself."[21] This is not an idle, casual comment nor an unsupported personal opinion of its author, Mary M. Roberts, editor-emeritus of the *American Journal of Nursing*. All signs point to what Dr. Thomas Parran has called an "emergency of opportunity" for nursing service. The responsibility for realizing our professional potentialities does not rest with any one group, community plan, hospital organization, Federal aid, or insurance program, though all these will have a part in future service to the sick. It rests fundamentally upon the best utilization of nurse power and its distribution where

[19] *American Journal of Nursing*, p. 74, February, 1950.
[20] RAYMOND, ROSSITER WORTHINGTON.
[21] Editorial, *American Journal of Nursing*, p. 985, December, 1945.

most needed. If, however, nurse power is weak and unprepared, if the individual nurses who compose the profession have not developed their skills and added to their knowledge in sufficient degree to fill the new demands, then the opportunities will be lost and there will be no future growth. Emergencies have a disconcerting way of being met by substitutes who leap to fill the temporary need and remain by virtue of their firsthand experience rather than because they have acquired a broad and deep understanding of the job and its future. Every professional nurse and student reading this book has a personal responsibility for developing her capacities to the utmost to be ready for the unpredictable demands for service on a professional level which will "transcend anything we have ever known." Not only will the nursing profession be the richer in well-prepared, adequate members and leaders, but the nursing care of the sick will grow into something better than the world has ever known.

BIBLIOGRAPHY[22]

1. ADDAMS, RUTH, and RUTH B. SCOTT: After Graduation, Growth, *American Journal of Nursing*, p. 328, June, 1950.
2. AMERICAN NURSES ASSOCIATION: State-wide Minimum Employment Standards, *American Journal of Nursing*, p. 514, August, 1948.
3. BINGHAM, WALTER V., and BRUCE V. MOORE: "How to Interview," 3d rev. ed., Harper & Brothers, New York, 1941.
4. CAFFEE, F. B.: Cost of Living, A Decade of Changes and Trends, *Public Health Nursing*, p. 373, July, 1949.
5. CORNLEY, PAUL B.: A Study of Negro Nursing, *Public Health Nursing*, p. 449, August, 1942.
6. CRAIG, LEROY N.: Opportunities for Men Nurses, *American Journal of Nursing*, p. 667, June, 1940.
7. DEMING, DOROTHY: Annuities Planned for Nurses by Nurses, *American Journal of Nursing*, p. 175, March, 1948.
8. DEMING, DOROTHY: "Pam Wilson, Registered Nurse," Dodd, Mead & Company, Inc., New York, 1946.
9. DINES, ALTA E.: What Her Employer Wanted to Know, *American Journal of Nursing*, p. 616, June, 1939; p. 303 (editorial), March, 1940.
10. *Facts about Nursing*, American Nurses Association, New York. (Published yearly.)
11. FILLMORE, ANNA: It's Your Career, Why Not Plan for It? *American Journal of Nursing*, p. 36, January, 1946.
12. FINK, ELIZABETH E.: It Works Both Ways, *American Journal of Nursing*, p. 421, July, 1950.

[22] These references concern job selection, general factors affecting job selection, and the personal application for positions. For reading on guidance and counseling, chiefly for counselors, see Appendix B.

13. FRASHER, CHARLES B.: ABC's of the Merit System, *Public Health Nursing*, p. 273, May, 1950.
14. GARDNER, MARY S.: "So Build We," The Macmillan Company, New York, 1942.
15. GELINAS, AGNES: "Nursing and Nursing Education," Commonwealth Fund, Division of Publication, New York, 1946.
16. HARRELL, VIRGINIA: Annuities and Retirement Plans, *R.N.*, March, April, 1948.
17. HARRISON, GENE: "The Nurse and the Law," F. A. Davis Company, Philadelphia, 1945. (See especially sections relating to contracts.)
18. HEINTZLEMAN, RUTH, and DOROTHY DEMING: How Federal Civil Service Works, *American Journal of Nursing*, p. 319, May, 1946; p. 379, June, 1946.
19. HILBERT, HORTENSE: Maternity Leaves in Public Health Nursing Agencies, *Public Health Nursing*, p. 602, November, 1942.
20. LESNIK, MILTON J., and BERNICE E. ANDERSON: "Legal Aspects of Nursing," J. B. Lippincott Company, Philadelphia, 1947.
21. LEWIS, FRANCES: R.N. Speaks—After Retirement What? *R.N.*, p. 26, August, 1950.
22. Looking for a Job? ANA Professional Counseling and Placement Service, *American Journal of Nursing*, p. 413, July, 1950.
23. MANNINO, ANTHONY J.: Men in Nursing, *American Journal of Nursing*, p. 198, March, 1951.
24. "Professional Nurses, The Outlook for Women in Occupations in the Medical Services," Women's Bureau, Department of Labor, Washington, D.C., Bulletin 203, No. 3, 1945.
25. ROSNAGLE, LAURA E.: Business Ethics for Nurses, *American Journal of Nursing*, p. 19, January, 1949.
26. Salaries of Professional Registered Nurses, *American Journal of Nursing*, p. 329, June, 1950.
27. SCHEELE, LEONARD A.: Looking Ahead with the Nursing Profession, *American Journal of Nursing*, p. 631, October, 1950.
28. SCHULZ, C. L., "Your Career in Nursing," McGraw-Hill Book Company, Inc., New York, 1941.
29. SCOTT, RUTH B.: Before You Move to Another State, *R.N.*, p. 61, October, 1948.
30. SCOTT, WILLIAM C., and DONALD W. SMITH: Workmen's Compensation and the Nurse, *American Journal of Nursing*, p. 136, March, 1950.
31. SMITH, EDITH H.: References, *American Journal of Nursing*, p. 633, October, 1948.
32. SPALDING, EUGENIA K.: "Professional Adjustments," rev. ed., J. B. Lippincott Company, Philadelphia, 1950.
33. STEWART, MAXWELL S.: "Buying Your Own Life," Public Affairs Committee, Pamphlet No. 134, New York, 1948.
34. "Survey of Men Nurses," New York State Nurses Association, Albany, N. Y., 1948.

35. TRIGGS, FRANCES O.: A Counseling and Placement Service for Nurses, *Occupations* (Vocational Guidance Association), p. 211, January, 1946.
36. TRIGGS, FRANCES O.: The Preparation of Counselors, *American Journal of Nursing*, p. 545, July, 1945.
37. Unions, discussions as they relate to nurses, *American Journal of Nursing*, p. 1122, November, 1936; p. 766, July, 1937; p. 733, June, 1938; p. 934, August, 1938; p. 231, March, 1944. *Public Health Nursing*, p. 700, November, 1944.
38. U.S. PUBLIC HEALTH SERVICE. "Study of Nursing School Health Practices and a Recommended Health Program for Student Nurses," Public Health Reports, Supplement No. 189, Washington, D.C., 1945.
39. WEST, MARGARET D.: Estimating the Future Supply of Professional Nurses, *American Journal of Nursing*, p. 656, October, 1950.
40. WICKENDEN, HOMER: Will You Have a Monthly Income When You Reach Old Age? *New York State Nurse, p.* 10, April, 1949.
41. WOLFE, LULU K.: The Nurse as a Person, *American Journal of Nursing*, p. 176, March, 1931.

Personal Appearance

1. BEARD, SARAH ALLEN: "Vocational Rehabilitation," New York University, New York, Occupational Abstract No. 71. (Vocational rehabilitation as a career.)
2. DIEHL, HAROLD S., and RUTH E. BOYNTON: "Healthful Living," 3d ed., McGraw-Hill Book Company, Inc., New York, 1949.
3. ERICKSON, CLIFFORD E., and MARION C. HAPP: "Guidance Practices at Work," McGraw-Hill Book Company, Inc., New York, 1946.
4. HAMILTON, KENNETH W.: "Counseling the Handicapped," The Ronald Press Company, New York, 1948.
5. LANE, JANET: "Your Carriage, Madam," John Wiley & Sons, Inc., New York, 1947.
6. LEWIN, PHILIP: Selection and Care of Shoes, *American Journal of Nursing*, p. 580, September, 1948.
7. LINCOLN, MIRIAM: "Danger! Curves Ahead," The Macmillan Company, New York, 1948.
8. MIDGELY, MARION: Your Speaking Voice, *American Journal of Nursing*, p. 411, April, 1941.
9. SPENCER, PAUL J.: Employee Health and Morale, *American Journal of Nursing*, p. 288, May, 1947.
10. WENIGER, CHARLES E.: Speech—A Nurse's Qualification, *Public Health Nursing*, p. 136, March, 1946.
11. "When You Grow Older," Public Affairs Committee, Pamphlet No. 131, New York, 1947.

See also List of Visual Aids, Appendix D.

CHAPTER II

Hospital Nursing

Of all the fields of nursing, hospitals employ the highest number of professional nurses. In 1949, there were 6,572 registered hospitals of all varieties, of which 61.6 per cent were classed as general hospitals.[1] They cared for 16,659,973 admissions. The number of patients in general hospitals has been rising steadily since 1935. Prepayment plans of one sort or another account for some of the increase. The Blue Cross hospitalization plan alone, now covers nearly forty million persons. A higher birth rate with greatly increased hospitalization of deliveries also added to the patient load.

Hospital (institutional) nursing, including schools of nursing, constitutes an occupation of almost half of the active professional nurses. Exclusive of private duty nurses (65,022), 232,625 professional nurses were employed in all hospitals in 1949. Of those in general hospitals, the distribution was as follows.[2]

Total	232,625
As nurse superintendents and assistants of hospitals and directors of nurses	9,281
Full-time instructors	5,259
Supervisors and assistants	20,970
Head nurses and assistants	31,352
General duty	106,508
Part-time and private duty	51,822
Not classified	7,433

Opportunities for advanced positions as administrators in many fields are highly attractive to nurses, and the field is relatively free from com-

[1] *Journal of the American Medical Association*, pp. 23, 26, 28, May 7, 1949.
[2] *Facts about Nursing*, p. 15, American Nurses Association, 1950. Includes schools of nursing.

petition by men. The top positions are the directorships of schools of nursing and of nursing services, and superintendencies of small hospitals. Professional nurses manage more than a third of the registered hospitals in the United States.

According to the rough estimates of future needs in the various fields of nursing, hospitals of all types will need 300,000 professional nurses by 1952. This is probably an underestimate as the population will be 154,-000,000 by 1952. The student nurse considering the hospital field for her future career is therefore fairly safe in counting on steady employment.

The field of hospital nursing is the most familiar to you.[3] You have seen professional nurses at work all around you, as private duty or "special nurses," floor nurses, clinical specialists, supervisors, teachers, and administrators. Perhaps you have already made up your mind which position you would like and know how to attain it. It is usually not difficult to find a job right in your own hospital and to keep on working up the ladder of promotion there. On the other hand, you may feel the need of a change, for a few years at least. You know that your experience will be broader if you seek work in a totally different kind of hospital from your own—a smaller one, a larger one, one in another part of the country. Some nurses find that they develop confidence faster, learn self-reliance and initiative, and are promoted sooner in a new environment.

The following are the usual positions filled by registered nurses in general hospitals. There are few hospitals that have all the positions listed, and there will probably be new positions developed every year to suit the need of the times. The list given is simply suggestive of the fields of interest.

> General duty or staff nurse
> Special duty or private practice nurse (may or may not be paid by the hospital)
> Head nurse
> Assistant head nurse
> Supervisor
> Assistant supervisor
> Instructor of clinical specialty or of special nursing group—students, aides, volunteers[4]

[3] For this reason a job description is omitted in this chapter.

[4] In some hospitals with schools of nursing, supervisors and instructors may combine educational and service responsibilities. For faculty requirements, see Chap. XV.

Director of nurses
Associate director of nurses ⎫   May be in charge of a depart-
Assistant director of nurses ⎭   ment or division of the hospital
Superintendent of the hospital
Assistant superintendent of the hospital

In the small hospital, a nurse in an administrative position often combines supervisory duties, while a supervisor may take on head-nurse duties or act as assistant to the director, or both. In emergencies or shortages, any nurse may be called on to substitute for another, or to take charge and direct. Special training and advanced clinical courses are necessary for all the positions above head-nurse level.

Other hospital positions sometimes filled by nurses are[5]

Anesthetist   Physical therapist (hydrotherapy,
Dietitian   electrotherapy, diathermy, mas-
Housemother   sage)
Laboratory technician   Receptionist
Medical social worker   Record historian or librarian
Occupational therapist   Recreation director
Pharmacist   Statistician
                                      X-ray technician

For most of these positions, some special preparation is required, in some cases a year or more of study and practice. A license to practice is necessary for many of them. A few are suitable for elderly nurses.

Hospital Service in Other Institutions

Positions open to nurses in other institutions where the hospital type of service is expected (not described in detail in other chapters of this book) are in the infirmaries or small hospital units of children's shelters, prisons, reformatories, very large industries (see Industrial Nursing, Chap. XIII), and private nursing homes of all types. In accepting a position in any one of these institutions, the applicant must assure herself that the institution is registered or at least licensed by the state and in good standing. She must have her position, responsibility, and hours of work clearly understood and the terms of her employment in writing. It is well to inquire how many other professional nurses are employed and

[5] See also Chap. XVII.

to whom you will be responsible. Of all the opportunities open to nurses, this group presents the least well-defined conditions of work and offers the greatest possibilities of disappointment, if the situation is not observed and clearly understood before employment is accepted. It is unwise to accept a position in a nonregistered hospital without a visit to the place and a personal interview with your employer.

GENERAL DUTY OR STAFF NURSING

As you have seen general staff (floor duty) nurses working about you all during training, it is hardly necessary to describe their functions. Your basic curriculum in the school of nursing should prepare you for this position.

The position of general duty nurse in a well-organized service offers highly satisfactory preliminary or first experience for the young graduate in preparation for head-nurse or supervisory responsibilities. A year or two of such experience in medical, surgical, or other hospital services enriches the all-too-brief patient contacts of student days. It strengthens a nurse's confidence in herself, her skills, and her knowledge and develops her capacity for leadership. This first year after graduation may be the one to determine your future choice of a specialty. It is especially recommended to the nurse who cannot make up her mind what she wants to do when she graduates. Some counselors believe the nurse should seek this general staff experience in a hospital other than the one connected with her school of nursing. The change is especially beneficial if satisfactory supervised experience can be secured in a hospital of a different size or type from the one the nurse has known as a student. A nurse familiar with a large public hospital of several hundred beds would find work in a private hospital of 100 to 200 beds a very enlightening experience, while the nurse who has graduated from a rurally situated, average-sized school of nursing—100 students—would enjoy a year in a large city. However, there are advisers who believe that young graduates should be urged to remain a year in the employment of their parent hospital before going elsewhere or undertaking advanced study. It is obviously to the advantage of the hospital or school of nursing to retain as staff nurses those familiar with their situation.

Counselors do not advise young graduates to seek the first year of hospital experience in a highly specialized field,[6] a proprietary hospital,

[6] Such, for example, as a hospital for drug addicts or alcoholic patients, epilepsy, incurable diseases, and eye, ear, nose, and throat specialties.

or an institution in which no qualified supervision is available from a professional nurse.

Whether you continue to work in your own hospital or seek a position elsewhere, it is advisable to try to live outside the institution if you can possibly afford it, and can find comfortable accommodations within your means. This is an acute problem in some areas today. You have probably discovered already how unwholesome it is—and, in the long run, how boring—to spend your free time talking shop, rehashing events on the ward, or complaining about thoughtless doctors, strict head nurses, or "difficult" patients. It will become more boring as time goes on. Therefore, as a graduate nurse, if you are "living in" and still connected with your own hospital, you will do well if you make it a rule to drop hospital gossip when off duty. Indirectly, you will benefit your patients, too. It may be hard at first, but if you do not make the effort you will soon find your small talk disappearing, your awareness of current events dulling. You will be in the embarrassing position of the operating-room nurse who, on dining with friends one Sunday, could not reply to a question about a current "best seller"—which she had not read—because she was obsessed by the urge to tell her host how beautifully Dr. Blank could remove the pigmented mole on his chin!

Staff nursing is a rewarding and absorbing career in itself and for itself. There are many nurses who find ample opportunity to perfect their skills, increase their knowledge, and develop unusual ability in this field, and who prefer it to all others. Here one never loses touch with patients and can see the latest victories of medical and surgical science. There is also the refreshing atmosphere of the students' world if there is a medical or a nursing school connected with the institution. Hospitals are beginning to encourage the growth and recognize the competence of an experienced staff of general duty nurses, both by promotional opportunities and by graded salary scales.

Hours of duty in general, non-Federal hospitals still continue to be longer than the recommended standard of the 8-hour day and 40-hour week. Many hospitals do not pay for overtime; many still allow but 2 weeks' vacation, although this limit is frowned upon and 4 weeks is recommended by the state and national nurses associations. It is expected that more and more hospitals will establish the 8-hour day, the 40-hour week, and 3 to 4 weeks of vacation annually with pay, as well as sick leave with pay. "Broken hours" are less common than formerly and will shortly be entirely abolished, it is thought. Personnel policies recommend that overtime be paid for at the rate of time and a half, or that compensating over-duty time be given. It is also recommended that night duty receive higher compensation than day duty.

The full white uniform of the graduate registered nurse is worn when on duty in the hospital. Administrators do not wear it continuously.

ADVANCED POSITIONS

SUPERVISION

Positions as head nurse, supervisor, educational director, and director of departments or divisional services, although they may be secured occasionally simply through satisfactory performance on the job over the years, are usually open only to those nurses who have taken advanced courses in ward, clinic, or unit administration teaching and supervision, and who have had at least a year—preferably 3 years—of experience in ward (or other unit) management. The greater the variety of experience, the richer will be the supervisor's or administrator's contribution to the program and, other personal factors being favorable, the faster will be her advancement.

HEAD NURSES

You are familiar, also, with the work of head nurses. Their functions differ somewhat, depending on the type of service to which they are assigned. The New York State Nurses Association[7] states that

"A head nurse is usually responsible for the administration of the nursing service and the supervision of nursing personnel in a single unit of a clinical department. She functions as an assistant supervisor in the hospital nursing staff and usually, also, as assistant clinical instructor in the nursing school staff. Her principal functions as a head nurse are

(1) Making adequate provisions for the nursing care of patients in her unit and maintaining good relationships with them, and also, with their medical attendants, relatives and friends.

(2) Arranging for the assistance required by the members of the medical staff and other professional personnel and co-operating with them in providing for the patient's total needs.

(3) Providing for accurately descriptive records of the medical treatment and nursing care of patients.

[7] *New York State Nurse*, p. 21, October, 1947.

(4) Defining the responsibilities and assigning the specific duties of assistant head nurse, staff nurses, and student nurses.

(5) Planning the ward teaching program (in co-operation with clinical instructors) and utilizing all opportunities to enrich the clinical experience afforded students, evaluating and recording results, and guiding students on the basis of findings.

(6) Assisting in the study of methods of nursing care (including total nursing service) for the purpose of promoting its continuous improvement.

(7) Directing, co-ordinating, and supervising the activities of the non-professional nursing personnel.

(8) Directing in co-operation with the housekeeping staff, the housekeeping activities which insure a safe and comfortable physical environment for the patients.

(9) Securing and distributing supplies and equipment necessary to the maintenance of the nursing service.

(10) Co-ordinating the services rendered by other departments of the hospital in the interests of effective management and patient welfare.

NURSING ADMINISTRATION

At the present time, the widest field of opportunity for nurse administrators is offered by hospitals and the schools of nursing connected with them.[8]

Positions for nurses in hospital administration are

Superintendent, assistant superintendent
Director of nursing service and assistant director
Supervisor of a department and assistants[9]
Head nurse and assistants (part-time administrative duties in small hospitals)

As a rule, general duty nurses do not have many or continuous administrative duties. In small hospitals, however, they may relieve in any of the positions listed above (see Chap. III).

[8] For administrative positions in public health nursing agencies, see Chap. XI.
[9] A variety of teaching and supervisory responsibilities may be assigned to nurses on this level. For example, operating-room supervisor, out-patient service director, or supervisor of the private pavilion.

In the small hospitals the superintendent may combine the duties of director of nurses, or her assistant may have that responsibility.[10]

One of the recently developed consultant positions is that of hospital nursing consultant at state level. Some of these consultant positions are connected with special divisions of the state health departments. For instance, the hospital nursing consultant would be under the professional guidance of the state director of public health nursing, but would be assigned to the administrative direction of the director of the division of hospitals. The hospital consultant positions have developed in connection with the activities governing the administration of the Hospital Survey and Construction Act (Public Health Law No. 725). The consultant assists in visiting hospitals, reviewing their design, and studying the physical facilities from the point of view of efficient and adequate nursing care and types of service. She consults with the hospital nursing staffs, recommends standards of service and kinds of personnel, and cooperates with the other state divisions in the furtherance of joint plans for improved public health protection.

Requirements for the hospital nursing consultant positions usually state that the nurse must have a B.S. degree, have taken advanced studies in the field of hospital administration, and give evidence of at least 6 years of experience, 3 of which must have been in positions above the general staff-nurse level and in which responsibilities in teaching, supervision, or administration were included. Ability to make studies, surveys, write reports, and speak in public is expected. Willingness to travel widely over a state is, of course, taken for granted.

In schools of nursing, typical administrative positions are

Director, assistant director
Supervisor (may have instructor's duties)
Instructor
Head nurse, assistant head nurse (part-time duties as instructors in small schools)

Occasionally, all these individuals are also instructors. This is especially true in the small schools. The public health coordinator is frequently a shared position with the hospital (see Chaps. XI and XV).

Administrators must be well-prepared persons. Administrators in

[10] Authorities agree that the director of nursing service is a full-time job in itself. A combination of the duties of superintendent and director can be a killing and entirely inefficient arrangement for all concerned.

schools of nursing probably must be the best prepared of all nursing personnel because of the grave responsibility which is theirs in directing, guiding, and leading young women into the profession of nursing.

It is difficult to generalize the desirable preparation for administrative positions, and practically impossible to define personal qualifications. Executive ability, capacity for leadership, imagination, adaptability, and skill in public relations—all necessary—may be developed through years of experience and still not assure administrative success. Similarly, academic degrees and outstanding scholarship, although adding prestige, do not make an administrator. To the young nurse who confidently hopes to direct and administer nursing service to the sick, the best advice appears to be: Obtain solid, broad, fundamental, firsthand experience in *nursing* under qualified supervisors; secure the best university courses you can find in administration, supervision, and personnel management, acquiring a master's degree within 5 years of graduation if you are already a college graduate and within 10 years if you are not; expect to offer at least 5 and probably 8 years of nursing experience in well-recognized institutions before receiving promotion to the top positions. The broader the base, the higher your ladder can reach. Bright young college graduates who have found the theoretical work in their schools of nursing easy are tempted to apply for advanced administrative positions in the first year or two after graduation. Occasionally they land on their feet in good positions. More often, they are given responsible jobs in mediocre institutions, paid well, and lured into thinking that they know it all. They then remain in that same position for many years through lack of the broad, basic experience that would have qualified them for the bigger jobs elsewhere. Too late they discover that one cannot skip the first grades and expect to qualify for the highest jobs. Army generals were not privates yesterday. In all your planning, seek the advice of the best administrators you know.[11]

SALARIES IN HOSPITALS

These vary with the size and character of the hospital, the area of the country, and the qualifications of the applicant. Maintenance (laundry, board, and room) is usually included, but lately more and more hospitals are arranging for the graduate staff to "live out," permitting the purchase of hospital meals, if desired, on a cost basis, and room allowance. If the

[11] For job descriptions of advanced positions, see Bibliography at the end of this chapter.

hospital is far from town, and transportation inadequate, the staff nurse may prefer to live at the hospital. Authorities agree, however, that separation from the hospital atmosphere, the change of scene, and the more normal life permitted by living in one's own home, even if it be only a rented room, are more wholesome for the graduate nurse and result in a more interesting companion for patients. The choice is often left to the nurse.

The allowance granted by the hospital for living out must be carefully stretched if it is to cover all expenses, including transportation and telephone. At the present writing, the cost of living out is not covered by the allowance made by many institutions. The day is not far off when all hospital administrators must look upon their nurse employees as other businesswomen are looked upon and give them salaries commensurate with their professional status and an "outside" life of their own. Living-out allowances must be adjusted to the cost-of-living standard for the area.

For general staff nurses in non-Federal hospitals, salaries have been in the neighborhood of $2,000 to $2,500; for head nurses and supervisors, $2,500 to $3,600; for hospital consultant nurses, $3,300 to $5,000; while those with executive and administrative duties receive up to $8,500.[12] How largely salary scales are affected by area differences can be seen when one compares California with New England. In the former, $2,600 is a minimum for staff nurses; in the latter $1,800 is still usual in urban areas, and even less in rural hospitals.

Superintendents of large hospitals—public hospitals in state or Federal services—are usually men, frequently doctors. However, 80 per cent of the hospitals under 100 beds were run by professional nurses in 1946. Their salaries now range from $4,000 to $8,000.

Although it is extremely unwise to generalize salary rates in this way, probably the following conclusions may be safely drawn by the young nurse:

1. A beginning salary may be low but, if qualified supervision is offered and promotional opportunities are in evidence, it would be better to accept such a position than one in which a high salary is paid but no provision made for supervision, in-service training, educational and promotional activities.

[12] Unless otherwise stated, the salaries quoted in this book do not include maintenance. It should also be remembered that they represent the prevailing levels at the time of writing (1951), and that the trend was then upward. The latest figures should be obtained from the appropriate organization listed in Appendix A.

2. Beware the job involving supervisory duties which offers a high salary to a beginner and states, "No experience necessary."
3. If a beginning salary seems very much out of line with what you know about the work, make inquiries before accepting it. If it is unusually low, you must be assured of compensating factors, such as a high quality of experience and supervision, rate of promotion, or chances to carry outside courses. If it is unusually high, be sure you understand just what is expected of you, what your hours of duty are, holidays, vacation, and sick leave. Sometimes a nurse finds she is expected to more than earn a high salary by relieving during evening hours or on holidays.

Inquiry as to prevailing salary rates in hospitals can always be made of your state nurses association or the ANA; or the index of the *American Journal of Nursing* may be consulted for reports of the latest salary studies. Also, read over the salaries quoted in the advertisement section of the *Journal*.

OPPORTUNITIES FOR EMPLOYMENT IN HOSPITAL POSITIONS[13]

1. Professional registries and placement bureaus (see official directory of these in the *American Journal of Nursing*)
2. General and special hospitals: Federal, state, local, public, and voluntary. The hospital connected with one's own school of nursing is a natural, though not necessarily the best, source of employment information. For the names of registered hospitals in the United States, refer to the American Medical Association,[14] or see the hospital census of the American Hospital Association and the AMA, published annually in the journal of the AMA.
3. Federal hospitals (write to the U.S. Civil Service Commission, Washington, D.C., or inquire at one of the regional bureaus of the Commission; see also Chap. XVI)
4. State employment services (for local offices, see telephone directory)
5. The university where you have taken courses: someone there may be able to put you in touch with desirable openings.
6. Advertisements in professional journals

[13] See also Chap. III, Rural Hospital Nursing.
[14] The addresses of all organizations mentioned in this chapter will be found in Appendix A.

Check to see that the hospital is registered and that you may practice in the state in which it is located if you are not registered there.

BIBLIOGRAPHY

1. Administration—A Bibliography, *American Journal of Nursing*, p. 368, May, 1945.
2. BECK, Sister M. BERENICE: General Staff Nursing, *American Journal of Nursing*, p. 57, January, 1937.
3. DEMING, DOROTHY: "Pam Wilson, Registered Nurse," Dodd, Mead & Company, Inc., New York, 1946. (Last chapters relate to nursing in a small hospital.)
4. DEMING, DOROTHY: "Sharon's Nursing Diary," Dodd, Mead & Company, Inc., New York, 1948.
5. FLORENCE, Sister MARY: Is Medical Nursing for You? *American Journal of Nursing*, p. 373, June, 1949.
6. The General Staff Nurse, *American Journal of Nursing*, pp. 1221–1229, November, 1938; pp. 300–301, May, 1946.
7. MORRISON, PEARL L.: The Nurse in Hospital Administration, *Canadian Nurse*, p. 672, October, 1940.
8. "Personnel Practices for General Staff Nurses," pp. 32–46, American Nurses Association and National League of Nursing Education, New York, 1944.
9. PETERSON, FREDA A.: Eleven to Seven, *American Journal of Nursing*, p. 127, February, 1951.
10. PHANEUF, MADELEINE: Preparation of a Hospital Nursing Consultant, *American Journal of Nursing*, p. 311, May, 1948.
11. POLATIN, PHILLIP: The Mental Hygiene Aspects of Full Maintenance, *American Journal of Nursing*, p. 254, March, 1942.
12. "Problems of Hospital Administration," Joint Commission on Education, Chicago, 1948.
13. Recommended Standards for General Staff Nursing (Hospitals), *American Journal of Nursing*, p. 897, September, 1944.
14. STEFFEN, ANNA M.: Field Experience in Head Nursing, *American Journal of Nursing*, p. 465, July, 1949.
15. Suggested Minimum Qualifications—Nursing Schools and Hospital Nursing Services, *American Journal of Nursing*, p. 80, January, 1943.
16. TSCHUDIN, MARY S.: A Plan for Preparing Head Nurses and Supervisors, *American Journal of Nursing*, p. 213, March, 1945.
17. Types of Clinical Courses for Graduate Nurses, *American Journal of Nursing*, p. 1162, December, 1944.
18. WILLIAMS, JANETTE SPURRIER: My Orientation to a New Job, *American Journal of Nursing*, p. 42, January, 1951.

CHAPTER III

Rural Hospital Nursing

Not all small hospitals are rural and not all rural hospitals are small. One may say with considerable truth, however, that small registered hospitals are usually located in centers of less than 25,000 population.[1] Hospitals of less than 25 beds in large cities are apt to be proprietary hospitals, while those of more than 300 beds in strictly rural areas are usually governmental—Federal, state, or county supported.

The small or rural hospital presents quite a different scope of work for the professional nurse from that in the hospital of 100 or more beds. A small rural hospital is not just a large hospital on a small scale. It has its peculiar problems of meeting community needs; of offering care for every ailment and accident known to man, with limited equipment; of struggling to raise enough money to keep going at all; and of overnight shortages which may send the superintendent into the kitchen, the maid to help in the nursery! In proportion, small hospitals have greater problems than large ones. Actually, 4,000 hospitals, or more than half of those registered in 1949, had less than 100 beds. Of these, 2,849 had less than 50 beds.[2] So hospitals of this size deserve special consideration, and nurses planning to look for positions there should understand the situation, appreciate the differences, and be ready to take advantage of the many opportunities for promotion that may come their way, for this is a field of nursing where there is great need of young, well-qualified, and ambitious nurses. They will find rapid advancement awaiting them if they will stick to the job and prepare for its special demands. It is often in the rural hospital that a nurse discovers for the first time that she has aptitude for and an interest in hospital administration.

[1] See *Journal of the American Medical Association*, p. 26, May 6, 1950.
[2] *Facts about Nursing*, p. 74, American Nurses Association, 1950.

The salaried positions open to nurses in small hospitals are

Superintendent
Assistant superintendent
Supervisor or head nurse
General duty[3]

In addition, if the small hospital is serving as a field of experience for student nurses, an educational director or clinical instructor may be added to the staff. Hospitals with a census of less than 50 patients, daily average, do not—and should not—conduct schools of professional nursing. Rural hospital experience, however, as an affiliation for the senior student nurse or as a part of postgraduate study in ward and hospital administration, is a recent development that bears watching. Desirable teaching positions are available where these educational programs are under way.

As it is not usually easy to secure special duty nurses in rural areas in the same quantity as in the cities, general duty nurses are frequently called upon to "special" very ill patients. Adequacy of general duty staff, therefore, is especially important, as well as flexibility and willingness on the part of all members of the staff to carry any duty assigned. Work with volunteers, both lay and professional, will be a part of the rural nurse's experience.

Most nurses soon discover whether or not they like nursing in rural hospitals. A few find they miss the rush and bustle of a large hospital, the ever-present resources for care and treatment, and the proximity of every form of urban recreation. Others, however, like Miss Bohn, whose story follows, welcome the friendliness and letup in pressure of the small hospital. They enjoy the less formal life of the country and come to develop a real sense of shared ownership in every activity of the hospital. One of the great compensations in nursing in a small community is that it becomes home in the real meaning of that word, and more and more rural nurses are acquiring their own homes and gardens near their place of work.

Qualifications for work in a small hospital stress adaptability, self-reliance, and thorough preparation in general duty. A nurse who has graduated from a small hospital is advised to secure experience in a large

[3] In small hospitals there are apt to be part-time general duty nurses who come in for emergencies. Married nurses take advantage of these opportunities. These are in addition to "special duty" nurses.

hospital *before* specializing in rural hospital nursing. Just because a hospital can accommodate only 30 patients at a time is no guarantee that the nurse can "get by" with superficial preparation in any one of the basic clinical areas. She is as likely as not to be in sole charge of all 30 patients, representing as many conditions, within a few months of her appointment. In emergencies she may replace temporarily the operating-room supervisor, the superintendent, or the obstetrician! The more thorough and sound her nursing education, the better are her chances for success and promotion in the rural hospital.

Rural hospitals do not as a rule have very large medical staffs of specialists and sometimes send long distances for consultation service. On the other hand, doctors from a wide area may use the hospital for diagnostic and treatment services for their private patients; the out-patient and clinic service may be far more varied and interesting than in a congested city area; and the hospital nursing staff is necessarily much more aware of the public health activities—including the public health nurses—functioning in the surrounding country. It is usual for the public health nurses to visit the hospital frequently and freely, even relieving for a few hours in times of shortages, and there is a growing acceptance of the community hospital as the health center for one or more counties. A few hospitals and county health departments have combined headquarters.[4] It is thought that such combinations strengthen the position of both agencies, broaden their service, and provide a higher quality of trained personnel. They make rich teaching fields for student experience for doctors and nurses and will probably increase in number as time goes on. A nurse seeking a position in a rural hospital would be wise to choose one that has an affiliation of this sort. Nor can she go far wrong if she selects a hospital being used as a teaching center by a university or medical school.

Other qualifications needed for staff work in the small hospital are described in Miss Bohn's sketch. Miss Dina Bremness, the present superintendent of the hospital, has been kind enough to supply enough information to bring the account up to date.

Nursing in a Rural Hospital

Five years ago I was graduated from an accredited school of nursing in a large city. After passing my state board examinations and acquiring

[4] For example, Bremerton, Kitsap County, Washington.

state registration I was ready for my first position. I had had good professional education but no advanced preparation and I knew I needed experience before choosing a definite field of work, so I decided to do general nursing in my home community. Here I thought I would find the experience I was seeking and a variety of nursing practice.

My home is in a small town of 2,600 population in rural Minnesota. While I was away at school, this community had planned and completed a new 35-bed municipal hospital. The community was very proud of this hospital. It was a symbol of progress and a means, at last, of providing adequate medical and nursing care for the sick in the surrounding area.

A few days after my return home I went over to the attractive brick building and introduced myself at the business office. I explained that I was a new graduate and asked if there was a position open for a general staff nurse. Like all hospitals at that time they were in need of more registered nurses. The superintendent, therefore, was glad to welcome me, but there were quite a few preliminaries to be settled. Before filling out the application, there were facts that I wanted to know: What was expected of me as a general staff nurse, what would be my salary, the salary increase, vacation, hours of duty, and opportunities for promotion? The superintendent, in her turn, explained that as an applicant I must be in sound physical health and that a physical examination was required at the time of employment. An annual checkup was advised, more often if indicated.

I learned that my beginning monthly salary would be $100, paid semi-monthly, with full maintenance which included room, board, and laundry.[5] I wished to live at home and was delighted to hear it could be arranged, with a cash allowance for my room. The first salary increase could be anticipated in 6 months and each year thereafter. Salary increases were based upon ability, satisfactory service, and promotions.

My working day would be $8\frac{1}{2}$ hours, inclusive of mealtime, straight or broken shift for those on day duty. I would have 1 day off each week and a half day on Sundays and holidays, alternating weekly morning and evening hours.[6] A weekly time schedule was always posted so plans for time off could be made in advance. A period of 12 months' service must intervene before a 2 weeks' vacation with pay would be granted, otherwise 1 day for each month after 6 months was allowed.

The superintendent then went on to tell me something of the personnel.

[5] In 1951, salaries were $220 a month.
[6] In 1951, hours were 40 per week, straight shifts.

There were nine registered nurses including the superintendent, seven nurses' aides, and a registered laboratory and x-ray technician. There were a few married nurses, who were called in for relief or part-time work when extra help was needed. This constituted the nursing staff. How small the staff seemed after the great hospital where I had worked! But then there were only 35 beds! We were responsible for the supervision of the nurses' aides, carefully teaching them their duties and nursing routines for the best and safest nursing care.

Naturally, I was anxious to see the hospital and the different departments. I wondered what facilities a nurse was expected to work with and under what conditions. We began our tour on the main floor, which is divided into two sections. To the left of the lobby is the segregated obstetric department, to the right is the clean medical division. The nurse's station, medicine cabinet, utility rooms, and small diet kitchen are centrally located so that the distance is not too far to any patient's room. The nurse sitting at the desk has full view of the corridor.

The nursery is viewed through a large double-plated window. There are ten bassinets and two incubators. I was impressed with the simplicity of the plan, the anteroom with sink and shelf for masks, hooks for gowns, and a swinging door into the nursery proper. Here I was sure a good nursery technique could be carried out. Next, along the left of the corridor is the labor room directly connected with a well-equipped delivery room. The rooms on this side of the corridor all have soundproof walls.

The second floor is for medical and surgical cases. The nurse's station, utility room, and diet kitchen are in the same relative position as on the main floor. At the head of the stairway is a fracture room with a large closet for fracture equipment and supplies. The windows have darkroom curtains so that fluoroscopy can be done with the portable x-ray machine. Next to this room, at the left, is the x-ray room which has a large machine for diagnostic purposes. Off this is a small darkroom for developing films. Across the hall is the laboratory with the registered technician in charge. At the end of the hall you come to the central supply room. At the time of my first visit, a nurse and a nurse's aide were busy packaging gloves and sterilizing supplies for the next day's schedule. The operating room is a large bright room with the usual gleaming fixtures, windows on two sides, and glass-enclosed instrument cupboards. Adjoining this is the scrub room. At the end of the hall is the doctors' lounge with lockers and shower. Each week, staff meetings are held there. Another small room is the library and record room.

We took the elevator to the ground or basement floor. At the end of the corridor is an isolation suite, consisting of two private rooms, utility room, small kitchen, and closet. Here was safe isolation for a patient with a communicable disease or questionable diagnosis. To the right are the ambulance entrance, store rooms, main kitchen, and dining room. Laundry and engine room are in the subbasement.

I was really surprised at the completeness, compactness, and convenience of this small hospital. It was spotless, and the friendliness of the staff and the smiling patients made me feel at home already. Much of the rush and confusion which a stranger sometimes feels in a big institution were absent here. Things were happening, everyone was busy but not too busy to be interested in the visitor. I felt eager to be a member of the staff.

Returning to the office, I quickly filled out my application, giving my qualifications, registration number, and references. A week later I reported for work.

I am glad to record here that I made a good choice! I discovered that standard techniques and nursing procedures were in use which enable a new nurse to adjust herself readily. I appreciated more and more the services of the well-trained nurses' aides, who carry out the daily routines and simpler nursing duties, leaving the more important procedures for the professional nurse.

This hospital affords good educational as well as emergency experience for the "generalist." I became familiar with many problems present in a small hospital which you never meet in large institutions. It isn't long before you feel the hospital belongs to you, rather than you to the hospital! Our hospital is like a beautiful little machine. It is our pride to keep it running smoothly.

It was not long before I was advanced to the head of the obstetric department, adding more responsibility and experience. I was then given the chance to go to the continuation center at the state university for a brief study course. These courses are attended each year by the head of one of the departments in our hospital who brings back information on new developments and methods in nursing. These are discussed at our nurses' conferences. The conferences are held once a month for informal discussion of nursing problems, new techniques, and medications. They stimulate better nursing service. Three years ago, student practical nurse affiliates from one of the state-accredited schools of practical nursing were sent to this rural hospital to get their practical experience in the care of mothers and babies, thus adding another interesting service for the staff.

I favor the pleasant experiences in the obstetric department. I like to see that each case is individualized and not treated as a routine affair. It is satisfying to be able to recognize the emotional upset, the fears or anxiety that sometimes accompany a young mother in this condition, to talk with her and help her initiate a happier mental attitude. I enjoy giving demonstration baby baths to a group of two or three mothers, giving them outlines and leaflets to take home, with a few elementary rules on infant care and formula making. If a mother leaves the hospital early with insufficient help at home, we report the case and she is visited daily by the county public health nurse until she is strong enough to care for herself and family again. Thus hospital and community come close together.

Our hospital is recognized by the American Medical Association, is a member of the state and American Hospital Associations, and is fully approved by the American College of Surgeons. It is also a member of the Blue Cross hospital plan. In 1947, Glenwood Hospital joined the Public Employees Retirement Association making available a retirement plan which gives at age sixty-five a monthly annuity for life of half the average monthly earned salary. This annuity, along with the monthly payments under Social Security (just starting), promises real security on retirement from the staff.

Little did I realize before coming here the significance to a community of having a hospital that meets the standards of these organizations and of having safe hospital service available to all its people! Never before had I appreciated the interest the people of the community have in their hospitals. This is a very good thing because it helps to keep up our standards.

The women of the community have a hospital auxiliary. They hold meetings once a month, help to raise funds for new equipment, and sew layettes for the nursery. Hospital employees have an opportunity to speak before this group and explain the work of the different departments. In this way we have a chance to help in the public education and interpretation program of the hospital. Our hospital has had a very successful public education program—so successful, in fact, that we have won state and national awards for 6 successive years. Each employee feels she has had a real share in contributing to its success.

The community has patronized the hospital so well that it is full to capacity most of the time. There are seven doctors on the staff. We draw from an area of 1,296 square miles in which there is an estimated population of 23,085. Because of the rapidly increasing number of patients we find our hospital too small and are planning an addition as soon as labor and materials are available.

I like our small hospital and I like our community. For the first time in my life, like the other girls who come here to work, I feel like a citizen and a part of the community. We are included in many social functions and participate actively in them. There are numerous clubs, church organizations, and a hospital bowling league. I have become vitally interested in community politics, and getting out to vote was a real privilege for I personally knew the candidates, their office, and what they stood for. The welfare of the community has become one of my major interests.

Life in a small community offers many diversions to release the tension of a weary mind and body. Every nurse here is urged to have a hobby. Most of us manage several, one or more for each season: golfing, tennis, and swimming in summer, skating, fishing, and skiing in winter. Many of the girls indulge in sports and recreations that they have never tried before and love it! City nurses are inclined to sleep too much on their hours off, leaving little time for anything else. This produces a feeling of irritability and dissatisfaction, of nothing accomplished and a monotonous life. We say, "Give your job the best you have while you are working and forget all about it when you are off—get out and have fun!" The carefree, outdoor life is excellent for us. Some of us like hunting, ice skating in winter, and horseback riding. We go into the woods and try new barbecue recipes.

For those who like less strenuous recreation, we have literary and musical clubs and church organizations. Two of the girls planted and cared for a garden last year, while two others successfully raised 50 chickens, sold the products, and divided the proceeds! Some have a talent and like to paint, write, dance, or sing. The choice of a hobby, of course, depends on your personal make-up and interest, but everyone can find a satisfactory one, there are so many to choose from at little cost. No matter what the hobby, there is a chance to develop it here. It is an invitation to a more stimulating and happier life. The ways in which the staff of this hospital use their vacations would make interesting reading. The girls have traveled into practically all sections of the United States and have visited Mexico, Canada, and Europe. Vacations may be extended a bit for the longer trips, if relief nursing service is available.

No young nurse should hesitate to do nursing in a small community hospital. The wholesome life and friendly atmosphere will do much for the development of her personality. She will find herself rich in experience that will prove valuable no matter what future field of work she may choose.

ELSYE BOHN, R.N.
Glenwood Community Hospital
Glenwood, Minnesota

The following is the report of an actual day's activities of a nurse who is both the director of nursing service and in charge of a school of practical nursing in a hospital in a rural area.

A Typical Day of The Directress of Nurses of The Henry W. Putnam Memorial Hospital, Bennington, Vermont

MONDAY

5:30 A.M. Out of bed after a pleasant week end at home.

6:00 A.M. Visit with night supervisor. Help her solve her problems of the night.

Go to drug room to find special drug order needed for use at 7:00 A.M.

Night report from night supervisor.

Visit critically ill patients.

Review time sheet.

Check admissions for the day.

7:30 A.M. Now for breakfast!

8:00 A.M. Chapel—prayers with student practical nurses.

8:15 A.M. Supervisors' meeting.

8:45 A.M. Complete visiting patients, at the same time consulting with floor supervisors about problems that confront them with regard to the patients' care.

10:45 A.M. Conference with the administrator of the hospital, interrupted by two telephone calls about booking a patient and an appointment with a prospective student.

11:15 A.M. Conference with pharmacist: problem of the nursing department's not getting requisitions into drug room so that proper charges can be made to patient.

11:30 A.M. Interview with instructor: going over curriculum for students and planning what should be accomplished during the coming week. Also arrangements for my assistant and instructor to attend meeting in Albany tomorrow.

11:45 A.M. Appointment with one of the graduate practical nurses who asks if she may see me for a few minutes—she is leaving for Arizona to be married but will be back in a few months and would like to know if she may still have her job and room when she returns.

11:50 A.M. A salesman has been waiting for half an hour to demonstrate his special kind of sheets with corners already made.

12:15 P.M. Luncheon with my assistant, interrupted by a phone call for the ambulance for a bad accident.

12:45 P.M. Back to the office! Chief of staff calls and wishes to make a suggestion about a procedure in the operating room and registers a complaint about a patient's diet.

1:00 P.M. Appointment with prospective student from out of town.

1:30 P.M. Appointment downtown with the administrator and chief of maintenance to see if it would be better to have our laundry done outside as we need to invest in new equipment. We must decide whether this plan is economical or not.

3:00 P.M. Back to office and in uniform again. Revisit critically ill patients.

4:00 P.M. The afternoon has vanished and the evening supervisor has arrived and it is time for the evening report.

4:30 P.M. Meeting with the student program commitee to make plans for card party to earn money to defray expenses for the lobbyist and lawyer for the Practical Nurses' Bill, and make arrangements for an orchestra for the student dance.

5:15 P.M. Suppertime—enjoy eating with the evening supervisor and one of the doctors who is waiting for an obstetrical patient.

5:45 P.M. Appointment with a graduate nurse regarding a position here—bad bus connections made it impossible for her to arrive earlier.

6:30 P.M. Call from the administrator stating he has out-of-town hospital friends visiting him and asking me if I would take them on a tour of the hospital and grounds.

8:00 P.M. Final good-night check with evening supervisor.

8:15 P.M. Back to my apartment—I forgot to check with the housemother, who comes on duty at 7:00 P.M., about the study hour for the students—decide to call her on the phone.

A rush to get ready for Bennington County Nurses' Meeting at 8:30 P.M. Guest speaker is Norman Rockwell. I must be ready to introduce him to the group.

10:30 P.M. Ready to retire—tomorrow is another day.

11:30 P.M. Awakened by telephone—a long-distance call from Montpelier from the lawyer. There is to be a special public hearing on the Practical Nurses' Bill. He feels it is very important that I attend. Conversation is finally ended with my promise that I will be there rain or shine.

11:45 P.M. Wearily to bed, having this time actually finished the "Day Report" for Miss Deming's book!

PHYLLIS COBURN, R.N.
Superintendent of Nurses

Miss Coburn adds:

The director of nurses must not only be on duty her 8 or more hours a day but must be on call most of the remaining hours. She must make decisions and keep things running smoothly. She is generally the assistant director of the hospital and takes complete charge when her executive is away. She must be capable of taking over any department in the hospital from diet kitchen to maintenance. She must be "the in-between person" for doctors and nurses and patients and be ever-interested in the welfare of her patients.

Many small hospitals have schools for practical nurses. The director plans the school program and curriculum and interviews all applicants; and it is her responsibility to arrange, oversee, and—many times—teach the classes in order to turn out nurses of whom she and her hospital may be proud.

It would seem, in the face of all this, that the director of nurses of any type of hospital has a very busy and full life, but her job is one which can bring her and her associates a great deal of happiness and satisfaction.

SALARIES

In small hospitals in rural areas, initial general duty salaries for staff nurses usually range (1951) from $150 to $250 a month with maintenance. In larger or urban hospitals, they range from $160 to $300, the higher salary being without maintenance. It must be remembered that living costs are higher in the cities and that money does not go so far as in the country.

Salaries for clinical specialists range from $160 to $250; for supervisors, to $300; for instructors, from $200 to $300. (For administrators, see Salaries of Administrators in Small Hospitals, below.)

ADMINISTRATION: SUPERINTENDENTS OF SMALL HOSPITALS

Of all the positions in small and rural hospitals, that of superintendent is most attractive to nurses who can offer experience, training, and evidence of executive ability. The superintendent in these hospitals is the administrator of the hospital and usually of the nursing service. In 1940, nurses were superintendents in 80 per cent of the registered hospitals of less than 100 beds. The responsibilities of this position are fascinating to many nurses, combining as they do business knowledge and acumen, love of homemaking, nursing, and personnel administration.

The management of a hospital is a business. The more talent and training a nurse has for this field, the more successful she will be in developing her product, balancing her books, and succeeding. As superintendent, she has oversight of every department, maintains the plant, purchases supplies, and sells the service to the public. She is responsible to the board of trustees for the economical use of equipment, the installation of up-to-date and safe appliances, and pleasing the customers, which in this instance are two groups—patients and doctors.

Her homemaking duties involve hospital housekeeping—a special field in itself—acting as hostess, much as does the manager of a hotel, to an ever-changing roster of guests and their families, and overseeing the general appearance, atmosphere, and spirit of the institution and the staff, which should give the impression of a cordial, friendly welcome to patients while maintaining efficiency and prompt service.

As a nurse, the superintendent must understand how to make it possible for the medical staff to function to capacity, to have all necessary equipment and facilities and, in short, to make the hospital the best place to which to take and serve their patients. A knowledge of the needs of patients in all types and stages of illness, of what constitutes good nursing care and where to secure it, of the routines that promote comfort and efficient service, and the physical surroundings conducive to recovery— these are a part of the superintendent's armamentarium.

The superintendent is the administrator. Under her are the business, housekeeping, nursing, and custodial staffs. Their "hiring and firing," training, promotion, and supervision are under her general direction. Records and accounts must be kept or supervised. Although each department may have its own head responsible to the superintendent, the board of trustees holds her responsible for the over-all management of the personnel and the delegation of duties. Indeed, one of the superintendent's most important functions is to carry out the decisions of the board, to secure directive policies for the running of the hospital, and to report results.

In a small community or county, the hospital is a prominent institution, and its superintendent has many social and business connections. She must develop skill in handling public relations and publicity—two quite different things—and maneuver to keep the hospital in a position in which it deserves and wins public support and approval. As a small hospital is not often wealthy, its superintendent must usually be thrifty and imaginative in ways to save and raise money.

Superintendents of rural hospitals agree that readiness to deal with emergencies great and small is the ever-recurrent test facing each administrator. Actual emergencies reported to the writer on the day of her visit to six small hospitals widely scattered geographically were as follows:

1. Midnight flooding of the furnace room from broken water main
2. Admission of six persons badly injured in an automobile accident, with hospital already full to capacity
3. Fire in wastebasket in nurse's room, spreading to draperies and bed before discovered
4. Walkout of chef just as patients' dinner was about to be served (Superintendent carved lamb for 40 patients)
5. Failure of electric power delayed laundry for 4 days. Another local laundry refused to take the hospital linen which was finally sent to a city 30 miles away.
6. Shortage of nurses necessitated the closing of a whole floor on 2 days' notice.

In general, other desirable aptitudes in a superintendent include ability to speak in public, write clear business letters, appraise materials and equipment, deal with salesmen, and organize committees. The wise superintendent takes time to share in community activities, and it is most important for her to know how—and when—to delegate work and to recognize the place of the specialist and the volunteer.

A hospital administrator who is not responsible for nursing service need not be a registered nurse. If she is a nurse, the board of trustees must understand that her primary responsibility is an administrator. She must not be expected to pinch-hit in the delivery or operating room or on the wards.

Not all these qualifications can be developed without study and practice. It is necessary for a nurse planning to enter this field to take advanced courses in hospital administration, following several years of experience on wards and divisions as head or supervisory nurse. If possible, experience should be gained as an assistant before taking over the full duties of superintendent. Courses in hospital administration and personnel management are becoming more essential and more available every year.

For information regarding advanced courses in this field, write to the American Hospital Association, Chicago, Illinois, and to the American Nurses Association.[7]

SALARIES OF ADMINISTRATORS IN SMALL HOSPITALS

The superintendent in a small hospital is provided with full maintenance, which usually means a small apartment in the nurses' home, meals, and laundry. Her car may be garaged free. It is desirable that she be furnished with a separate house or that sufficient allowance be added to her salary in lieu of maintenance to provide for a separate apartment. The habit of expecting the superintendent of a hospital to serve as housemother or director of the nurses' home has been decried and is not popular with the group. Salaries ranged in 1951 from $3,500 to $7,000, with the larger ones in hospitals of over 75 beds.

Sources of Employment

For general duty nurses, openings may be found by direct approach —like Miss Bohn's—or through the agencies listed under Opportunities for Employment in Hospital Positions.

Advanced positions may be secured through

Professional placement agencies
American Hospital Association

[7] For the addresses of organizations mentioned in this chapter, see Appendix A.

Colleges and universities where courses have been taken
State hospital associations
Hospitals themselves by direct application
Other hospital superintendents
Advertising sections of medical, nursing, and hospital journals
Commercial agencies

Be sure that the hospital is registered and that you are permitted to practice in the state, if you are not registered in it.

BIBLIOGRAPHY

1. BOYLE, RENA, and EFFIE LARSON: Rural Hospitals Attract Nurses, *American Journal of Nursing*, p. 742, December, 1948. See also p. 786.
2. Consider the Predicament of the Rural Hospital, *New York State Nurse*, p. 15, January, 1948. (Quoted from *Nursing News*, Connecticut.)
3. DAERS, MICHAEL M.: The Nurse in Hospital Administration, *American Journal of Nursing*, p. 561, June, 1936. (For point of view.)
4. DENSFORD, KATHARINE J., and MARGERY LOW: Student Experience in Rural Nursing, *American Journal of Nursing*, p. 732, November, 1949.
5. GELINAS, AGNES: A Rural Hospital Administrator, *American Journal of Nursing*, p. 650, June, 1940.
6. Nursing in Small Hospitals, *American Journal of Nursing*, p. 1372, December, 1940.
7. RYBERG, IDA C.: Rural Nursing Is for Me, *American Journal of Nursing*, p. 40, January, 1951.
8. SLOAN, RAYMOND P.: These Small Hospitals Can Take It, *Modern Hospital*, p. 46, January, 1944.
9. The Small Hospital Supervisor, *American Journal of Nursing*, p. 315, March, 1941.
10. SOUTHMAYD, HENRY J., and GEDDES SMITH: "Small Community Hospitals," Commonwealth Fund, Division of Publication, New York, 1944.
11. WALTERS, NELLIE W., MARY J. WHITESELL, and OLIVE M. BENN: A Rural Nursing Affiliation, *American Journal of Nursing*, p. 270, April, 1951.

See also Bibliography at the end of Chap. II.

CHAPTER IV

Out-patient Department and Clinic Services

Nursing service in the out-patient department of a hospital or in a dispensary, health center, or other institution offering medical care through organized clinics, offers a happy combination of public health practice and general duty nursing, with emphasis on teaching. Amelia H. Grant, commenting on this subject at a state nurses' meeting (New York, 1934), once said, "The nurse serving in a clinic or health conference is hostess, nurse, teacher, and social worker rolled into one." In small out-patient departments or clinics offering highly specialized services where the case load is light, the nurse in charge is especially aware of this fourfold function, while in hospitals conducting 40 or 50 clinics a week, she may be functioning chiefly as a nurse, the other roles being filled by receptionists, admitting clerks, medical social-service workers, medical secretaries, health educators, and volunteers—to name a few of the nurse's teammates.

Directors of nursing service and supervisors in out-patient services and clinics should be qualified public health nurses. When public health background is not required, the nurses are usually drawn from the hospital staff. Because of the daytime hours and freedom from duty over week ends, these are popular positions and in great demand.

Positions in out-patient and clinic services connected with rural community hospitals are especially varied in their scope and responsibilities and will in all probability develop in greater numbers as the national rural health and hospital program gets under way. Rural clinics usually receive a greater variety of cases over a wider economic range than city clinics because they may serve a total population unit of 30,000 or more scattered over several counties,[1] while the out-patient service of an urban

[1] For example, the Hitchcock Clinic in Hanover, N.H.

hospital may be only one of half a dozen local hospitals in a congested area serving a fairly homogeneous population. The public health nurse employed in a rural area is frequently expected to organize and serve in clinics and health conferences of all varieties (see Chap. XI). These may include itinerant clinics sponsored by the state health department.

The use of rural hospital clinics for diagnostic and treatment services by local physicians for their private patients, usually on a fee basis, is becoming an increasingly familiar practice of advantage to all three parties—the country physician, who cannot afford to provide the expensive equipment for all necessary tests and treatments; the patient, who finds skilled service and up-to-date facilities centered in one place; and the hospital, which thus takes its rightful place as a community health center and meets the cost of its services.

Group medical service, which provides pooled examining, diagnostic, and treatment facilities to patients, is also expanding with the encouragement of various prepayment and insurance plans. It is not unusual to find several specialists housed in a professional building or health center, offering a wide range of diagnostic and treatment services to paying patients. Under this type of arrangement, the physicians may share waiting rooms, record and secretarial services, x-ray, diathermy, metabolism, and other clinic facilities, while nursing service may be drawn from a "pool" or assigned by a head nurse. Professional nurses are finding these opportunities of growing importance and interest.

When, as occasionally happens, the out-patient department, health center, clinic, or dispensary provides nursing service in homes, the nurses should be qualified public health nurses or, if this is a student-nurse project, be under the close supervision of a fully qualified public health nurse (see Chap. XI).

Maternity clinics and out-patient departments sometimes conduct home delivery services in which nurses and student nurses share. In this case, the nurse in charge is required to have advanced clinical preparation in obstetric nursing (see Chap. V).

A nurse usually wears a hospital uniform, smock, or over-all gown when on duty in a clinic; the public health nurse's uniform or business suit for home visiting; a washable gown or public health nurse's uniform and gown for home delivery service.[2]

[2] Many of the duties of clinic nurses are described in a study by HILBERT, HORTENSE: "Public Health Nursing Services in Clinics," National Organization for Public Health Nursing, 1944.

The supervisors of nursing service in out-patient departments are in a strategic position to share their knowledge of the community and family backgrounds with other nurses of the hospital staff and, if there is a school of nursing connected with the hospital, to interpret the social, economic, and public health aspects of illness to the students. The supervisor takes part in staff conferences and in curriculum planning, guides the students' clinic experience, and offers suggestions for educational opportunities among the community health and social agencies. Positions of this type are distinctly stimulating and absorbing. Their variety and scope are well and truly described by Martha Johnson in her letter below.[3]

It is "on the books" of the future that the out-patient departments of hospitals will offer more educational opportunities of two types: health education of patients under the direction of a qualified health educator, and education in the general aspects of and approach to community health for student nurses under the supervision of qualified public health nurses.

Out-patient Nursing Service

Baltimore, Maryland

Dear Gretchen:

What to choose now! Nursing has opened up so many possible areas of activity that it is difficult to decide in which field you will be able to contribute the most and find the greatest happiness. Remember how just being a nurse seemed an end in itself when you were contemplating nursing as a career? You ask me about out-patient nursing. I shall try to give you a realistic picture of what it is like but because it has given me such deep satisfaction, I shall not be able to be completely impartial in my comments.

The out-patient department really is like a doctor's office on a huge scale. The patients are ambulatory and for the most part are able to carry on their usual activities of going to work and taking care of their homes and families. This does not mean, however, that they are not in need of nursing care. They very often need the same kind of nursing and medical care as those patients whom you have cared for in the hospital, although their illness has not been completely incapacitating. The nursing problems are the same but the approach to them is different.

[3] See also reference to her article in the Bibliography at the end of this chapter.

On the wards, if a patient needs a particular medication, you give it to him; if he needs a special treatment, you do it for him; or if he should require a certain diet, you offer it to him. In the out-patient department he may need these same things, but you do not control the situation. It becomes necessary to depend upon him to do these things for himself. He must first want to do them, which necessitates his understanding his illness and how he can help in its management. He needs to learn what to do, and it is our responsibility to teach him. This is, perhaps, what makes out-patient nursing so much fun. Each patient has his own problems, and helping him to face and meet these problems is a constant challenge. Asking a mother with three children and a home to manage to apply hot compresses to a leg ulcer every 4 hours for 30 minutes becomes a problem of gigantic proportions compared to doing it yourself on the wards.

Then too, your interest is not entirely centered on the condition which brought the patient to the clinic. You become interested in the patient's total health needs—in fact, in those of the entire family. You are concerned with helping this family attain optimum physical and emotional health, to add to their feeling of adequacy and security, to share with them your wealth of knowledge about health, and to bring community resources to their attention. Not long ago, a six-year-old boy came into the surgical clinic to have his finger dressed. He had caught it in a door. The nurse asked the mother about how it had happened—incidentally, thinking the opportunity to talk about home accidents might present itself—and the mother burst into a torrent of complaints about how this youngster was always getting into trouble and having accidents. The nurse interested the boy in looking at some pictures of airplanes to get him out of earshot of the conversation, and then found out that the mother considered this child of hers stupid, willful, and not at all like his older brother, who was clever and amiable. The nurse watched the boy while he was playing in one corner of the clinic and observed that his fingernails were bitten down to the quick and that he seemed tense and high-strung. After the doctor finished the dressing, the nurse told him about her conversation with the mother. He suggested that the boy be referred to the child guidance clinic and spoke to the mother about it. As you see, this youngster got more than a finger dressing, and this nurse, because she was interested and alert, opened up an avenue of help for this family which gives promise of making life much happier for all of them.

You have heard and practiced all through your course that you should approach and nurse each patient as an individual and try to understand his individual problems. At times this was, perhaps, difficult because with a group of patients all dressed alike in hospital gowns and robes and surrounded by similar hospital equipment, their individuality was submerged in the general hospital atmosphere. It becomes easier to approach this goal in the out-patient department where each patient is dressed in his own clothes and very often has a relative or a friend along. There is more evidence of his individuality and he wears his personality more obviously. Then too, the patients often return to the clinic quite frequently and over long periods of time. You have the opportunity to get to know them very well and they to know you. The clinic almost takes on the character of open house every day—having your friends come in, hearing the latest news, and getting caught up on what's happening, even to the color chosen for the new dining-room wallpaper.

This isn't all there is to out-patient nursing, but I do think that the nurse-patient relationships that you build up and the satisfaction you get from working with each patient is one of the fascinations of this type of nursing.

You are, I know, interested in adding to your clinical and nursing knowledge, and the out-patient department will offer you ample opportunity to do this. New diagnostic measures and new methods of treatment are constantly being introduced and practiced here. You will be able to keep up with what is going on in medicine. Although the clinics are segregated according to particular specialties (this is becoming less and less rigid), there is so much overlapping that you will be able to keep an eye on what is happening in the other clinics. If you are particularly interested in obstetrics, pediatrics, or what have you, you can concentrate in these areas, but it will be almost impossible for you to restrict your interest to any particular clinical field. Your patients will be referred to other clinics and you will want to know what is happening to them.

Research is an important part of the activities of the out-patient department, especially if it is situated in a teaching institution. Helping with research problems becomes an interesting part of the nurse's activities. Research requires the observation of patients over a long period of time and she can be of immeasurable value by maintaining a warm friendly atmosphere in the clinic, making it one to which patients want to return. Her attitude and interest in making the clinic visit meaningful to the patient, making him feel welcome, and arranging for him to be seen expeditiously, go a long way in sustaining his interest. Very often, she also helps to keep records and data that can be used for analysis. Sharing in research and medical investigation is very stimulating.

Another aspect of out-patient nursing that makes it interesting is that it reaches out into the community. The activities are not circumscribed or restricted. Through the out-patient department the hospital extends its services to the community. It cooperates with other social and health agencies for the welfare of the patient and the family. The nurse becomes familiar with the purposes and functions of these agencies and, together with other workers in the clinic, helps to coordinate services to patients. It makes one feel a part of a large inclusive program.

The working conditions one finds in the out-patient department are usually good. There are times during the day when the clinic is in full session and the nurse is very busy, but these peak periods are not sustained. At the end of the day, when the patients have gone home and the clinic has to be straightened up and put in order for the next day, all becomes very peaceful. You have a feeling of having finished a day's job. You make plans for the morrow but you don't have the feeling of leaving loose ends dangling. The hours are usually from 8 A.M to 5 P.M. with Sundays and holidays off. Where there is a 40-hour week, you might have all or a part of Saturday off too. This might sound ideal, but don't let the hours alone influence you! Getting dental appointments or having your hair done sometimes creates quite a problem. Most other workers have these hours also, and you run into complications. In some organizations, the out-patient nurses relieve on the wards for week ends, but this is usually well regulated and you will know how often it is expected. This has advantages and disadvantages. It is interesting to work with bed patients and to keep your hand in; it is also difficult to work on a strange ward for a few hours, not knowing the patients well and having to share responsibility of a different kind.

However, the clinic hours do give you an opportunity to have a full life outside of your work. Having regular hours makes it easier to have your own apartment. Brushing shoulders with other people who are going to and coming from work makes one feel in tune. You can plan on evening activities and know you will be free. If you are located near a university where evening classes are offered, you will find time to attend them without having to make special arrangements for time off duty.

There is a certain amount of routine work that must be done in any job, and out-patient nursing is no exception. Setting up clinics, keeping up supplies, and maintaining equipment in good order, or supervising the workers responsible for these duties, is apt to become dull if one does not see beyond the monotonous mechanism of it. Everything must be seen in its relationship to something else, and it does give one a sense of pride to have a clinic that moves smoothly and efficiently. The aim is to give good service to patients, and this is accomplished best if the doctors and other workers in the clinic find things ready and in order. Efficiency, however, is not an end in itself. An assembly line is efficient, but that is not what we are looking for in managing patients in a clinic.

To be a good out-patient nurse, I think one of the most important qualities to have is an understanding of and a real liking and respect for people. The nurse in an out-patient meets so many people of varying temperaments, backgrounds, and interests that if she is prejudiced or has strong feelings about certain individuals she will be unable to give them the care they need. Understanding comes with experience, with an attitude of open-mindedness, and with willingness to know people. To get it takes study and a bit of living. I know of no better experience to help develop it than by doing public health nursing for a time. It is here we see the families in their own environment, to see problems as they see them, to learn why they solve problems as they do, and to develop appreciation of their ways of thinking and living. The out-patient nurse with public health experience is better equipped to help the patient in the clinic with his problems because she knows something of what these problems mean to him. She sees his problems in better perspective. So I urge you to keep this in mind should you choose to do out-patient nursing.

If you like administration, you will be happy in a clinic. The out-patient nurse needs to keep several pots boiling at a time—giving treatments in one spot, getting patients ready for examinations in another, providing assistance to the doctors, and keeping an eye on the registration and appointment desks. It takes a person who can plan well to avoid chaos and have time to devote to individual patients.

Liking to teach is also a must for the out-patient nurse, but it is the informal, conversational type of teaching which is so much fun to do. Sharing your knowledge with someone else is a privilege; we should be generous with it—and seeing the patients leave the clinic better equipped to take care of themselves is really gratifying. Recently a nurse told me about teaching a mother how to read a thermometer and how proud the mother was to call in the next day to report that the baby's temperature was down. It isn't only nursing techniques that we teach, however, but health measures in general. Our aim is to keep people well and to help them maintain optimum health. I wish I could tell you of the many opportunities that out-patient nursing affords in health teaching—the use of visual aids, for instance; the appropriate selection and distribution of health literature; group teaching—but that would take volumes.

The field of out-patient nursing is an expanding one. Clinic facilities are being enlarged and new ones are being added for which well-qualified nurses will be needed. The impetus of medical-care programs to give better medical care to a greater number of people, the extensive use of antibiotics and chemotherapy which allow patients who were formerly hospitalized to be treated on an ambulatory basis, the rich field they provide for teaching and research are factors affecting the expansion of out-patient services. There is a dearth of well-qualified nurses to carry on teaching programs for student nurses in the out-patient department, so if you are contemplating teaching, this would be a good field to investigate.

I am sure there are many questions in your mind that I have left unanswered. I might suggest that you read Harriet Frost's book "Nursing in Sickness and in Health," a classic of its kind, and Robinson's "Patients Have Families." Much of the source material in these books has been from the out-patient department.

Success in whatever you do!

Sincerely,

MARTHA JOHNSON, R.N.
Head, Out-patient Department
The Johns Hopkins Hospital
Baltimore, Md.

SALARIES

Salaries for general duty in out-patient services are usually on the same scale as for the rest of the hospital nursing staff (see Chap. II). Those who hold supervisory positions in the clinics or who can present advanced clinical or public health nursing preparation receive higher salaries. (For those in public health nursing, see Chap. XI.) At the present time (1951) the general trend of all salaries for specially prepared nurses is upward.

Sources of Employment

1. Professional placement bureaus
2. The large general hospital with an out-patient department—this is the most obvious source of employment in the field. Smaller hospitals, special hospitals, and those known as "community hospitals" serving wide rural areas may conduct active out-patient and clinic services. A background of public health nursing experience will prove a worthwhile acquisition, and is prerequisite for work in rural areas or where home visiting is expected of the nursing staff.
3. Local, county, and state health departments. There are a few positions open to professional nurses without public health training in clinics connected with health departments. Some of these are under Civil Service. Rapid-treatment centers, venereal disease clinics, tuberculosis and maternity services are also employing these "clinic nurses."
4. Group medical clinics, diagnostic centers, and organized health services for paying patients are increasing, assisted by various forms of prepayment and insurance plans. A list of these in your community can be secured from American Medical Care Plans,[4] or the classified telephone directory can supply a recent list. It is well to check with the state department of health or local medical society as to the standing of the group clinic with which you plan to connect yourself, unless this group is already under the auspices of a university or large general registered hospital or health department.
5. The other sources of information regarding out-patient or clinic positions are professional and commercial registries, the advertising sections of nursing journals, and state employment services. (See also lists at the end of Chaps. II and XI.)

BIBLIOGRAPHY

1. ALBERT, SISTER MARY, and MYRNA G. CAMPBELL: Viewing the Community through the Out-patient Department, *American Journal of Nursing*, p. 801, December, 1949.
2. BUTLER, MYRTLE HORNBUCKLE: Public Health Nurses in a V.A. Clinic, *Public Health Nursing*, p. 535, October, 1949.
3. COLMERS, ELIZABETH P.: United Nations Health Clinic, *American Journal of Nursing*, p. 452, July, 1947.
4. FROST, HARRIET: "Nursing in Sickness and in Health," The Macmillan Company, New York, 1939.

[4] For the addresses of organizations mentioned in this chapter, see Appendix A.

5. GOLDMAN, FRANZ: Nursing in Health Insurance Plans, *Public Health Nursing*, p. 405, September, 1948.
6. JOHNSON, MARTHA, and Committee: Student Experience in the Out Patient Department, *Public Health Nursing*, p. 478, September, 1950.
7. KLEM, MARGARET C.: Is Prepaid Nursing Care Possible? *American Journal of Nursing*, p. 1155, December, 1944. (Approximately two thousand nurses were employed in various types of agencies in group medical-care programs in 1945.)
8. KLEM. MARGARET C.: Nursing Opportunities in Medical Care Insurance, *Public Health Nursing*, p. 8, January, 1951.
9. ROBINSON, G. CANBY: "Patients Have Families," Commonwealth Fund, Division of Publication, New York, 1945.
10. STRAUSS, HENRIETTE: Health Education in Hospitals and Out Patient Departments, *American Journal of Public Health*, p. 1175, November, 1945.
11. WEAVER, ABBIE H.: Statewide Immunization Program, *Public Health Nursing*, p. 578, November, 1944. (Use of professional nurses without public health nursing preparation for selected clinic services.)

CHAPTER V

Maternity Nursing and Nurse-midwifery

Maternity is one of our country's largest "industries" and, by all possible standards of measurement, the most important. If you are caring for mothers and babies, you are nursing the world of tomorrow. There is no field of nursing where you can make your knowledge and skill count for more than right at the gateway of life itself. All that happens after an infant's birth cry may be affected by a nurse's quick thinking, quick action, and common sense. There are few professional nurses who after spending a year or two in the field of obstetrics cannot say, "I saved a baby's—or mother's—life." The United States is still losing too many mothers in childbirth—many of them needlessly, authorities say—and while infant mortality has declined dramatically in the last 25 years, thousands of babies still die in the first few weeks of life, and deaths throughout the first year are too numerous in the Southern area of the nation. Many could be saved by the right care at the right time.

MATERNITY NURSING

Maternity nursing, in the sense of being a service separated from general medical and surgical patients, is one of the oldest "specialties" in hospital nursing. In earlier days, this separation was probably for purposes of convenience, to give privacy to a noisy group of patients. Today, the physical separation of the obstetric department from the rest of the hospital is chiefly for the purpose of keeping cross-infections at a minimum. At the same time, the modern techniques of delivery, infant care, and the care of premature babies have reached a degree of specialization demanding not only elaborate equipment but also special basic preparation of at least 12 weeks for student nurses and additional study and practice to qualify nurses for advanced positions as graduates. The results of better obstetric practice, more knowledge of the prevention of infections, better nutrition, wider hospitalization of deliveries, and better maternal health information among expectant parents and the general public have resulted in marked decreases in both the maternal and infant mortality rates. It is a magnificent record, especially as the birth rate rose sharply in the postwar years. It is estimated that 30,000 professional nurses will be needed in maternity hospitals in the next 10 years.[1]

Maternity nursing, then, can be viewed as a special field of service, in which there will always be a steady demand, in which improvement in techniques and adequacy of personnel bring results in lives saved. It is a field in which a combination of teaching and skilled nursing care is needed in homes, clinics, hospitals, and doctors' offices. Maternity nursing knows no geographical boundaries or seasonal fluctuations and, as Miss Dustan remarks in discussing the field (below), it is a "happy service." There are opportunities in maternity nursing for those who undertake advanced study and supervised experience, in universities, schools of nursing, schools for nurse-midwives, general and maternity hospitals, clinics, out-patient services, visiting nurse associations, state, national, and Federal health and hospital agencies. About the only fields in which nurses specially qualified by maternity courses would not be apt to find employment would be in industry, in school nursing, and in hospitals devoted to other entirely distinct specialties—such as communicable diseases, care of the aged, chronic diseases, or convalescent patients—and in children's institutions.

Because the opportunities are so varied, a sampling of typical positions held by specially prepared nurses is listed here.

Typical positions held by nurses who have had advanced preparation in obstetric nursing:[2]

1. Superintendent of small maternity hospital
2. Director of nurses in maternity hospital (or division), offering both undergraduate affiliation and supervised graduate experience to students

[1] "Building the Future for Children and Youth," p. 15, Children's Bureau, Social Security Administration, Federal Security Agency, Washington, D.C., 1945. For addresses of all organizations mentioned in this chapter, see Appendix A.
[2] For information regarding nurse-midwives, see Nurse-midwifery, below.

3. Consultant in maternity and child health, state department of health
4. Consultant in maternity nursing of large visiting nurse association, giving some home delivery service
5. Instructor of student nurses and medical students, out-patient maternity service, including home deliveries
6. Chief nurse in labor and delivery rooms, in large city hospital
7. Nurse-midwife in rural county in the South, includes supervision of untrained midwives
8. Nurse in charge of maternity home, such as a Florence Crittenden Home
9. Director in school of nurse-midwifery
10. Director or supervisor of special program for the care of premature babies
11. Consultant under national (voluntary) agency or Federal auspices
12. Instructor in university course, or instructor in obstetric division of a general hospital
13. Service in private obstetrician's office
14. Maternity service in private practice

Of these positions the most usual are supervisors, instructors, and head nurses of the various divisions or departments in hospitals. One of the newer positions is that of maternity hospital consultant. This consultant nurse, working at state level under the guidance of the division of maternal and child health and with the division of hospitals, is expected to consult with and advise nurses and hospital authorities regarding nursing facilities, personnel, procedures, and equipment. She assists in surveying hospitals and new plans for hospitals, visits maternity homes and sometimes day nurseries, assists in setting up special services—such as the care of premature infants—and cooperates with the various local public health nursing agencies in promoting continuity of nursing service for mothers and babies. This consultant is expected to make surveys, carry on studies, make reports, and speak in public. Familiarity with the rules and regulations of the state as they relate to maternity and child care and the ability to develop good public relations in her travels over the state, while interpreting the law, are included in the description of duties of this position.

The responsibilities of an instructor in the obstetric division of a hospital are described in the following sketch.

A Supervisor and Instructor in Obstetric Nursing
Talks about Her Work

Members of the Alumnae Association:

It is a genuine pleasure to have this opportunity to tell you about my work. Teaching and supervision in a large maternity hospital are particularly absorbing if you like to be in at the beginning of things. When you realize that 85 per cent of all babies born in the United States open their eyes in hospital delivery rooms, is it any wonder that we, who have made obstetric nursing our specialty, feel that we have a vital role in getting the next generation off to a good start? You, too, can join our ranks if you are especially interested in this—to me—happiest phase of nursing.

I am only one of a number of teaching supervisors in this large institution. We, as a group, are responsible for the nursing care of about three thousand patients, the supervision of the graduate nurses on the staff, and the obstetrical education of approximately a hundred student nurses in the course of a 12-month period. Does that sound challenging? It is!

There have been many changes in our field during the last few years. We are more and more concerned with teaching women how to prepare themselves for the advent of their babies, and then for the care of themselves and their babies following delivery. In the past we thought that teaching a mother-to-be how her body reacted to pregnancy, how her baby grew inside the uterus, and how to care for the physical needs of her infant was sufficiently enlightening. Now many obstetricians believe an expectant mother should prepare her body for the physical exertion of labor by practicing carefully taught exercises and relaxation techniques.

The doctors in charge of obstetric patients used to feel that no newly delivered woman should be allowed out of bed for 8 or 10 days. Now, in most instances, these women are up in 12 to 24 hours. They go to the bathroom under their own power, take showers, and call their homes to keep a check on family affairs. By the time they are ready to leave the hospital they are feeling spry and full of pep and energy.

Perhaps the greatest progress can be seen in the preparation of mothers to care for their babies at home. This is furthered by placing the baby's bassinet at the mother's bedside for the last part of the hospital stay which gives her an opporutnity to practice the fine art of folding and changing a diaper, to judge when her baby is hungry, and to feed him herself, whether by breast or bottle. With the nurse standing by to guide and help, think what confidence this must give a young mother who has never handled a newborn baby. At present this type of experience is available in a limited number of hospitals, but more and more doctors and hospital administrators are realizing its importance. Let us hope that in the future all interested mothers and nurses will have an opportunity to participate in such a plan.

Let us take Miss Jay as our first example of how a teaching supervisor fits into the present-day maternity program in our hospital. Only a short time ago her responsibilities were confined to the nursing supervision of patients in labor and to teaching students that very important phase of obstetric nursing. Her work, and that of her staff, began *after* the patient came to the hospital. Now she is also teaching interested mothers-to-be to prepare themselves during the period of pregnancy for the natural phenomenon of giving birth. As a result, when an expectant mother enters the hospital in labor, she knows Miss Jay or someone on the nursing staff who has assisted with her preparation. She is confident that the nurses will give the kind of support needed during her delivery. The nurses, too, benefit, for they both learn and gain great satisfaction from helping a mother achieve a happy ending to 9 months of expectation. There are those women who say that to be awake to see their babies born is the most joyous experience of a lifetime! Any contribution the nurse makes to this happiness is bound to bring her reflected glory and an inner glow of pleasure in a job well done.

As a second example of the duties of an instructor, let us consider Miss Kay, who is responsible for the nurseries. Newborn infants used to be considered practically untouchable. Now we feel that babies need love and attention as much as they need food, a change of diapers, and protection from germs. Gone are the days when the nurse complained bitterly of a broken back and aching feet because she spent her entire day bending over cribs, keeping the babies at arm's length. Because of our new philosophy of care she now sits down and holds the babies when they are being fed or comforts them when they are in distress. Miss Kay spends much of her time guiding students who are learning baby care, not only in the nurseries, but at the mother's bedside. Here is the best school for both mother and nurse. Is there a better way for a student to gain an appreciation of the interdependence of mother and baby than to observe them in a unit where they can be together from morning till night?

Our working hours cover many activities besides those mentioned above. All of us participate in providing a constant supply of nursing service for all parts of our department, and in training an auxiliary staff to assist in the simpler activities of patient care. Recognition of the importance of staff education has added another aspect to our work which involves assistance in planning programs of interest to all nurses in our hospital, with particular emphasis on activities and subject matter related to our specialty. Nor can we forget our responsibility to the visitors who come from all parts of the United States and some foreign countries to review our methods. We find the exchange of ideas with these nurses and doctors of vital interest, for all of us are working toward the same goal of better care for mothers and babies.

The education of the students assigned to our division involves not only supervision on the pavilions but many hours spent in the classroom. Clinical instruction is not like teaching an abstract science, a foreign language, or history. We are helping our students acquire both knowledge and nursing skill in this particular phase of their learning. The fact that they have immediate need of the material discussed in class guarantees their interest. By passing on to them the information which we have gathered through experience and formal education we gain the satisfaction of contributing to the over-all pattern of student-nurse education as a whole and the advancement of maternity nursing as a specialty.

You are interested, I know, in the type of preparation which is considered prerequisite to such positions as I have described. One does not step directly from training into them, that I can assure you. Personally, I believe it is well to do general duty first in your chosen or a related field. The next step is to acquire a B.S. degree, unless you already acquired a degree before entering nursing or graduated from a collegiate school. Then comes head nursing so that you may gain experience in ward management and ward teaching. Even then you are not ready, for you need advanced study in your chosen field.

Many schools of nursing connected with universities throughout the country have courses to offer graduate nurses who are desirous of further training in the various nursing specialties. The advisers in your school can assist you to decide which type of advanced work will best suit your needs. Personally, I derived great satisfaction and benefit from my course in nurse-midwifery given by the Maternity Center Association in New York City. There is nothing like delivering babies with your own hands to help you to a firsthand knowledge of the birth process.

This happened to be the kind of advanced work which I chose to give me more complete preparation in my specialty.

If you like people—and their babies—and if you like to help people who are eager to learn, perhaps you too will choose maternity nursing.

> LAURA C. DUSTAN, R.N.
> *Instructor-Supervisor*
> *Obstetric and Gynecological Nursing*
> *Cornell University—New York*
> *Hospital School of*
> *Nursing, New York, N.Y.*

QUALIFICATIONS

To qualify as an advanced clinical instructor, consultant, or supervisor in maternity nursing, the following qualifications should be met:[3]

1. At least a year of supervised nursing experience following graduation. This may be in a hospital or in public health nursing. It should include contact with maternity patients and newborn infants.
2. Advanced clinical study and supervised experience in maternity nursing. Nurses who intend to teach should have a college degree— a master's degree if possible—and courses in nursing education, public health nursing, or ward administration. Advice should be sought regarding advanced courses in maternity nursing and the related subjects desirable for a nurse planning to be an administrator or consultant in this field.

SALARIES

In maternity nursing, as in other specialized fields, the salaries for nurses who have completed advanced study in the subject and who have had satisfactory supervised experience are higher than for general duty and staff nurses. They range (1951) from $2,800 to $4,500 per year, with maximums as high as $6,000 for those in administrative positions or directing academic courses. Salaries for maternity hospital consultants range from $3,300 to $5,000.

[3] For qualifications of a nurse-midwife, see Qualifications for Nurse-midwives, below.

NURSE-MIDWIFERY

Because in many rural areas the services of physicians are not available for the delivery of mothers in their homes, and because many foreign-born women, following their native customs, prefer the services of a midwife, the need persists for a well-trained person, a nurse-midwife, to consult with pregnant mothers and to attend normal deliveries, calling on the physician for physical examinations, for consultation, and for deliveries that may present complications.[4]

There are fewer untrained midwives now than there were 25 years ago. In 1947:

There were 15 states and the District of Columbia in which midwives were not practicing at all or had delivered fewer than 0.05 per cent of the live-born. In 15 additional states they attended no more than 1 per cent of the deliveries. All 30 of these states are located in the northern and western regions.

The midwife is concentrating her work in the rural areas of the South, particularly among the Negro population. In 1947, there were approximately 20,200 midwives, 93 per cent of the country's total, practicing in the 18 states of the South and Southwest. Midwives delivered 174,470 live births, or 13.8 per cent of the total in these states. . . . In only 3 states—Kentucky, Texas, New Mexico—do midwives now deliver more than 5 per cent of the white babies. Among the nonwhite population there are still 11 southern states in which from one-third to two-thirds of the mothers are delivered by midwives. . . .

It is clear from these figures that many American mothers do not yet have the benefit of medical attendance at confinement. The prospects are that the situation will improve as the hospital building program, particularly in rural areas, goes forward. In the meantime, the midwife remains indispensable in areas where medical and hospital facilities are lacking. Therefore, the midwife should be adequately trained, supervised, licensed, and controlled.[5]

There are not a great many practicing nurse-midwives in this country, probably fewer than a thousand, but the value of preparation as a nurse-

[4] "Professional Nurses, The Outlook for Women in Occupations in the Medical Services," Women's Bureau, Department of Labor, Washington, D.C., Bulletin 203, No. 3, p. 41, 1945.

[5] What's Happening to the Midwife? *Public Health Nursing*, p. 451, August, 1949.

midwife as a basis for skilled obstetric nursing care, in teaching, for consultant and public health nursing positions, and for work in rural areas, cannot be overestimated. Nurses planning to be missionaries, or enjoying the challange of rural emergencies, will find great satisfaction in the contribution which they can make to this much-needed service.

The Maternity Center Association, which has conducted a famous school of nurse-midwifery for over 20 years, points out that

Many of the Association's nurse-midwife graduates are now consultants in Federal, state and local health departments or are obstetric supervisors in hospitals or professors of nursing education in university schools of nursing. Some are carrying on home delivery services in conjunction with county health departments.

Others are working in far-away places of the earth where medical and hospital facilities are woefully inadequate, often non-existent. Nurse-midwife graduates have successfully carried on obstetric services in the African bush, in the mountain fastnesses of Canada, on the islands of the South Pacific and the jungles of Central and South America.[6]

A nurse-midwife has been defined as

. . . a professional nurse who has had a recognized course in midwifery which qualifies her to function as a clinical specialist in the team of professional obstetric workers. With the appropriate medical relationship, and with a midwife's license from the local authority, she may teach, examine, and care for pregnant women, attend normal deliveries, give postpartal care, and care to the newborn baby. When she detects complications or abnormalities, she functions with the physician as any other professional nurse.

She combines

. . . the knowledge and skills of obstetric nursing with the art and judgment of midwifery in the care and education of the pregnant, parturient, and nursing mother, and her baby so long as progress is normal. Preparation in nurse-midwifery qualifies the professional nurse to function as a specialist in the team of professional and other workers

[6] Quoted from *Briefs*, p. 8, Maternity Center Association, New York, Winter, 1950–1951.

concerned with the care of childbearing women; and, after licensure, to manage the antepartal, intrapartal, and postpartal phases of childbearing, under medical guidance so long as progress continues normal; and to give and supervise the care of newborn babies.[7]

QUALIFICATIONS FOR NURSE-MIDWIVES

Preparation for the field of nurse-midwifery calls for an advanced program of study at a recognized school for nurse-midwives. At the present time, there are four such schools, one of them for Negro nurses.[8] Information regarding the curriculums in these schools, the costs, etc., may be secured from the Children's Bureau. Only about forty-two students in all can be accommodated at one time in these four courses for the 6 months' program of study and practice.

One of the most picturesque rural areas served by nurse-midwives is in the Kentucky mountains—a program under the direction of the Frontier Nursing Service, Wendover, Kentucky (see Bibliography at the end of this chapter, section on Maternity Nursing).

The nurse-midwife student at the Maternity Center Association's school must be

. . . a graduate of an accredited school of nursing and eligible for college matriculation. She should be between twenty-five and forty years of age and in good health. The public health nurse must have had two years of professional experience and at least one of these in public health work, under supervision. Teachers from schools of nursing and hospital staffs are exempt from the year of public health nursing experience. They may substitute work in teaching and supervision in hospitals, provided this has been done under supervision. It is preferable that a student be sponsored by an agency interested in her services when she graduates.[9]

The tuition fee is $150, and at least that amount should be allowed for living costs.

The impressions of a student taking the course in midwifery at the Maternity Center Association are shared with us in the following account.

[7] These quotations are taken from a tentative report of the National Organization for Public Health Nursing, Section on Nurse-Midwifery.

[8] Tuskegee, Ala.

[9] Quoted from the Association's announcement, 1951.

I Like It!

R-r-r-ing! That clamoring telephone! Groping for consciousness, I wondered why any right-thinking baby would want to arrive in the world at such an unearthly hour as 3:00 A.M. Furthermore, whatever had made me think I needed a course in nurse-midwifery anyway? . . . Must have been temporary madness! Pulling clothes on, adding last-minute contents to the delivery bag, and striding through the dark, deserted streets with the staff member, I was, at first, only thinking of the cozy bed I had left behind. After a few minutes I felt more alert; and we talked in low tones about Mrs. A's good antepartal progress, her expressed wish for a girl, and the possibility of a breech presentation . . . .

Six hours later, as I lowered the dark shade over my window and crawled back into bed, I knew my decision to learn nurse-midwifery had been a good one. The events that I had been able to share in that night would deepen and refine not only my nursing abilities, but my capacities as a human being. The mutual love and support of Mr. and Mrs. A. throughout the labor, their satisfaction in being able to use their own efforts to achieve their wanted daughter, and their grateful, but very humbling (to me) thanks for the nurses' help, were impressive experiences indeed. The careful and expert instruction of the staff member helped me to apply previous classroom teaching in the very practical and skill-demanding task of delivering little Maria.

I drowsily remembered the time last year when I was arguing with myself about the advisability of applying for enrollment as a student here. I'd been practicing as a maternity nurse for several years and seriously questioned my need for further preparation. During student days, I'd heard of Maternity Center Association and of the midwifery school it operated as one of its many activities. But *I* didn't want to be a midwife! I had no plans for working in any area where such skills might be vital. I thought it a wonderful idea for nurses in remote rural spots, or in foreign service, but I would never have to deliver babies myself!

It took a few years before I really gained a perspective on the scope of maternity nursing, and came to realize how midwifery fits into the picture. A fortunate opportunity to see the M.C.A. clinic in action, and the roles played by graduate and student nurse-midwives, crystallized my decision to take the course. Only here would I have the chance to give total care to a woman before, during, and after the birth of her baby. Here I would see the whole picture of good obstetric care—not isolated segments or blocks of it, as I had previously. Though I'd worked in antepartal clinics, I had never really been responsible for conducting visits, giving individual guidance and instruction, conducting group classes, and evaluating the mothers' progress. I would be under the supervision of outstanding obstetricians and experienced nurse-midwives as I worked, and spend half of every day in classroom and laboratory learning the theory, skills, and techniques for improving my care to patients.

Similarly, though I'd worked in labor and delivery rooms, I had never really stayed with a woman throughout labor, and come to grips with the nursing problems involved in truly helping her. Certainly, I had never learned exactly how to deliver a baby with maximum safety to mother and child, though I had seen thousands delivered! Having with help faced and solved some of the problems met when conducting a delivery, I felt I would be a far more understanding teammate to women in labor and to their doctors.

My postpartal and newborn experience also had always been rather separate entities before. Here, I would not only care for mother and baby together, I'd do it within the family setting of the mother's own home, a natural focus of all good maternity care.

I decided that even though I might never wish to practice as a nurse-midwife, *anything* I'd choose to do in maternity nursing would be improved by having this preparation. Whether in antepartal clinic, hospital delivery room, or visiting nurse service to new mothers and babies, I'd have more and better equipment with which to meet patients' needs. If I wished to become an instructor for basic students in obstetrics, what better tool could I have than the solid, concrete background acquired in midwifery? Supervision and consultant responsibilities in the maternity field made such a course vitally necessary, I had learned. Local, state, national, and international health services were more and more requiring midwifery training from these specialists, so that, aside from immediate personal values, completion of the course would enable me to advance into these fields, if I should later choose to do so.

I was not disappointed in my expectations. Classroom instruction from obstetrician and nurse-midwife includes not only a comprehensive background in obstetrical theory, but detailed demonstrations of all the practical skills needed in giving expert care to mothers and babies. Classes are small enough so that each student's personal needs are known and met. Individual tutoring is carried on by experienced nurse-midwives and obstetricians in the ante- and postpartal clinics, and in the home during labor, delivery, and immediate postpartal period. The student first learns *what* to do, and *why;* then actually carries this out, under supervision. For example, classroom practice in pelvic examination technique is followed by actual examination of patients in clinic, with an instructor beside the student to interpret, correct, and guide her performance. During each of the 15 to 20 deliveries which the student herself conducts in the patients' homes, an expert nurse-midwife accompanies her and guides her, step by step, in the safe care of mother and baby. To any nurse at all interested in obstetrics, each experience provided is challenging and zestful, and there are no dull spots.

The course is not an "all work and no play" arrangement, either. Since she is on call approximately two to three nights every week, the student is, at these times, confined to the clinic, and actually sleeps there. Though at first this appears to curtail her social life, it also gives her opportunity to make new and lasting friendships with other students and staff members. The close, warm, family atmosphere that pervades the entire place greatly enhances the evenings spent together. Frequent parties, excursions, and "get-togethers" in off-duty time soon make her feel that her social life has expanded in new directions that are satisfying.

Candidates are accepted at the school on an individual basis, when prerequisites are considered, so . . . don't hesitate to apply, if you're interested. I'm sure you'll never regret it!

VERA KEANE, R.N.
Student Nurse-Midwife
Maternity Center Association
New York, N.Y.

The firsthand experience of a nurse-midwife working in a rural state in 1944 (quoted in part from the first edition of this book) gives a unique picture of the demands on a nurse trained in this field. Positions of the type Miss Wamsley held in New Mexico when this account was written are rare in the United States. However, the conditions do exist.

Catching Babies at Home[10]

At midnight, my neighbor rang the bell again. Maria had been feeling her pains for almost 3 hours, and she was sure that her baby would be there soon. My special training and experience with patients in labor

[10] For the longer story of this delivery see the first edition of this book, p. 100.

told me that the contractions which the patient was having were not of the character needed to push the baby along the birth canal. The two older women, the neighbor and the mother-in-law, could not appreciate the delicate operations of nature. They wished to hurry things, to save time, to shorten the hours the patient must endure her pains. They insisted that the patient "Push, push, push!"

But the moment to "push" was not yet. During the night the patient must rest, must take nourishment, must walk about a bit, must have another enema for stimulation, before her uterus, tired from so many previous babies, could change the poor contractions to good ones. This is what the modern science of obstetrics teaches the nurse-midwife.

The patient in the adobe house in the New Mexico village was asleep again and so were the two other women, as I thought of and tried to put into practice all the arts and science I had learned as a student nurse-midwife at the Maternity Center Association. But in New York the doctors who had taught me, specialists in obstetrics, were never more than half an hour away should a supposedly normal patient prove to have not so normal a labor as expected. A nurse-midwife may attend only patients who have been examined by a doctor and found to be, at least presumably, normal. For those who are not normal, nothing less than a doctor's, preferably a specialist's, care is needed. Maria's doctor had expected a normal delivery.

After 2 hours of sleep, my patient was awake. Her contractions had started again and within an hour the "good" contractions for which the nurse-midwife had waited so long, really commenced.

Usually the patient would have delivered by this time, and had I been back in New York, I would have called a doctor by now, to check my findings. But this was New Mexico, and I could only be grateful for the experience I had had in delivering babies in the rural homes of Maryland before coming here. There I had learned to depend upon my own judgment, and not to call a doctor unless absolutely necessary. So, watching and timing the contractions, I waited hopefully, praying that nature would follow a smooth course.

In the morning, just about the time I would ordinarily have been going on duty (8:30 A.M.), the baby was born. But there was a troublesome amount of bleeding from the mother's uterus right after the birth, and the baby was blue. The mucus had to be suctioned from his nose and throat with a small rubber tube, boiled previously for such a contingency.

The baby's breathing was finally established, but the mother was still bleeding briskly and her uterus had not yet expelled the placenta. Our obstetrician had ordered that medicine be given into a vein in a condition such as this—one of the real obstetric emergencies. But, as so often happens in hemorrhages, the veins had collapsed and I had to use the slower route into a muscle. There was nothing to do but send a member of the family hurrying for the other nurse-midwife. I could not leave Maria alone even to make a telephone call to the doctor.

Still there was no sign of the placenta. Bleeding continued. After what seemed like an hour—but really a matter of minutes—my partner arrived and we two nurse-midwives went to work. The placenta was finally expelled. Other emergency medications were given, as well as plenty of liquids, warm blankets, and hot-water bottles. Even on a warm June morning a patient who is hemorrhaging is cold.

When everything possible had been done, the second nurse-midwife left me to notify the doctor, and I stayed, continuing to give coffee and medicine, until at last I saw a look of relaxation replace that of anxiety on Maria's face. A checkup of her pulse and blood pressure revealed that, sure enough, the danger period had passed. Shortly, she fell asleep, but not without a murmured prayer of thanks to the Spanish saints whose images and pictures adorned the room.

Even so, we dared not leave the patient for fear the bleeding should start again. The second nurse-midwife having sent the message to the doctor, who could not be reached directly, returned and relieved me. I had been on duty from midnight to noon.

Late that afternoon the doctor came and I returned to see my patient. To the delight of all, the doctor pronounced Maria's condition so satisfactory that no transfusion was needed, and little Juan Antonio, the new arrival, was found to be a perfect specimen. Six months afterward, as this is being written, Juan comes to the clinic to see the baby specialist once a month along with all the other babies whom the nurse-midwives have assisted into the world since the new health center opened.

But when all is done and a very tired nurse-midwife goes to bed at last, she does not have to worry about being on duty at 8:30 the next morning. Unless she has made a definite appointment with a patient, she can sleep all the morning to make up for the overtime she has worked.

When the work of the day or night is done, whether it has been an obstetric emergency, an immunization clinic, or a day of visits to homes, New Mexico offers us a variety of extraprofessional activities to refresh our minds and deepen our interest in this remarkable country. There is the opportunity and fun of a Spanish lesson, for it is much easier to learn a language when it is practiced every day, both on duty and off. There are riding, picnicking, fishing, and hunting. New Mexico is a tourists' mecca, with the residents just as eager as the tourists to see and do everything. Most of the towns are small—villages, really—but each seems to have a distinct atmosphere and allure all its own. Each has one or more annual fiestas, and these are events visited and enjoyed by everyone who can possibly get to them. In the summer, a rodeo is nearly always part of the fiesta. Innumerable rodeos are also held independent of the fiestas.

Rural nursing and midwifery are not easy; neither are they all grim and unrelieved work and responsibility. There is much about the work, especially in a gay place like New Mexico, to beckon the young in heart.

NANCY WAMSLEY, R.N.

El Rito Health Center[11]

Another, quite different situation, is quoted with permission from *Briefs:*[12]

New Life in Liberia

. . . The significant fact is that, be it under the most up-to-date facilities in a modern American university hospital or in a crude Indian hogan by a glacier in remote Alaska or in a native grass hut in the steaming African bush, the nurse-midwife is delivering mothers successfully and helping parents to welcome their new babies with joy.

Here is Ellen Moore, for instance.

She is a native of Liberia on the coast of West Africa, an area of the world once called *the white man's grave.* One day she read in an American religious paper that Bishop Samuel Grimes of Richmond, Virginia, was interested in Liberia and its people. She, too, wanted to help her people, many of whom live under conditions virtually untouched by modern civilization. So she sat down and wrote a letter to the Bishop. In it she asked him to pay her expenses to come to America to study nursing. It was a big request, but as she so graphically described it, "I prayed to God and as I prayed, God grew smaller and smaller. When he got small enough, I put him into the letter and sent him to Bishop Grimes.

[11] Conducted in 1944 by the Maternal and Child Health Division, Department of Public Health, New Mexico.

[12] *Briefs,* pp. 11*ff.,* Maternity Center Association, New York, Winter, 1950–1951.

When the Bishop opened the letter, God jumped out." Strangely enough, the Bishop *was* interested in this letter from across the sea. He *did* send her the money to come. He helped Miss Moore to get her basic education and assisted her as she studied at the Lincoln School for Nurses in New York. After completing her university course in public health nursing, she came to the Association's School for nurse-midwifery. She applied herself diligently and when she went back to Liberia she had with her the coveted nurse-midwife diploma.

She settled in the small town of Kakata, less than one hundred miles from Monrovia, the capital. This village was miles from the nearest doctor and hospital and the road in and out was barely passable during the rainy season. With wisdom she determined to discover the resistance to her new ways of doing things among the people before she began her work. She found her chief difficulty in the severe antagonism and mistrust of the native midwives. She decided that before she could help the families in this remote and primitive community, she had to win over these midwives. Days were spent in making purely social calls upon them. Then she made it clear that she wanted to work *with* them. She said, "*You know the people, and I have some new knowledge about catching babies from America. Let's do the job together.*" This approach melted the reserve and distrust which she first felt. She waited for days, however, for her first call for help. Then one night a messenger came to her house in great haste. A mother had been in labor for many hours. The midwife had been unable to deliver her. The mother was now in convulsions. Would Miss Moore come?

She found the mother lying on the dirt floor of the hut beside a hot fire. The midwife was pouring cold water upon her to stop her convulsions. Calmly Miss Moore took out her stethoscope, a new and frightening instrument to these people, and she listened to the baby's heart tone. Yes, the baby was still alive. She let the midwife listen, too. Then she said, "We are going to have to turn the baby. I want *you* to help me." So she guided the native midwife's hands in the maneuver. They delivered the child together. Fortunately, both mother and baby lived and her fame spread through the surrounding town and forest. The bars of resistance were broken.

As the work grew, a leading merchant of Kakata helped her to secure from the American army, when it abandoned Roberts Field after the war, an old army barracks. With native help, they dismantled the building, board by board and nail by nail, and carried it through the tropical forest to Kakata where it was re-erected as the first unit of a hospital which Miss Moore hopes to see developed. The hospital was furnished with beds and cribs made from old packing cases, much of the wood given by the people at the Firestone Rubber plantation. The American doctor at the plantation hospital, many miles away, offered to be Miss Moore's medical consultant. In an emergency, he frequently drove his jeep through rivers of mud to reach her primitive hospital at Kakata. "The Firestone people have been very good to me," she said. "Whenever we had a person in need, they gladly took care of my patients." . . .

Miss Moore recently came to this country for a refresher course and to enlist support for her work in Liberia. "It is our belief," she says, "that with adequate funds and equipment to work with, a more permanent maternity building for mothers, with a well-equipped nursery and pediatric unit, we would be able to serve a greater number of our people in a more satisfactory way." . . . Miss Moore, with her self-sacrificing efforts and her obstetric knowledge gained from America, plus a natural ability to understand people, has carried on a successful maternity service under extremely adverse conditions.

SALARIES

Salaries for qualified nurse-midwives are higher than for generalized supervisors and consultants—$3,800 to $4,800. Consultants and teachers in this field receive the higher salaries within this range; administrators, $4,000 to $7,000.

SOURCES OF EMPLOYMENT

Nurses with advanced clinical preparation in maternity nursing or qualified as nurse-midwives may find positions by inquiring at the following agencies:[13]

1. Professional placement agencies
2. Maternity hospitals or obstetric divisions of general hospitals
3. Out-patient services, clinics, visiting nurse associations, or health departments conducting home delivery services, special maternity pro-

[13] Nurse-midwives will be most likely to hear of openings through the schools where they received their training as midwives. See also lists of missionary societies, in Chap. XVII, Sources of Employment.

grams, or supervising midwives (there are a few maternity centers combining field service, teaching, and delivery programs)
4. Frontier Nursing Service, Wendover, Ky.
5. Organizations promoting maternal-health programs (for example, the Planned Parenthood Federation of America, Inc., New York, N.Y.)

For consultant or teaching positions:

1. Maternity Center Association, 654 Madison Ave., New York, N.Y.
2. State health departments
3. Universities and schools of nursing
4. Children's Bureau, Social Security Administration, Federal Security Agency, Washington, D.C.
5. U.S. Public Health Service, Federal Security Agency, Washington, D.C.
6. Bureau of Indian Affairs, Department of the Interior, Washington, D.C.

BIBLIOGRAPHY

Maternity Nursing

1. BOYLE, FRANCES: Public Health Nursing in an Obstetrical Clinic, *Public Health Nursing*, p. 253, May, 1949.
2. CORBIN, HAZEL: Changing Maternity Services in a Changing World, *Public Health Nursing*, p. 427, August, 1950.
3. "Guide for an Advanced Maternity Nursing Course," National League of Nursing Education, New York, 1948.
4. HICKOX, VERDA F.: Maternity Care, *American Journal of Nursing*, p. 59, January, 1940.
5. HILBERT, HORTENSE: Nursing in the Maternal Health Program, *Public Health Nursing*, p. 176, March, 1940.
6. LOSTY, MARGARET A., and others: What the Hospital Nursing Consultant Does, *American Journal of Nursing*, p. 158, March, 1948.
7. POTTER, EDITH L.: Maternal Health in Relation to Infant Mortality, *American Journal of Nursing*, pp. 122, 155, February, 1945.
8. Prenatal Care, *The Child*, p. 108, January, 1946.
9. RUBBELKE, LEONA: Home Delivery Service in a Generalized Program (Rural), *Public Health Nursing*, p. 34, January, 1944.
10. TAYLOR, RUTH G.: Trends in Maternity Nursing Service and Education, *Public Health Nursing*, p. 455, September, 1948.
11. What about the Future in Obstetric Nursing? *New York State Nurse*, p. 26, May, 1948.
12. WORREL, KATHRYN E.: The Maternal and Child Health Consultant in the Hospital Program, *Public Health Nursing*, p. 329, June, 1950.

Nurse-midwifery

1. BUCK, DOROTHY F.: The Nurses on Horseback Ride On, *American Journal of Nursing*, p. 993, September, 1940.
2. COURT, JOAN: A New Citizen Arrives in Calcutta, *American Journal of Nursing*, p. 38, January, 1951.
3. DEMING, DOROTHY: "Anne Snow—Mountain Nurse," Dodd, Mead & Company, Inc., New York, 1947.
4. FELL, FRANCES: A Midwifery Delivery Service, *American Journal of Nursing*, p. 220, March, 1945.
5. HEMSCHEMEYER, HATTIE: The Nurse Midwife Is Here to Stay, *American Journal of Nursing*, p. 220, March, 1945.
6. LANGE, DEOLA A.: Plantation Granny—A Necessity, *Public Health Nursing*, p. 603, November, 1949.
7. Nurse Midwifery Today, *Public Health Nursing*, p. 278, May, 1949.
8. Nurse-Midwives in the Mountains, *American Journal of Nursing*, p. 102, February, 1951.
9. POOLE, ERNEST: "Nurses on Horseback," The Macmillan Company, New York, 1932. (Out of print, try public libraries.)
10. SHOEMAKER, Sister M. THEOPHANE: "History of Nurse-Midwifery in the United States," The Catholic University of America Press, Washington, D.C., 1947.
11. What's Happening to the Midwife? *Public Health Nursing*, p. 451, August, 1950.

See also *Briefs* (quarterly bulletin), Maternity Center Association, New York; and articles in *The Child* (monthly bulletin), Children's Bureau, Social Security Administration, Federal Security Agency, Washington, D.C.

CHAPTER VI

Pediatric Nursing

America's children need specially trained pediatric nurses. Among the many handicaps from which they suffer, besides the commonly called "diseases of childhood," are tuberculosis (400,000 children have it), congenital syphilis (980,000 cases), and rheumatic fever and heart disease (500,000 sufferers). In lesser numbers, but no less serious, are poliomyelitis, cancer, diabetes, and nephritis. About 20,000,000 children need dental care.[1]

Some of the service needed by children comes from public health nurses, some from school nurses, and much of the acute illness is cared for by general staff nurses in children's hospitals and children's wards of general hospitals. There are many children in schools for the handicapped, nurseries, and children's shelters of one kind or another. Nearly 100,000 children are inmates of institutions for the dependent. Many in the latter are in the care of untrained or semitrained attendants. It is not hard to find places where children need the care of professional nurses!

In 1931, the White House Conference on Child Care and Protection urged that professional nurses be better prepared in the care of well children, emphasis being placed on child development, parent education, nutrition, mental and social hygiene, and sociology. The effort to follow these suggestions has been an earnest one and the content of the advanced clinical course in pediatric nursing outlined by the National League of Nursing Education covers instruction in all these points.

Although several of the communicable diseases of childhood are pre-

[1] Figures from Children's Bureau, Social Security Administration, Federal Security Agency, Washington, D.C.

ventable or capable of being shortened in duration or lightened in their severity through the use of appropriate serums and vaccines, nevertheless a thorough knowledge of the early symptoms and possible complications of all communicable diseases to which children are susceptible is necessary in this field of pediatrics, together with an ability to explain preventive measures and isolation procedures to parents and teachers. Special preparation is needed for the treatment of poliomyelitis (see Chap. VIII).

Rheumatic fever, about which more is known every year, and the various types of heart disease frequent in children also call for special attention from the nurse who plans to devote her service to children. Cancer and the leukemias are in the spotlight at the present time.

The field of child development and parent education is a promising one for the nurse who wishes to take advanced university courses in psychology and education.[2] Study in any of the fields related to childhood should be accompanied by observation, preferably in selected activities, of the various services for children, such as child guidance clinics, nursery schools, juvenile courts, etc. A knowledge of the community resources for child care and development is essential.

To enter this specialty, a nurse should enjoy being with children. It is true that some nurses think they do not like children because they have never lived with them or worked with them. Part of their failure to enjoy nursing them is unfamiliarity with children, possibly even fear of handling them. After the right introduction to their basic needs and an interpretation of their childish motives of behavior, many nurses quickly lose their sense of strangeness with children and become not only at home with them but greatly intrigued with their special problems.

Miss Cameron, author of Pediatric Nursing—A Fascinating Experience, which follows, had a slightly different experience, in that the potential opportunities for becoming a specialist in this field had not been made clear to her in her basic course. The basic course should obviously give a nurse sufficient acquaintance with children to enable her to know whether she will like to be with them. It is the rare nurse who really dislikes sick children—if she is in good health herself! Children *are* trying to overtired, sickly nurses and do "make them nervous."

Pediatrists frequently remark that the most essential quality in a success-

[2] See the story of these changes over 50 years as told by Goostray, Stella: Pediatric Nursing at the Turn of the Century, *American Journal of Nursing*, p. 624, October, 1950. See also the reports of the Mid Century White House Conference on Children and Youth, 1940.

ful pediatric nurse is an ability to put herself in the child's place and see the world, the ward, and the crib through a child's eyes. If you remember your childhood vividly, this is easier to do—some adults don't! You can learn from books what will please, scare, or amuse a child, but it is much better to have an "understanding heart."

A child, even more than an adult, needs to be viewed in his home setting. The parental influences there need to be understood. A nurse with no interest in backgrounds, no curiosity as to what makes the "wheels go round" the way they do in a child's mind, and no patience with the first fumbling attempts of a child to do something for himself, will not be happy among children, sick or well.

On the other hand, there are a few nurses whose maternal instinct is so strong and all-consuming that they find it difficult not to let their emotions get the better of their judgment. Tragic cases wring their hearts, and the temptation to spoil all the helpless children proves to be too great. There is a happy medium between the impatient, short-tempered nurse and the overdevoted, emotional one, and the nurse who achieves that happy medium makes a successful companion for children.

As Miss Cameron points out, however, it takes more than a happy relationship with children and a liking for them to become a head nurse or instructor in a children's ward. Advanced clinical study, observation, and practice are necessary. It is a great advantage to have special knowledge of children if you plan to enter the field of public health nursing.

The demand for professional nurses with special training in pediatrics is steady and, with the high birth rate of the last 5 years, many doctors predict a busy time with the school age group in the next 5 years.

It is probable that private duty nurses with special pediatric experience will find employment in homes at higher rates than do professional nurses without this specialty. Children are more apt to be at home when sick, unless acutely ill or in need of surgery. Doctors who have a large practice among children prefer pediatrically trained nurses.

In the public health field, consultants in maternity usually include child health, at least up to school age (see Chap. XI). The Children's Bureau program has given impetus to these services and there are a good many consultants in maternity and child health employed in state health departments, as well as in city health departments and visiting nurse associations.[3] It would be well to look into the availability of scholarship in this field. Other opportunities are listed by Miss Cameron.

[3] For the addresses of all organizations mentioned in this chapter, see Appendix A.

Pediatric Nursing—A Fascinating Experience

On the threshold of graduation the student nurse of today stands in an enviable and unique position. At no other time in nursing history has such a variety of opportunity for careers in nursing presented itself for her appraisal. Such variety may make it difficult for her to choose a specific field in which she, as a graduate, would like to work. To those who are in this quandary, I shall attempt to present pediatric nursing as I have found it—a fascinating experience.

At present, I have a supervisory position in a large children's hospital. How I arrived there may be of interest. Like all of you, I had my basic pediatric course during nursing-school days. Unfortunately this left me with little desire to further my knowledge in this field. As I look back, I feel the reason can be attributed to the fact that this course was taught by people who were themselves insufficiently equipped to make me aware of its intrinsic values. Although this situation has improved, it is still far from ideal. If you have shared my experiences and a natural enthusiasm to work with children has been dampened, do not be discouraged.

Considerable time elapsed before realization of my own limitations turned my interest to pediatrics again. An increasing desire to know more about children brought me to the decision to work in a hospital which was devoted entirely to the care of children. I have never regretted this decision. The next few years spent as a general duty nurse and an assistant head nurse wholly dispelled any of my former apathy. They were years of constant stimulation. It is true, I acquired a more certain knowledge of the diseases of children and skills in pediatric techniques than I had ever thought to master, but my most important discovery was how unlike nursing children in a pediatric hospital is nursing children in a general hospital! Too often in the latter, the children's service is merely a side issue, and the child is more or less expected to fit an adult environment.

One of the most amazing and attractive qualities of children is their resiliency. One day may find the child prostrate, the next finds him alert and interested in all his surroundings. The modern pediatric hospital is well aware of this factor. Personnel are in accord in making the child's hospital life as natural as possible. The innovation of playrooms in charge of trained workers for convalescent children, occupational therapy, and bedside teachers for little rheumatics and chronic patients, story hours, the cooperation of the dietitians in making holidays and individual birthdays festive occasions, all these were new to my experience. But perhaps the most startling revelation was the day I discovered an order for "Extra T.L.C." (T.L.C. is, being interpreted, tender, loving care) for one of our little eczema patients who spent his days restrained lest, in his agony, he scratch himself to pieces. To be encouraged to pick a child up for the sole purpose of giving him affection was revolution to any teaching I had hitherto encountered. It was forcibly brought home to me not only that the care of children required that they be fed, bathed, and treated for their physical ailments but that they needed other things equally important for their well-being, which I as a nurse should recognize and be able to supply.

"Visiting hour" was a constant reminder that children have parents. As all of you have participated in this occasion, even the memory will evoke a smile. The questions that one anxious parent could think of filled me with amazement. How to answer them filled me with alarm. If I were Mary's mother should I be unduly worried because I cannot get Mary to drink milk? Is it natural for Johnny to fight with his baby sister? Can anything be done about Sammy's thumb sucking? Too often I found that I was not prepared to give any advice with confidence.

Not only visiting hour but the ordinary day produced its puzzling situations. How should I discipline Tommy who, regardless of the fact that he is likely to break his neck, insists on swinging on the curtain bars? What should I do about Sally's temper tantrums? Often what worked with one child would not work with another. That children were individuals, even as you and I, became more and more apparent.

I was constantly troubled by my own inadequacy, and I was sure this was obvious, not only to myself but to the student nurses who looked to me for guidance. Frequently my knowledge was no greater than theirs. These problems could undoubtedly have been clarified by those whose experience had given them more insight, but in the tension and business of hospital life, there never seemed to be the desired leisure to discuss them. When someone suggested the advanced clinical course in pediatrics, I accepted the idea readily. The next 4 months were the most stimulating in my life.

Practical experience provided for us in nursery schools, visiting nurse services, and well-child clinics gave to many of us, myself included, our first real opportunity to view the well child in normal surroundings. Class discussion of our observations and an attempt to interpret the children's behavior in various situations gave us a down-to-earth basis of understanding not only the children but, incidentally, ourselves. From this understanding evolved an increasing awareness of the "family" and parental problems, the development and fundamental needs of the child, his interests at the different phases of his development, and finally, the principles and techniques for his care from prematurity to adolescence.

This study of the well child was followed by discussions of the sick child, at home and in the hospital, the physical and psychological factors which enter into his illness, and the appreciation of the fundamental needs of all children in sickness. In addition, we became familiar with legislation pertaining to maternal and child health and the function of agencies concerned with child welfare. Our study brought to our attention many resources which should be part of every pediatric nurse's background. Field trips to a milk bureau, a children's dental clinic—where the children were amazingly well-behaved—a children's library, and other child-welfare agencies were of the greatest interest. However, it was our visit to a foundling home that left an indelible impression upon me. The dearth of people specifically trained in the care of children, as evidenced here, is an arresting challenge to any graduate nurse, pediatrically inclined. Although adoption and foster homes solve much of this problem, the fate of the less fortunate is pathetic. As we were being shown through the various dormitories, the phrase, "unadoptable material" was repeatedly applied to some little child. Later our hostess explained that this meant that, because of the child's heredity or individual limitations, he was not considered suitable for adoption. The best he could hope for was to be boarded in a foster home, where he might be rejected by his foster parents, as very often happens, only to spend his entire childhood within the walls of an institution.

To those of you who may be chiefly interested in teaching basic pediatrics to student nurses, I can report that the course offered lectures in special problems of pediatric nursing, in the planning and evaluation of pediatric courses, in methods of instruction and demonstration of nursing procedures from the point of view of making them interesting to student nurses. This phase of the subject was rounded out by practical field work and observation in well-chosen pediatric services.

All of which brings me back to the beginning. At the completion of the 4 months' course, I returned to hospital life, not with all my problems solved by any means, nor with all my education complete, but with the confidence that in using what I had learned I had a greater contribution to make to the children, the parents, and the student nurses with whom

I would come in contact. Let me say here that I am convinced that, if the graduate nurse is to take her place with the members of other professions concerned with child life, she must acquire an understanding of the needs and care of children, well or sick, in the home and in the hospital. Not only is this knowledge in itself necessary, but she must have the ability to interpret these needs to parents and students. She should spend some time under supervision in a nursery school and a public health agency, such as a visiting nurse service or a well-child clinic. As this type of activity is not usually possible in a basic program, she will require additional postgraduate experience. To those who are contemplating such a step, I recommend the advanced clinical course in pediatrics now given at many universities throughout the country.

Isabel Cameron, R.N.
Babies' Hospital
New York, N. Y.

Salaries

Salaries paid to head nurses, supervisors, instructors, consultants, and directors in the field of pediatrics do not differ greatly from those in other specialties. Head nurses and supervisors receive (1951) from $2,000 to $3,500; instructors and consultants, $3,000 to $4,500; and directors, $3,500 to $5,500. These are cash salaries without maintenance. Public health agencies pay about the same amounts.

Sources of Employment

With the realization that pediatrics cannot be limited to the care of sick children but must essentially be concerned with the care of the child wherever there is child life, there have developed many openings for the well-qualified pediatric nurse, some of which are listed below:

Children's hospitals
Children's wards in general hospitals
Health departments—state, county, and local
Day nurseries, day-care centers, nursery schools
Orthopedic hospitals (see Chap. VIII)
Other hospitals for handicapped children
Child-care institutions

Visiting nurse associations (Chap. XI)
Child health stations
School nursing services (see Chap. XII)
Foster-home agencies
Federal agencies
Summer camps
Offices of child specialists

For other general sources of employment, see Chaps. XII and XVII. Professional placement agencies can assist you in finding positions of this type.

BIBLIOGRAPHY

1. "Advanced Clinical Course in Pediatric Nursing," National League of Nursing Education, New York, 1946.
2. ALDRICH, CHARLES C.: "Babies Are Human Beings," The Macmillan Company, New York, 1938.
3. ALDRICH, CHARLES C.: "Feeding Our Old Fashioned Children," The Macmillan Company, New York, 1941.
4. BENZ, GLADYS S.: "Pediatric Nursing," The C. V. Mosby Company, Medical Publishers, St. Louis, 1948.
5. CHILD STUDY ASSOCIATION: "Parents' Questions," Harper & Brothers, New York, 1936.
6. Evaluation of Advanced Clinical Courses in Pediatric Nursing, University of Chicago, *American Journal of Nursing*, p. 129, February, 1948.
7. GARRISON, CHARLOTTE G., and EMMA D. SHEEHY: "At Home with Children," Henry Holt and Company, Inc., New York, 1943.
8. GESELL, ARNOLD L.: "Infant and Child in the Culture of Today," Harper & Brothers, New York, 1943.
9. GRUENBERG, SIDONIE: "We the Parents," Harper & Brothers, New York, 1940.
10. NATIONAL LEAGUE OF NURSING EDUCATION: Guide for Nursery School Experience, *American Journal of Nursing*, January, 1948. See also NLNE bibliography on Care of Children, and "A Study of Pediatric Nursing," Department of Studies, 1947.
11. SELLEW, GLADYS: "Nursing of Children," 6th ed., W. B. Saunders Company, Philadelphia, 1948.
12. WASHBURN, RUTH: "Children Have Their Reasons," Appleton-Century-Crofts, Inc., New York, 1942.

See also *The Child* (monthly bulletin), Children's Bureau, Social Security Administration, Federal Security Agency, Washington, D.C.

Psychiatric Nursing

The attention of the public and of professional people has been centered recently on the growing case load of mental patients. No fewer than 2,000,000 people are mentally ill and their care costs our nation $500,-000,000 a year. Authorities estimate that there are 125,000 new cases yearly. More than half of all the available hospital beds are for mental patients. The Veterans Administration alone maintains more than 50,000 beds for neuropsychiatric patients.[1] The number of patients in state mental hospitals in 1948 was 466,496.[2]

The disproportionate number of registered nurses available and employed for this type of nursing staggers credulity, until one realizes that a large number of these patients require only custodial care and that another fairly large group can get along with attendant or practical nursing service under professional nursing supervision. Nevertheless, the shortage of professional nurses in mental hospitals existed before the war and has grown steadily. A hoped-for ratio of 1 professional nurse to 25 patients as compared with 1 to 7 patients in a general hospital is nothing to be proud of, but the actual ratio in state hospitals is, all too frequently, 1 to 100 patients.

It was estimated in 1943 that 30,800 nurses would be needed in mental hospitals when our population reached 138,000,000. As the population is already over 150,000,000 the need is even greater—more than 10 per cent of all professional nurses. At the present writing, there is no prediction that the admissions of patients to mental hospitals will decrease; quite the opposite, as the public becomes better informed and more hopeful

---

[1] *Facts about Nursing,* p. 75, American Nurses Association, 1950.
[2] *World Almanac,* p. 439, New York *World-Telegram,* N. Y., 1951.

regarding the early recognition of mental illness and its treatment and cure. It is thought that higher salaries and better working conditions for nurses will grow out of this understanding and more generous public support of mental-care programs. This, then, appears to be a sure field of future employment for *prepared* nurses.

The positions open to nurses with psychiatric training and experience are mainly in mental hospitals—Federally supported, state, or county institutions—and psychiatric divisions of general hospitals. There are comparatively few voluntary hospitals for mental patients; some of them, however, are of very high quality and offer the best in early treatment. Psychiatrically trained nurses are in demand as teachers, instructors, and consultants. The consultants are needed on Federal, national, and state levels, and in public health agencies as well as in hospitals. Child guidance clinics,[3] out-patient services, and psychiatrists in private practice prefer to employ nurses with experience in this field.

Psychiatric nursing should be a very promising field for registered men nurses. Before the war, men nurses were employed largely in institutional and industrial nursing, a smaller number in private practice. It is thought that nursing in mental hospitals and in the heavy industries will continue to offer particularly suitable and desirable fields for men. It is pressingly important to raise the level of nursing care on the wards for male patients in the mental hospitals. Studies have shown that in many institutions men are cared for by nonprofessional male attendants—some trained only on the job; no women are permitted on the wards. The standard of service on the "men's side" should, of course, be as high as on the "women's side" and should always be under the supervision of a registered professional nurse with experience in psychiatric nursing.

Many nurses, especially those who have not had the advantages of psychiatric nursing experience under qualified supervision, think of this field as dreary, discouraging, monotonous, and unrewarding. It is true that the cases of senile psychoses, the congenitally deficient (who should not be on wards with the mentally ill) and those who have reached the hospital too late for psychiatric help have discouraging prognoses. Still, modern methods in treating mental illness bring hundreds of patients back to normal living, and some cures, among young people especially, are both dramatic and complete. The workings of the normal human

---

[3] The National Association for Mental Health publishes an annual directory of psychiatric clinics in the United States. For the addresses of all organizations mentioned in this chapter, see Appendix A.

mind become fascinating to those who study the abnormal, while the fundamental principle of treating every mental patient as an individual case, when applied to normal patients, improves one's whole understanding and handling of illness. It is a very common occurrence to hear a nurse remark, "My psychiatric experience has given me a much deeper insight into all illness and I feel much more confident in handling my patients. I really understand them now!" Nurses in the armed forces found this branch of nursing essential to effective care of their patients, and many bewailed their failure to secure an "affiliation" in a psychiatric hospital during training. Both the Army and the Navy attempted to remedy the situation by arranging for intensive psychiatric nursing experience for selected members of the corps.

Perhaps the greatest asset to success in this field is a genuine interest in it. Nurses who think they will not like it or who say they get the jitters when they think about the mentally ill only reveal their lack of knowledge of the field and their total unfamiliarity with actual conditions. A month of service in an up-to-date mental hospital under capable supervision and directed study cannot fail to rouse the thoughtful nurse to a keen awareness of her opportunity to help these unfortunate patients. It will change her reluctance to be with them to an informed and confident knowledge as to how to conduct herself and observe their conditions. The second month usually brings an entirely new conception of what is meant by *nursing*—formerly almost entirely limited to the physical care of the body. In the presence of mental patients, the psychiatric nursing student suddenly realizes that here she is dealing with the most fundamental illness of all—the sick mind—and its effect on the body carries a new meaning to every procedure she has learned. "I will never see a sick person again without wondering what is happening to his mind and vice versa— how his mind is affecting his body," a student nurse said to the writer. "Half my nursing course would have been missed, if I'd skipped psychiatry."

Public health nurses are especially grateful when they are able to add psychiatric nursing to their general preparation, as one of their most valuable assets in being able to recognize the early deviations from normal behavior among the families they see in their homes, the children in clinics and schools, and the breadwinners at work. Many of the larger public health nursing agencies have added psychiatric nurse-consultants to their staffs or are sharing such service with other community agencies.

It takes time to make a good psychiatric nurse—one who develops a degree of control and firmness with patients, at the same time never cowing or estranging them. The nurse's attitude and approach to one schizophrenic patient may be quite different from the treatment needed by another. Only with practice, experience, and keen observation can a nurse learn to trust her judgment in dealing with the mentally ill. When she reaches that point, however, the work will become of absorbing interest and no longer monotonous or something for which she holds a hidden fear.

More than three-fourths of the schools of nursing now arrange for 2 to 4 months' experience in psychiatric nursing for their students.[4] Since 1940 there have been several advanced clinical courses in psychiatric and neurological nursing established at colleges and universities with practice in mental institutions. These courses range from 6 to 12 months.[5] It is thought that the past tendency of graduate nurses to shun this field after graduation will be largely counteracted by giving student nurses familiarity and confidence in nursing mental patients through a period of experience under supervision, by offering greatly improved living conditions and better salaries, and by the growing demand for instructors, head nurses, and consultants in highly desirable and well-paid positions.

The need for qualified nurses in this field cannot be exaggerated. Testimony to this statement follows:

The Career with a Future

As the last guest took her place at the long table, the chairman rapped for attention.

"Tonight our subject for the round-table discussion will be psychiatric nursing, and we are happy to have as our guests Dr. Newton, who is a psychiatrist, and a group of nurses who are actively engaged in the field. Miss Cox, would you like to explain the plan of the discussion?"

"Yes, indeed," responded Miss Cox. "Each of us is engaged in some type of psychiatric work. Some of us are administrators, some teachers, others general duty nurses, and still others are nursing students. We come to you from private hospitals and from tax-supported hospitals, from large units and from small units. So, you see, we hope to give you a bird's-eye view

---

[4] For information write the National League of Nursing Education.

[5] A very few mental hospitals maintain schools of nursing, giving affiliations elsewhere.

of psychiatric nursing and the opportunities it offers. We should like to describe our work for you, and we shall be glad to answer your questions —if we can! Dr. Newton," continued Miss Cox, "do you believe there is a real need for psychiatric nurses?"

Dr. Newton laughed, "In one word—*yes!* But don't let me start on that subject or I'll hold the floor all evening." His face sobered as he continued, "All the high hopes we may have for improving the mental health of the American people, for treating and rehabilitating our war casualties, and for effecting early cures will come to naught unless we can depend upon the assistance of well-trained and competent nurses—and the demand is constantly increasing."

"Thank you, Dr. Newton, that certainly renews our faith. And now," continued Miss Cox, turning to the nurse on her left, "Miss Blair, you are an administrator in one of our largest tax-supported psychiatric hospitals. Will you tell us about the nurse's opportunities for service in your institution?"

"Gladly," replied Miss Blair, "but I shall need the help of one of our students who has promised to jog my memory and help me to answer questions later. Where shall I begin?"

"Supposing you tell us about the types of work that the nurse performs," suggested Miss Cox.

"That would be a catalogue of the major activities carried on in the hospital, I'm afraid, but I can mention a few. Perhaps we should first understand that a knowledge of psychiatric nursing is a requisite for every nursing position in the hospital. Next, it is important to realize that all levels of nursing responsibility are represented—directors of nursing service, supervisors, head nurses, and general duty nurses. Of course, the duties of administrators in psychiatric hospitals closely resemble those of administrators in general hospitals. However, each graduate nurse employed in a hospital such as ours is an administrator and teacher, too."

"Could you tell us more about that?"

"Yes. With such large numbers of patients requiring care, it is necessary to employ many auxiliary workers, usually called attendants or nurses' aides. But the nurses are responsible for leading and directing these workers in caring for patients. I think experience as a general duty or head nurse in a large psychiatric hospital is a splendid training for administration."

"Now could we have an idea of what might constitute the duties of a general duty nurse? What does he or she do for the patient?"

"She nurses the 'whole' patient. Physical care may range from bedside care given the patient who is receiving special treatments or the patient who is physically ill or helpless, to the supportive care given the ambulatory patient who needs only to be reminded of his needs. However, this is only a part of our nursing care, the other part consists of giving the patient intelligent reassurance and what he needs most—a friend. Miss Quigley, you have had experience in many of our departments, would you tell us about some of them?"

"Yes, Miss Blair. I had my first experience on the admission ward where patients are received. I found that very interesting because there was such variety in the types of patients and because we were able to help them adjust to the hospital environment. We also learned to observe the patients' behavior accurately and to record our observations. We found that careful observation was a very important factor in psychiatric nursing."

"Indeed it is," maintained Miss Blair, "and I think Dr. Newton will agree that the nurse's observations are very helpful, in fact essential, to the physician."

"They certainly are," Dr. Newton affirmed. "The nurse spends much more time with the patient than does the doctor, and in psychiatry constant, accurate observation and recording are particularly essential. Now that the teamwork pattern in health care has gained such favor, the nurse is fast becoming a key member of the psychiatric team."[6]

"Then," continued Miss Quigley, "there were the special therapies such as electroshock, insulin shock, fever therapy, and hydrotherapy. In each of these we assisted with the care of the patient during the treatment and gave follow-up care throughout the remainder of the day. We also had experience in caring for patients immediately following psychosurgery—lobotomy and topectomy—and in helping with their rehabilitation programs. And," she laughed, "we learned that the nurse was not just 'playing' with the patients when she organized a bingo game or a sewing circle—occupations and recreation can be therapies, too."

"Quite true. Every game, every conversation is directed toward improving the patient's condition. Of course, there are other types of therapy which have not been mentioned. Perhaps others in the group are more familiar with them and can tell us about them," invited Miss Cox.

"Yes," spoke up Miss Munn. "We have a small private unit and we use

[6] See BARTON, WALTER E.: The Nurse as an Active Member of the Psychiatric Team, *American Journal of Nursing*, p. 714, November, 1950.

several types of treatment in addition to the psychotherapy which our physicians carry on with individual patients. We give electroshock and insulin shock therapy, and on occasion our doctors recommend psycho-surgery for the patient. I think, too, that, when the unit is small and each patient is under the private care of a therapist, the nurses find that more definite orders are given for the individual patient's care. The nursing care is directed along the lines on which the physician is treating the patient. Of course, that is much more difficult when the hospital staff must serve large numbers of patients."

"That's true," interposed Dr. Newton, "but we are finding new ways to spread the benefits of psychotherapy—even in the large tax-supported hospitals. Group psychotherapy is one example of this, and in some hos-pitals nurses, after being given special training, are serving as group leaders. They consult with the doctors, of course, and are guided by them."

"Our hospital is devoted entirely to research," Miss Shores said, "and many nurses find this type of psychiatric work both stimulating and rewarding."

"Is yours a private or a tax-supported research hospital?" inquired Miss Cox.

"It is connected with the state university and so is tax-supported. It has a maximum capacity of less than 100 beds."

"I think," suggested Miss Cox, "that it's time we heard about oppor-tunities in the military services and in the care and rehabilitation of our veterans. Miss Edwards, will you tell us about those?"

"The needs of the Army, Navy, and Air Force Nurse Corps for psychiatric nurses are most acute during periods of active warfare, of course. Even a limited knowledge of psychiatric nursing is valuable to the nurse in military service."

"In fact," Dr. Newton interrupted, "we have learned that some ex-perience in psychiatric nursing is invaluable in caring for the casualties of any emergency, whether the setting is military or civilian."

"The Veterans Administration," continued Miss Edwards, "provides many different kinds of psychiatric care, with special emphasis on re-habilitation. Our particular unit treats only psychoneurotic cases and we have a very high rate of turnover. Some of the patients are residents, while others simply come in for consultation. We follow definite orders written by the physician and our nurses may have to assume a variety of roles in caring for the different patients."

"Just what do you mean?"

"For instance, while one patient may need someone to lean on and to take responsibility for him, another may need to be 'put on his own.' The nurse must learn how this is accomplished. I think Miss Munn was referring to this sort of psychiatric nursing care when she spoke of the private unit."

"That's right," corroborated Miss Munn.

"Also, in rehabilitation there is a great deal of work to be done along occupational and recreational lines. Of course, we have trained therapists who direct these activities, but the nurse must participate, too. As Miss Quigley said, they learn that 'playing' can also be nursing, and sometimes hard work."

"There are other types of hospitals for the mentally ill veterans, are there not?" asked Miss Cox.

"Yes, there are much larger units which care for all types of mental illness. Those units are constructed along the same general lines as the large mental hospitals for civilians. In fact, some veterans are cared for in units directly connected with state hospitals."

"I think we must also remember the large private hospitals for the mentally ill, and the hospitals caring for the aged and infirm," suggested Dr. Newton.

"Yes, they must not be overlooked when cataloguing the opportunities for psychiatric nursing," agreed Miss Cox.

"Our student representative, Miss Quigley, has contributed to our discussion tonight. Shouldn't we hear something about opportunities in the educational department? Miss Grant, can you help us out?"

"I've been wondering," laughed Miss Grant, "how we were going to provide Dr. Newton with all the well-trained and competent nurses he wants unless we turn out well-trained and competent instructors. Nurses qualified as instructors in psychiatric nursing will find almost unlimited opportunities. You see, more and more schools of nursing are asking for affiliations in psychiatric nursing. These requests cannot be granted until new affiliate schools are opened, and new schools cannot be opened until qualified directors and instructors are available."

"That brings up the matter of educational qualifications for the positions we have already mentioned," suggested Miss Cox.

"I believe," replied Miss Grant, "that every nurse employed in caring for the mentally ill should have some special preparation for her work. For the general duty nurse, this may be obtained through affiliation or a supplemental course following her graduation, or even, in some cases, through an in-service training program. The nurse who aspires to an administrative position such as head nurse, supervisor, or director of nursing service will do well to take one of the advanced courses in psychiatric nursing now being sponsored at more than a dozen universities by the National Institute of Mental Health. Study at the university level, of administrative techniques, should be included in these courses or added by the nurse later.

"The nurse who wishes to teach psychiatric nursing should plan to obtain a university or college degree in nursing education with a major in psychiatric nursing."

"Doesn't the National Mental Health Act make funds available for advanced study in psychiatric nursing?" asked Miss Cox.

"Yes, stipends have been provided, and although the educational standards I have described have not been attained in some psychiatric hospitals and affiliate schools, they are realistic goals. According to a study made by the National League of Nursing Education in 1950, an unusually large number of psychiatric nurses had taken college or university work in their specialty during the preceding 5 years. More than 180 had obtained baccalaureate degrees, about 60 had completed work for their master's, and more than 400 others had earned credits towards a degree. Even larger numbers had obtained degrees or university credits outside their special field. Unquestionably the nurse preparing for a career in psychiatric nursing must remember that the trend here, or elsewhere, is toward higher educational requirements, and he or she should plan accordingly.

"Nursing education in psychiatry requires the same basic preparations as nursing education in the general school plus special study in psychiatric nursing. The nurse who wishes to teach psychiatric nursing should plan to obtain a degree in nursing education and a postgraduate course in psychiatric nursing. If the latter is taken at one of the schools connected with a college or university, the credits earned will help to fulfill the requirements for a degree.

"It should be understood, of course, that these are the desirable standards of education and as yet are not universal requirements."

"Thank you, Miss Grant. Now that we have the general principles in mind, supposing we open the meeting for questions. Please do not hesitate. If there is a question in your mind, it deserves an answer. Who will be first?"

There was a moment of silence, then a rather nervous voice asked, "Miss Cox, is it true that the work is dangerous?"

Miss Cox smiled as she turned to Miss Quigley. "I think I'll ask our student to answer that question."

"It's a good question," said Miss Quigley, "for it was uppermost in our minds when we reported for our affiliation in psychiatric nursing. We quickly learned, however, that our notions of mental illness were quite wrong. Very early we discovered that the popular misconceptions about mental illness and the behavior of 'insane' people had been responsible for our fears. The majority of the patients with whom we worked did not fit into our preconceived picture at all. We learned that there were many patterns of mental illness and that, as soon as we understood a little about these patterns, our fears promptly disappeared. Furthermore, we were taught how to cope with deviations from normal behavior."

"I'd like to add a word on that subject if I may," commented Miss Grant. "One of the most noteworthy achievements in psychiatry has been the substitution of skill for force in our care of the patient. The psychiatric nurse needs only average physique and average strength. Some of our best nurses in the field are small in stature but mighty in skill and understanding."

"Is it true that working with mentally ill patients affects the mental health of the nurse?" queried another listener.

"I think that question falls within my province as a mental hygienist," offered Dr. Newton. "It is not advisable for persons having severe emotional problems to undertake the care of psychiatric patients. However, the well-adjusted nurse, having an average degree of emotional stability, will find that she can leave her patients' emotional problems behind her at the close of her day's work just as she was able to leave her general hospital patients' physical problems behind. If she is able to do this and to attain a high degree of objectivity in her daily contacts with the patients, she need have no fear of emotional involvement."

"Isn't the work sometimes unpleasant, though?" persisted another girl. "I should think that it would be discouraging to work with patients who can't understand what is being done for them or don't appreciate it."

"That is a test of the objectivity mentioned by Dr. Newton," responded Miss Munn. "Many patients *do* understand and *do* appreciate what is done, although in many cases they are unable to express themselves adequately. But the nurse soon learns that even the complete unwillingness to accept any sort of treatment is a symptom of the patient's illness.

In fact," she laughed, "it is not far removed from the behavior of our 'normal' patient who knows better than the doctor or nurse what is best for him."

"Do mentally ill patients ever recover?"

"Yes," reassured Dr. Newton. "Many patients recover and many more could be returned to a useful place in society if they could be given prompt treatment. We must not think of the mentally ill as hopeless cases, and we must realize that there are as many degrees of severity in mental as there are in physical illness. Skilled nursing care can often mean the difference between chronic illness and the road to recovery."

"Also," added Miss Blair, "we should not forget that skillful treatment and nursing can help many a patient to make a more useful and a happier adjustment within the hospital, or enable him to return to his home for periods between episodes of illness."

"Are there opportunities for psychiatric nursing within the other branches of nursing?"

"There are numerous opportunities," answered Miss Cox. "Public health agencies are finding it advantageous to retain psychiatric nursing consultants on their staffs. Then there are opportunities for private duty nursing on psychiatric cases, and I might point out that the rate of pay for duty on such cases is usually somewhat higher than the rate set for general cases. Furthermore, the nurse with experience in the psychiatric field may find such experience a deciding factor in her employment as an industrial nurse, as an instructor in a school of nursing, or in other positions in which such a background is of special value. Finally, the nurse familiar with the principles of psychiatry and experienced in dealing with emotional as well as physical components of illness will find increasing opportunities in all fields of nursing as the close relationship between emotional and physical symptoms is more completely understood."

"And I'd like to add," contributed Dr. Newton, "that all nurses trained in psychiatry are well able to serve their communities and their profession by teaching their friends, their relatives, and their associates the truth about mental illness."

"Another point that should not be overlooked," suggested Miss Edwards, "is the need for men nurses in psychiatry. It offers them one of their very best employment opportunities."

"Where are most of the psychiatric hospitals located?"

"Do you mean are they located in the city or in the country?"

"Yes."

"Some of them are located in cities or towns," explained Miss Cox. "But country sites are usually chosen because that arrangement permits more freedom for the patients. Often the grounds are most attractive, and numerous outdoor recreational activities are available. In all cases some form of transportation is provided so that the nurse is not isolated from shopping and entertainment centers. In fact, a great deal of attention is being given the matter of providing better transportation facilities and more desirable housing for psychiatric hospital personnel."

"Could you please give us a summary of the advantages and satisfactions offered by each type of hospital?" asked the chairman.

"Certainly," replied Miss Cox. "Miss Munn, would you summarize for the private psychiatric hospital?"

"First of all, I think the nurse finds the rather rapid turnover of patients encouraging. Also, she has a close association with the individual patient and works under specific orders given her by the physician. In the private hospital she is likely to work in pleasant, attractive surroundings and is usually provided with more modern and adequate equipment than is available in the large tax-supported institutions. A portion of her time on duty may be spent in accompanying her patients to the theater and ball games, or in participating in other recreational activities. Finally, many units are connected with large general hospitals and are located in the centers of population."

"And, Miss Edwards, would you briefly outline the advantages of work with the military services and with veterans?"

"Nurses find a special kind of satisfaction—a sense of sharing—when they serve with the military, and a sense of having repaid at least a portion of society's debt to these men when they care for these veterans. Here again, the prognosis is good in large numbers of cases and the nurse plays a very active part in rehabilitation. As in the private unit, the nursing care is closely integrated with the physician's therapy."

"Now, what advantages are offered by the research hospital, Miss Shores?"

"Usually, the nursing service and physical plant of the research unit are similar to those found in the private psychiatric hospital. In addition, the nurse is given unique opportunities for assisting in research projects and for study. She has the very real satisfaction of participating in a most fundamental activity."

"And, Miss Blair, will you state the case for the large tax-supported hospitals?" asked Miss Cox, smiling.

"Most important, I believe, is the knowledge that her service reaches a very large number of patients whose needs are acute. She is able to assist in bringing the fruits of research to the mass of patients, and in giving the best possible care to those whose families are financially unable to maintain them in private hospitals. The variety of cases is unlimited, and the nurse is often given a large share of the responsibility for the care of the patients."

"Miss Grant, does psychiatric nursing education offer special satisfactions?"

"I think it does, Miss Cox, for the power of good teaching reaches far beyond the doors of the hospital. It sets the standards of psychiatric nursing care and molds attitudes toward the mentally ill wherever the nurse may go, whatever position she may attain."

"Thank you very much. And now, since our time is growing short, would you care to close the discussion, Dr. Newton?"

"There is little for me to add," replied the psychiatrist, "except to leave you with the thought that the frontiers of psychiatric nursing remain virtually untouched and offer a constant challenge to the nurse who is imbued with the pioneer spirit. To more than half a million victims of mental illness who are now hospitalized in our mental institutions, and to the one out of every 13 Americans who is likely to require care in a mental hospital at some time during his life, this spirit will be mighty important!"

JEANETTE V. WHITE, R.N.
Illinois School of Psychiatric Nursing
Chicago, Illinois[7]

SALARIES

General duty salaries in mental hospitals range from $2,200 to $3,600; the higher salaries are paid in Federal institutions under Civil Service. Head nurses, instructors, and consultants (including those in public health) start at $2,800 and rise to $5,400, while directors of nurses in psychiatric institutions are paid from $3,500 to $8,000. It should be pointed out that salaries in this field are definitely on the upgrade.

Private duty nurses caring for mental patients receive a higher wage than when nursing normal patients—usually $2 more per day.

[7] Miss White held this position when this account was first written. She has been kind enough to have it checked, and to reedit it herself (with the skill of a *Journal* staff member) for my use.

SOURCES OF EMPLOYMENT

1. Professional registries and placement bureaus
2. Federal, state, and county mental hospitals
3. Psychiatric wards of general hospitals, clinic services including guidance clinics
4. Private mental institutions
5. Universities where advanced work has been taken
6. Schools of nursing, as instructors
7. State health departments for consultant positions
8. Private psychiatrists
9. Advertising pages of professional journals

The National League of Nursing Education and the American Psychiatric Association provide general advice on employment trends and preparation. The National Association for Mental Health has information regarding community programs, psychiatric clinics, and preventive activities throughout the country. The National Institute of Mental Health should be consulted for administrative opportunities on the Federal level. For addresses see Appendix A.

BIBLIOGRAPHY

1. Advanced Course in Psychiatric Nursing, *American Journal of Nursing*, p. 683, July, 1944.
2. BEERS, C. W.: "A Mind That Found Itself," Doubleday & Company, Inc., New York, 1935.
3. CHARBONNEAU, LEON O.: Men Nurses in Psychiatric Nursing, *American Journal of Nursing*, p. 82, February, 1947.
4. CONNOR, MARY C.: Preparation of the Mental Hygiene Consultant, *Public Health Nursing*, p. 151, March, 1947. See also Functions and Qualifications, *Public Health Nursing*, p. 507, September, 1950.
5. FAVREAU, CLAIRE H.: Existing Needs in Psychiatric Nursing, *American Journal of Nursing*, p. 716, September, 1945.
6. FITZSIMMONS, LAURA W.: Facts and Trends in Psychiatric Nursing, *American Journal of Nursing*, p. 732, August, 1944.
7. GEISEL, WINIFRED M.: The Psychiatric Nurse in the Community, *American Journal of Nursing*, p. 25, January, 1949.
8. GILBERT, RUTH: "The Public Health Nurse and Her Patient," Commonwealth Fund, Division of Publication, New York, 1951.
9. HENDERSON, ADELE: The Nurse in a Mental Health Clinic, *Public Health Nursing*, p. 42, January, 1949.

10. LEMKAU, PAUL V.: What Can the Public Health Nurse Do in Mental Hygiene? *Public Health Nursing*, p. 299, June, 1948.

11. MORGAN, EDITH: This Chaotic World Needs More Psychiatric Nurses, *New York State Nurse*, p. 23, May, 1948.

12. NATIONAL LEAGUE OF NURSING EDUCATION, and NATIONAL ORGANIZATION FOR PUBLIC HEALTH NURSING: "Inventory and Qualifications of Psychiatric Nurses," 1950. See also *American Journal of Nursing*, p. 309, May, 1951.

13. "New Frontiers in Psychiatric Nursing Advanced by Universities and Community Nursing Services" (folder), National League of Nursing Education, New York, 1945.

14. ROBERTS, DOROTHY I.: Mental Hygiene in Public Health Nursing, *Public Health Nursing*, p. 63, February, 1944.

15. ROBINSON, ALICE M.: Changing of the Guard in Psychiatric Nursing, *American Journal of Nursing*, p. 152, March, 1950.

16. ROBINSON, ALICE M.: Why Not Psychiatry? *R.N.*, p. 44, February, 1949.

17. ROBINSON, G. CANBY: "The Patient As a Person," Commonwealth Fund, Division of Publication, New York, 1939.

18. ROWELL, JOHN T.: Psychiatric Nursing, A Specialty with So Few Specialists, *R.N.*, p. 37, October, 1947.

19. STERN, EDITH M.: "Mental Illness: A Guide for the Family," Commonwealth Fund, Division of Publication, New York, 1942.

20. U.S. PUBLIC HEALTH SERVICE, A Study of the Mental Hospitals in the United States, 1937–1939, p. 73, by HAMILTON, SAMUEL W., and others, Public Health Reports, Supplement No. 164, Washington, D.C., 1941.

21. WOLF, MARGUERITE: The Role of the Psychiatric Nurse, *American Journal of Nursing*, p. 1115, December, 1943.

CHAPTER VIII

Orthopedic Nursing

Anne Wiebe, orthopedic clinical instructor in the Children's Hospital, in Denver, Colorado, has given an appropriate introduction to the description of this specialized field. Starting with the student nurse, she gives a bird's-eye view of the steps from general nursing in an orthopedic service in a hospital to the advanced consultant positions in hospitals and other agencies.

A Happy, Rewarding Service

I find orthopedic nursing one of the most challenging and satisfying services! In the care and treatment of orthopedic conditions we often know that a patient cannot be cured of his disability or handicap and it becomes a challenge to help him adjust, to accept his condition, and to become an independent, happy individual making the best of the circumstances and becoming an asset to society.

Student nurses come to our service with a mixed feeling of fear and interest. We are all afraid of things we do not understand. The setup looks complicated but at the same time procedures and equipment fascinate students and graduates alike. Nothing is more satisfying in the teaching of orthopedics than to see a student's face light up with triumphant satisfaction when she has accomplished the "know how" of setting up a unit for traction. "Why, it's wonderful! I love it and it isn't half as complicated as I thought it would be." Once you understand and master the principles involved, you have accomplished the difficult part in orthopedics. After that the "principle remains the same; the procedures vary."

The orthopedic nurse becomes a very important part of the lives of these children who often spend more time here in our hospital than in their own homes. Children transfer their affection and trust to the nurse, thereby creating a wonderful opportunity for her to use her ingenuity in directing the children's activities. Here a nurse plays the part of mother, teacher, and nurse.

Orthopedic service lends itself most wonderfuly to actual teaching situations. Ward classes are patient-centered: set up to include actual patients and conditions on the service. Children love to come to the classroom for purposes of demonstration. The instructor has to be careful not to show partiality to certain patients. "Sammy went to class yesterday, it's my turn today!" or, "May I come to class today—please?" These are familiar remarks made by our children. Classwork makes them feel important and is a wonderful teaching device.

Teaching aids such as posters and models made by the students as orthopedic projects are very helpful in understanding procedures. If the needed type of traction is not actually in use on the ward, students often give return demonstrations by applying different types of traction on each other or on a model doll. Orthopedic equipment has been greatly improved. A nurse can assemble and set up equipment for all types of traction. The "Chick Smart" frames may be modified to meet many needs.

The orthopedic nursing instructor has her office and the ward classroom on the service so she is at hand to supervise procedures, to take advantage of the actual situations presented, and to assist and guide the student in her nursing problems. With the cooperation of the "Orthopods" and a flexible ward-class program, we often take advantage of a case coming in for treatment. If a patient with a congenitally dislocated hip comes in we call the students together and apply a putti splint or carry out other valuable procedures.

Students are assigned to selected patients for a period of one week. This enables a nurse to plan individual programs for each patient and to help him become a well-adjusted, happy child. She has an opportunity to direct activities, to stimulate good reading, to suggest and direct constructive games and other diversions. She is able also to teach good manners, to provide toilet training, to emphasize the importance of good body alignment, and to explain the necessity for eating certain foods and for accepting the rest periods.

Children on orthopedic service seem to adjust quickly, especially when with other children. We discourage the parents' desire to place children in private rooms. Children need friends and they do not want to be unlike the others. We make a great effort to be impartial because special privileges make children feel different.

The best method for aiding in the adjustment or in teaching of good posture and correct body mechanics is to be convinced of the need. We find that nurses who enjoy orthopedics are their own most enthusiastic disciples and this enthusiasm is reflected in the patients and coworkers.

It is impossible to give good orthopedic nursing care without an appreciation and understanding of the complex therapeutic service rendered by the various departments working as a team for the patient's physical and mental recovery. An explanation of the purposes of each of the correlated departments and their services is included in the nurse's basic introduction, running parallel, in a series of classroom lectures, with actual experience on orthopedic wards. Students also have an opportunity to observe and assist in the clinical services connected with orthopedics. For instance, a short period is spent in the speech clinic, in occupational therapy, physiotherapy, and in the cerebral palsy clinics.

After a student has learned the basic principles, and if she has mechanical aptitude, she usually loves this specialty. She soon learns to know intimately many of our patients and is moved by their ability to adjust happily to their handicaps. Their determination to succeed and make the best of their situations makes every effort in their behalf worth while. The satisfaction of seeing a little boy with Pott's disease put on his favorite cowboy boots and walk for the first time in two years has to be experienced to understand the thrill of this service. Then very suddenly all hard work and patient effort seem a small price to pay. Or, to see a seventeen-year-old basketball player who severed his spinal cord in a car accident the night before graduation, suddenly respond after months of despondence and bitterness and want to become a lawyer! Hundreds of incidents could be cited to show that there are many, many things much worse than a physical handicap. These are the experiences that make orthopedic service an exciting and challenging service.

After some general experience a nurse often wishes to advance in this field. She finds a wide-open field offering many opportunities. Teachers and supervisors are needed, and consultants are being used in public health services. General duty experience with patient-centered ward classes often attracts the graduate nurse and she decides to specialize in this field. We need happy, interested, and gentle nurses here. A graduate student can work for a B.S. degree and take courses in administration, supervision, and education!

Let us take a bird's-eye view of Miss James, a senior student, on her first and last days on orthopedic service here. Miss James came to us, a little nervous and afraid, not knowing just what to expect. As she stood waiting for further instructions, she noticed the models and posters in the ward classroom. She was fascinated by the model dolls on the shelves in various types of traction and casts. On another shelf she saw different types of braces with posters explaining their purpose and application. "Who made all of these miniature models?" she asks as the instructor comes to greet her. When she is told that the students made them as orthopedic projects she is immediately interested. The idea appeals to her imagination and mechanical aptitude, she has visions of working on a project of her own.

After receiving information on the requirements of the course and after the routine of the service is discussed, Miss James is shown the physical setup of the service. Suddenly, little Larry meets her in the corridor. He is helping the maid push a laundry hamper. Larry is a four-year-old with many congenital anomalies. He has no legs. His little feet are attached to the trunk of his otherwise normal body. He walks like a penguin but he is happy and smiling. When asked how long he has been here and what they are doing for him, Larry replies that the doctor is going to get him long legs like the other boys and take off these little feet. "I am helping with the laundry," he proudly adds, "and then I have to go to school. I go through the tunnel to the school across the road."

Upon entering the ward someone calls Miss James by name. It is Freddie, who was her patient when she was on this service as a freshman. Freddie was accidentally shot on a hunting trip and had a severed spinal cord. He has had several operations, has been home for several months, and is now learning to walk with braces and crutches. He proudly displays his progress. How can these children be so happy and well-adjusted?

As we walk into the girls' ward we meet Dorothy, a thirteen-year-old scoliosis patient. Dorothy, a month ago, was very discouraged and felt that life had little to offer and little purpose for her. One of the students appointed her hostess of the ward. She had been there the longest and it was her job as hostess to cheer up, introduce, orient, and look after new patients. From that day on Dorothy made progress. At last she felt needed and had a purpose in life. Many a time she would be found reading to a homesick child, or finding playthings for her, or attending to the trivial but very important conversation of a child. The whole ward was happier. She helped the student plan activities. Dorothy is proud and jealous of her job. She hardly finds time now to be sick or even to have her own treatments because the girls might need her.

In another ward our poliomyelitis patients are being given the Sister Kenny treatment, and Miss James notices the alignment of the body and is told that alignment and relaxation play a very important part in the prevention of deformity. A patient in a respirator smiles up at her as he brags about his progress: "I was out of the respirator for 30 minutes today." His prognosis is poor and he is a heartbreaking sight, but his radiant happiness is inspiring and we are convinced, as we move away, that there is much we can do—and with that confidence anything might be possible. Donny and Earl, two of the cutest little poliomyelitis patients, straighten their positions and push their little feet against the footboards. Oh, yes, they know that position and alignment are important but they have to be reminded! Every few days their beds are switched. This is necessary to prevent scoliosis because the children play together and curve toward each other. When the beds are changed they curve in the opposite direction.

At noon Miss James takes a tray to Sandy, a two-year-old arthrogryposis patient. Sandy fusses and scolds until she convinces Miss James that she should have a bib and a tray cloth and be placed in a high chair to eat!

Miss James is told that she will soon be assigned to a group of patients for a week at a time, giving her an opportunity to work out a whole program for nursing care. She is shown several rooms and closets with orthopedic equipment, and told that much of this can be used as an aid to her; for example, a trapeze is always an aid in lifting a patient, and at the same time is an exercise and muscle toner; a hammock for an injured or casted leg or arm aids in the comfort of the patient.

This is an interesting day, and tomorrow sounds equally exciting for she is assigned to care for a spinal fusion patient. She will go up and watch the surgery and then care for this patient. A spinal fusion requires all the skills of orthopedic nursing—care of a patient after major surgery, cast care, braces, traction, and mental adjustment. Mastering these skills means mastering the major principles of orthopedics.

Several days later in ward class Miss James goes into a respirator herself. Now she can teach from actual experience, she knows how it feels, what the problems are, and what adjustments are necessary.

During her time on this service, she makes several interdepartmental observations. The first clinical visit is to the physical therapy department.

The personnel there are very willing to answer questions and explain procedures. The key used in muscle check is explained and she discovers how to read muscle charts. The chart enables her to see what muscle involvement her patients have and helps her to give them support and protection while bathing or giving them care.

The interchange of ideas with this department is an incentive to continue the program on the service. They show Miss James how the determination of the children to succeed and the motivation to improve must be encouraged. Teamwork is highly stressed.

The second observation is in the occupational therapy department. This is the recovery period, which may cover a long period of time. Rehabilitation is a link in meeting the educational and vocational needs of the child.

Next Miss James sees the cerebral palsy patients. Just recently much research has been done to prove that about 70 per cent are capable of being taught. The degree of improvement for a child is recorded on a chart. The patient is taught to dress himself by learning to button clothes, dress dolls, lace practice shoes. The goal set for these patients must be something that can be obtained within a short period of time. Fundamental motions are taught, the keynote being relaxation.

As the orthopedic nurse is daily confronted with feeding problems, she may obtain many helpful suggestions from the occupational therapy department concerning feeding aids and recreational activities for keeping the child in a wholesome state of mind.

Next, the speech clinic. This is a service closely connected with all departments, and speech training with recordings is a valuable way to gauge progress. A visit to the out-patient department and cast room complete the picture of interrelated services. Miss James sees the importance of good cast care and adequate follow-up work.

Six weeks later, Miss James, now a confident nurse, walks into the office for her final conference. She hates to leave! She has become attached to many of our children and the time has been so short! She feels that she has learned and mastered much but that there is still so much more to learn. She has repaired, finished, and waterproofed casts, has helped with Rollier regime, and now understands the necessity of portional exposure to the sun. She has assisted and set up traction and cared for patients with Thomas splints, Pearson attachments, Dunlop's traction for supracondylar fractures, a Bryant's and Russell's traction used for fractured femurs. She has learned to turn a patient between frames. (Sammy laughed and called himself a Sammy sandwich when placed between these frames for turning.) She has figured out a method for exercising a hip with the leg in a Thomas splint. This was done by means of ropes and pulleys; by pulling the rope on one side the leg would swing back and forth or up and down.

As she leaves our service perhaps she is thinking especially of Celestino, a lonesome little boy with a tubercular hip, who, when scheduled for surgery sobbed brokenheartedly because he did not want to go to surgery alone. He wanted *someone* to care enough to go with him! Later he could brag to the boys in his ward that Miss James had gone up with him and watched and seen everything that was done for him. "You're my nurse, now, aren't you?" he said to her. Yes, she would remember Celestino.

ANNE WIEBE, R.N.
Orthopedic Clinical Instructor
Children's Hospital
Denver, Colorado

The field of orthopedics has expanded rapidly since the passage of the Social Security Act, which stimulated the development of official programs in all states for the care of "crippled children." The demand for nurses with broad preparation in orthopedics for these programs has far exceeded the supply. The Joint Orthopedic Nursing Advisory Service[1] has done much to promote interest, set standards, and assist universities in establishment of programs of study for graduate nurses. One has only to read Miss Wiebe's description of service to children suffering from orthopedic conditions to realize that in this service a nurse must have special preparation, but that all she learns about the application of the principles of posture and body mechanics will be of use to her in whatever field of nursing she ultimately enters. The private duty nurse, the public health nurse, and the nurse in school or industry will use this knowledge to promote efficient use of the body in rest and activity, in giving bedside care and in health teaching, and will learn to recognize the factors which cause crippling or physical disabilities. They will learn also to apply knowledges and skills in specific care of handicapped individuals. The increasing number of persons requiring care for orthopedic conditions

[1] This Service is under the sponsorship of the National Organization for Public Health Nursing and the National League of Nursing Education, aided by funds from the National Foundation for Infantile Paralysis. The author is indebted to the Service for assistance with this chapter. For the addresses of all organizations mentioned in this chapter, see Appendix A.

due to injury or disease, the continued prevalence of epidemics of polio-myelitis, the better recognition of crippling conditions, such as cerebral palsy, and the expansion of facilities for care of the patient have all given an important role to the nurse with special preparation in the orthopedic field. As the life expectancy of our population increases, continued expansion and development of new programs are necessary to meet the needs of those with chronic diseases, and more nurses will be needed to give appropriate care.

Orthopedic nursing, correctly speaking, does not mean physical therapy, although the terms are sometimes confused. Physical therapy is concerned primarily with the treatment of disease by physical means—heat, light, water, electricity, massage, and exercises. Some nurses, especially public health nurses, are qualified both as orthopedic nursing specialists and physical therapists. To apply the procedures of physical therapy, it is necessary to complete an approved course in the subject.

Once qualified as physical therapists, nurses will find many positions open to them in which the service required is physical therapy as distinct from nursing, while the nurse who can offer acceptable qualifications both as a physical therapist and as an orthopedic nurse is in the most fortunate position of all in relation to employment opportunities.

Many opportunities are open now for orthopedic nurses. Orthopedic wards and clinics all over the nation are urgently in need of staff nurses and head nurses with special skills and interests in giving a high quality of orthopedic nursing care. Qualified instructors are needed in universities and schools of nursing to plan and direct teaching programs in orthopedics and to act as consultants on problems of body mechanics for patients and students. Supervisors are needed for segregated and non-segregated services. Many consultant and administrative opportunities have developed in state programs for "crippled children," a term which in its broadest sense includes the cardiac, deaf, and blind, as well as children with rheumatic fever, epilepsy, or a physical handicap. The nurse working in a consultant capacity in this field works as a member of a team concerned with a variety of handicapping conditions among this age group.

Public health agencies—local, state, and national—are in search of public health nurses with preparation and experience in orthopedics and physical therapy, to plan and carry out a program of staff education to help nurses meet their responsibilities in prevention and care, and to give or supervise physical therapy in the home and in treatment centers.

Orthopedic nursing as a specialty may be described as that element in nursing which concerns itself with the preservation and restoration of the skeletal and neuromuscular systems. The orthopedic nurse needs a basic understanding of the principles underlying physical therapeutics in planning nursing care, just as she needs an understanding of the medical phases of her care.

Nurses planning to undertake advanced work in the field of orthopedics need to have an interest in patients who require long-term care. Improvement for the patient with an orthopedic condition is made by the attainment of small successive goals, and maximum rehabilitation may come about very slowly.

The nurse who enjoys working with children will find that a large proportion of orthopedic work is with this age group. For the nurse who especially likes the adult and older age group, there are many opportunities in adult fracture and reconstructive surgery wards, with arthritic and paraplegic patients, and with amputees.

Do you have a flair for working with appliances, adapting equipment to unusual conditions, and do you like improvising? Orthopedic nursing calls for ingenuity in contriving mechanical devices and adjusting them to meet individual needs.

As in so many fields of nursing this one demands a nurse who likes to teach. Individual and group teaching is an essential part of success with orthopedic patients and their families. Demonstrations, through actual work with one's hands, hold an important place in the program.

The nurse will work as a member of a team providing for all the needs of her patient—physical, emotional, economic, educational, and vocational. The physician, physical therapist, occupational therapist, speech therapist, social worker, teacher, patient, and family will share in the process of rehabilitation in the hospital and home.

Neither the theory in orthopedic nursing nor the practice in physical therapy is easy. A most thorough knowledge of applied anatomy, kinesiology, and physics is necessary. Nurses who dislike detail and have had poor averages in their science courses will find the program of study difficult. On the other hand, your working knowledge of body mechanics can make every physical task easier for you and may save a loved one from lifelong crippling. There is probably no field of nursing which gives a greater sense of satisfaction, none that proves to be of such long-lasting general usefulness. Here is a specialty that pays dividends in whatever job you undertake.

QUALIFICATIONS

Ideally, the nurse planning to study in the field of orthopedics on an advanced level should have had at least 1 year's experience as a head nurse or assistant head nurse in a nursing service which includes orthopedic patients. Nurses who are preparing for positions as clinical instructors should complete their basic preparation toward a college degree as well as a university program of study in orthopedic nursing. A period of supervised clinical practice following completion of studies is desirable.

Nurses preparing for positions in public health nursing agencies who are expected to assume responsibilities for physical therapy should be fully qualified in physical therapy as well as in public health.[2] In some state agencies with programs for crippled children, a university program of study in orthopedics is acceptable preparation, if the nurse's responsibilities do not include physical therapy. A period of supervised experience in a public health nursing agency with a physicial therapy service should follow an educational program in that specialty.

It will be of advantage in planning a program of study in this field if you know in advance whether you expect to nurse in a hospital, public health, or teaching position; whether your position will be in a hospital with a segregated service, or in a public health nursing agency with or without physical therapy service; and further, whether your teaching and supervisory function will be with undergraduate or graduate students, with staff nurses, or on a consultant level. Several universities have worked out a year's program in orthopedic nursing that is part of a degree program and designed for the nurse who wishes to become a supervisor, clinical instructor, or consultant in this specialty. Several shorter courses (up to now not for college credit) are offered by orthopedic medical centers and provide sound supplementary instruction and clinical practice in this special field of nursing. The nurse who plans to work with crippled children may find it advisable to combine special preparation in orthopedic nursing with pediatric nursing. Duplication in preparation can be avoided by selecting the program of study that will fit you best for the expected demands on your service. Questions as to desirable preparation and supervised experience may be referred to the Joint Orthopedic Nursing Advisory Service at nursing headquarters.

[2] For detailed information regarding physical therapy and schools offering courses in physical therapy approved by the American Medical Association, write to the American Physical Therapy Association or to the Joint Orthopedic Nursing Advisory Service.

Scholarships and grants-in-aid to help nurses secure preparation in the various branches of orthopedics are available from several sources. Federal funds available to state crippled children's services through the Social Security Act may be utilized to prepare hospital and public health nurses for orthopedic services. The National Foundation for Infantile Paralysis provides scholarships for courses in physical therapy approved by the Council on Medical Education and Hospitals of the American Medical Association for which nurses are eligible. The courses for which scholarships may be used depend on several factors in the applicant's qualifications and are decided upon after careful planning with the applicant. Candidates under forty years of age are preferred.

SALARIES

Salaries in hospitals correspond usually to those of other specialists, clinical instructors, and heads of departments. The entering salary is about $2,200 for staff duty, $3,000 for instructors' positions, and $6,000 for directorships.

The salaries in public health agencies for staff orthopedic nurses start at $2,200 and may go to $3,500; teaching positions may pay as high as $4,500. Salaries paid in consultant and administrative positions range from $3,500 to $6,800.

WHERE TO APPLY FOR A POSITION IN ORTHOPEDIC NURSING

1. Professional registries and placement services
2. Public health nursing agencies, city and state health departments
3. Local associations, clinics, or societies for the crippled or handicapped
4. Homes or schools for the handicapped
5. Special hospitals or hospitals with large divisions devoted to orthopedic conditions[3]
6. The university or school of physical therapy where you receive your preparation for this field

[3] Among the special hospitals, those supported by the Shriners are perhaps best known. The Shriners' hospitals (officially the Ancient Arabic Order of the Nobles of the Mystic Shrine) are located in Greenville, S.C.; Shreveport, La.; Honolulu, T.H.; Minneapolis–St. Paul, Minn.; San Francisco, Calif.; Portland, Ore.; St. Louis, Mo.; Spokane, Wash.; Salt Lake City, Utah; Montreal, Canada; Springfield, Mass.; Winnipeg, Canada; Chicago, Ill.; Philadelphia, Penn.; Lexington, Ky.

Tuberculosis hospitals may maintain small divisions for children or adults with bone tuberculosis.

Information may be sought from the Joint Orthopedic Nursing Advisory Service, the Children's Bureau, the Veterans Administration, or the National Society for Crippled Children and Adults of the United States.

BIBLIOGRAPHY

1. BARTON, BETSEY: "And Now to Live Again," Appleton-Century-Crofts, Inc., New York, 1944.
2. CARLSON, EARL R.: "Born That Way," The John Day Company, New York, 1941.
3. DIVISION OF NURSING EDUCATION, TEACHERS COLLEGE, COLUMBIA UNIVERSITY: "An Activity Analysis of Orthopedic Nursing," News Series, Bulletin V, July, 1943. (Provides an analysis of orthopedic activities of nurses in hospitals and public health nursing agencies.)
4. NATIONAL LEAGUE OF NURSING EDUCATION: "Guide for an Advanced Clinical Course in Orthopedic Nursing," 1948.
5. OLMSTEAD, LOIS: The Orthopedic Nurse Specialist in the Hospital, *American Journal of Nursing*, p. 838, October, 1945.
6. PHENIX, FLORENCE L.: Nursing and Physical Therapy Consultation in State Crippled Children's Programs, *Public Health Nursing*, p. 2, January, 1946.
7. Physical Therapy in Public Health Agencies (four comprehensive articles), *Public Health Nursing*, 1948–1949. (A free reprint may be obtained from the Joint Orthopedic Nursing Advisory Service.)
8. "Public Health Nursing Curriculum Guide," Chap. XVI, National Organization of Public Health Nursing, New York, 1942.
9. RUSK, HOWARD A.: Implications for Nursing in Rehabilitation, *American Journal of Nursing*, p. 74, February, 1948.
10. RUSK, HOWARD A., and EUGENE T. TAYLOR: "New Hope for the Handicapped," Harper & Brothers, New York, 1949.

CHAPTER IX

Communicable Disease Nursing

Great strides have been made in the last quarter century in the control and prevention of the communicable diseases. DDT and other insecticides, penicillin, the sulfa drugs, streptomycin, and gamma globulin, as well as new methods of treatment—such as rapid treatment in syphilis and gonorrhea—have all been added to the group of vaccines and serums in use in the control of smallpox, typhoid, diphtheria, scarlet fever, tetanus, and other diseases. Every year brings more knowledge in relation to the cause and the means of preventing these diseases. In no other field is it more important for nurses to keep up to date. The remedies, dosages, and methods in common use a year ago may be outdated today, and the detailed knowledge expected of the nurse by both her patients and the medical profession demands constant reading and observation.

The American Public Health Association[1] lists some 50 forms of communicable diseases, but of these about a dozen are rarely seen outside of tropical countries, and another dozen are those we think of as the communicable diseases of childhood although adults suffer from them occasionally. All may require nursing at some stage, even the light cases of chicken pox and impetigo, and all involve health teaching. As a result of war and of international travel by airplane, more attention is necessarily being devoted to such diseases as malaria, the dysenteries, and tropical fevers. Insect and rodent control are more important than ever, and the nurse on the Eastern seaboard must be able to answer questions about Rocky Mountain spotted fever, sleeping sickness, or typhus—diseases her older sisters seldom heard of. Thus, while our knowledge of preventing and lightening these diseases is greater and nurses see fewer very acute

[1] For the addresses of all organizations mentioned in this chapter, see Appendix A.

cases—indeed, can go through their schools of nursing without seeing diphtheria—the field of opportunity and the need for specializing are far more demanding of the nurse as a teacher and technician than formerly. Few schools of nursing give a wide and thorough grounding in the care and prevention of all the communicable diseases, and none can or should give preparation in this field as a specialty. It must of necessity be a subject for postgraduate study and practice.

Of most concern to the public, at the present time, are tuberculosis, syphilis, gonorrhea, poliomyelitis, rheumatic fever,[2] and the ever-present group of upper respiratory infections. Of these, tuberculosis, the venereal diseases, polio, and, recently, rheumatic fever call for intensive preparation on the part of both nurses and doctors. Special courses, institutes, and supervised practice have been developed for those planning to concentrate in the care of these infections. In this chapter, tuberculosis nursing is described in detail as fairly representative of the group requiring intensive preparation.

The nurse devoting her services to the *general* field of communicable disease nursing must understand the epidemiology of all the commonly occurring infections, know the aspects of control and prevention, the symptoms and especially the early signs of each disease, and be thoroughly familiar with the complications and typical sequelae of each. The public health nurse needs to know in addition the state and local regulations governing quarantine, available diagnostic and laboratory services, and the current public information programs. All nurses in this field must be able to improvise equipment and means of maintaining proper isolation for their patient and protective measures for themselves and the patient's family. Many of the hospital routines must be simplified and adapted to homes, and medical asepsis taught at a level that will be understood and followed by all those in contact with the patient. The nurse who plans to specialize in the home care of communicable disease or who is bound to come across it in the course of her day's work in homes, schools, or industry must be able to teach prevention and protection, and to answer questions with sound, workable information. Nurses working in clinics and hospitals must also be technically proficient, especially if they are responsible for the preparation of medications and for assisting with the various diagnostic tests.

[2] While not classified as communicable in the strictest sense, the preceding streptococcal infection which precipitates rheumatic fever is communicable, though it has usually subsided at the time rheumatic fever manifests itself.

A liking for children and the ability to handle and amuse them are important as so many cases are among children. School nurses need well-developed and alert powers of observation in detecting the first signs of a communicable disease and must, as their share in the control program, be able to explain and interpret it to families, teachers, and the pupils themselves. This means speaking in public as well as other avenues to public health education, such as radio broadcasts and writing for newspapers.

Both the institutional and home nursing care of communicable disease require persistent and untiring effort on the part of the nurse to control the spread of infection to others. Not only must a safe technique become second nature to the nurse, but she must never relax her supervision of others in contact with the patient. This requires tact and infinite patience. Firm persistence and watchfulness go with the nursing of every case, no matter where it is located, if the development of new cases and cross infections are to be avoided. For these reasons, a nurse planning to specialize in communicable disease nursing must have an extra well-developed sense of cleanliness or, speaking technically, an "aseptic conscience." She must like detail and never tire of the routine of technique so vital to the safe care of these patients.

It is obviously of first importance for the nurse to keep her own immunity up to date and to maintain good physical resistance toward those infections for which at the present time we have no immunizing agent. The nurse with sinus trouble, easy liability to colds, or a history of rheumatic fever should shun this field. Hospitals, clinics, and public health nursing agencies have rules regarding the health of those who care for patients, and supervisors see that nurses with colds, sore throats, etc., are relieved of duties in which they might infect others. This is not the case in private practice and in some industrial positions, in which the nurse must be her own judge.

Special courses in communicable disease nursing are available in nearly every section of the country. In many instances they are called "supplemental courses" and are taken by nurses whose basic preparation in their school of nursing was weak. Courses are from 3 to 6 months. Lists may be secured from the National League of Nursing Education. In enrolling for special work in this field, make sure that you are going to receive adequate grounding in the specialty and not just a review of what you had in your basic course.

SALARIES

Staff salaries for the care of communicable disease in hospitals are slightly higher than in the general wards, ranging from $2,500 to $3,000 without maintenance. Instructors' salaries are $300 to $800 more.

In private practice, nurses usually receive from 50 cents to $2 more per day (8 hours) than when caring for a patient with a noncommunicable disease. If there is more than one patient in a family, as sometimes happens, wages range from $8 to $12 per day. The higher salaries and wages are paid in the large cities and on the East and West Coasts.

Public health nurses and industrial nurses meet communicable diseases in their daily run of cases and are not paid more for their care, except in the case of public health nurses who have specialized and are employed in the special programs.

For nurses who have prepared in a specialty, such as tuberculosis or venereal disease nursing, staff salaries may be slightly higher than in a generalized program—that is, in the neighborhood of $2,800 without maintenance. Instructors, supervisors, and consultants in these fields receive from $3,000 to $5,000. Clinic nurses in the special fields are paid from $1,600 to $2,500, depending on training, experience, and ability; supervisors and directors of clinic services, $3,500 to $4,500.

SOURCES OF EMPLOYMENT

1. Professional placement agencies
2. Federal agencies, especially the U.S. Public Health Service, the Veterans Administration, and the Bureau of Indian Affairs
3. Hospitals with special divisions for the care of communicable diseases or specialized hospitals, such as tuberculosis sanatoria (the National Tuberculosis Association publishes a list of all sanatoria, giving size and superintendent's name)
4. National voluntary agencies interested in promoting the specialty, also state associations with similar objectives
5. State and local health departments
6. Clinic positions, usually in connection with hospitals and health departments. There are a few clinics under the auspices of local tuberculosis societies. Also, there are a few very good private hospitals for the care of tuberculosis. The standards in small, privately owned tubercu-

losis hospitals may not be of the best. Inquire of your state health department or state tuberculosis society. A professional placement agency usually has this information also

7. Local hospitals and schools of nursing
8. Assistance in the offices of private doctors specializing in one of these diseases. This forms an interesting position for the nurse who has had special experience. Professional registries and placement bureaus list such opportunities
9. "Want ads" in professional journals and local health bulletins

TUBERCULOSIS NURSING

Tuberculosis is still an unconquered disease, still one of the 10 leading causes of death in the United States. In 1948, nationally, 48,883 persons died of tuberculosis, and the toll over the nation among productive workers—the group of men and women between the ages of sixteen and forty-five—was heavier than for any other disease.

We have no sure immunizing agent against this insidious disease, no "rapid treatment" to cure it in a few days once it is discovered. Nurses working in homes, schools, clinics, and industries find it one of the most common and difficult problems to handle, entailing as it does disruption of the family, frequently a long absence of the breadwinner from home and work, and an exhausting search for the source of the disease through examinations of all contacts. Tuberculosis is no respecter of climate, age, season, or country. The disease was practically epidemic in the war-torn countries of Europe. Yet, so great has been our advance in recent years in reducing the death rate in this country through public education, early diagnosis, and proper care, that eradication of the disease is not an impossibility. There is still much work to be done. No small credit for partial victory is due to the untiring efforts of public health nurses, industrial nurses, and the nurses in tuberculosis and general hospitals. One more concerted coordinated attack on this enemy, with nurses specially trained leading the way in partnership with all the other medical, social, and educational forces, and the total victory should be won. Among the special activities in which nurses have participated that have revealed many unsuspected cases of tuberculosis, many in an early stage, are community-wide chest x-ray surveys, out-patient and industrial x-ray programs, studies of selected population groups, and the routine of chest x-ray on all patients admitted to general hospitals.

At the present time there are 72,560 acceptable hospital beds for tuberculosis patients in the United States. There is need for 154,836. Plans are under way for providing 60,000 new beds, so the number of tuberculosis nurses must be doubled to meet this need. (This information comes from 52 states and territories reporting data for the administrators of the Hospital Survey and Construction Act.)

The Joint Tuberculosis Nursing Advisory Service (which has been most helpful in preparing this chapter) reports that in 1950, 456 schools of nursing were offering experience in tuberculosis as part of the basic program. This, however, represents but 38 per cent of the state-accredited schools. It is therefore obvious that many nurses will graduate without significant knowledge of tuberculosis and little readiness for the job to be done. It will be necessary to secure special preparation through refresher courses or work conferences. The Advisory Service can be of assistance in suggesting sources of help.

If you have not had an affiliation in a tuberculosis hospital as a student, you may not know how highly developed and specialized is the care of patients suffering from tuberculosis. If you are interested in surgical nursing, this offers a rapidly growing field. Nursing tuberculosis patients demands skill, tact, cheerfulness, and a keen insight into human nature. A good working knowledge of how to apply the principles of psychology is needed to help the patient adjust to his situation and to face with courage the long-drawn-out "cure," or repeated surgery. Miss Schwier explains these points so convincingly in her Letter to Alice (p. 149) that no further comment is needed here.

Nurses with a thorough knowledge of tuberculosis nursing are especially in demand in industry, in schools of nursing as instructors, and for advanced consultant positions in public health agencies. Service with a mobile health unit is one of the newer fields. Our modern techniques in case finding and diagnosis, the increasing use of surgical procedures and with biotics in arresting the progress of the disease, and the very great need to teach patients, families, student nurses, teachers, and parents how to control the spread of tuberculosis, call for more and more nurses prepared to teach and supervise in this field. A course in tuberculosis nursing as an advanced clinical specialty is now regarded as a prerequisite for those intending to take supervisory, consultant, or teaching positions.

There are also new opportunities for well-prepared nurses to study, in schools of nursing and other institutions, activities with relation to preventing tuberculosis. Among other matters needing attention from nurses are investigations into the best use of nursing time in the care of patients, the promotion of in-service training programs, and better ways of designing hospitals to facilitate the care of patients and save nurses' steps! Cooperation with the very active rehabilitation agencies and personnel is also a comparatively new field for nurses, and an essential one.

If in the least uncertain about the standing of an institution or agency in which you have been offered a position, by all means consult or write one of the following organizations before accepting it.

1. A professional placement agency
2. The Joint Tuberculosis Nursing Advisory Service[3]
3. The tuberculosis nursing consultant in your state department of health, or the U.S. Public Health Service

SOURCES OF PREPARATION

Training[4] is offered in tuberculosis hospitals, in general hospitals with tuberculosis wards or divisions, and in formal postgraduate courses available in many institutions. At present, six universities are offering programs of study for would-be supervisors, consultants, and teachers.[5]

SALARIES

Salaries for general duty in institutions caring for tuberculosis patients range from $1,800 to $2,000 with maintenance; higher for supervisors and instructors.

In public health agencies,[6] salaries in the advanced supervisory and consultant positions range from $2,500 to $5,600 without maintenance. Various national agencies; the state health departments, universities, and colleges; and the U.S. Public Health Service are employing public health nurses (with advanced training and experience in tuberculosis) in consultant capacities to promote nursing interest in and preparation for this specialized field. Salaries usually start at about $4,000.

It is possible to specialize in the hospital care of tuberculosis in several

---

[3] Sponsored by the National Organization for Public Health Nursing and the National League of Nursing Education and made possible through a grant from the National Tuberculosis Association.

[4] Used in the sense of theoretical instruction and supervised practice.

[5] For a list of the approved courses and programs of study, write to the Joint Tuberculosis Nursing Advisory Service.

[6] For staff salaries in public health, see Chap. XI, and for industrial nurses, see Chap. XIII.

of the Federal services, especially the Veterans Administration; the U.S. Public Health Service, Bureau of Medical Services; and the Bureau of Indian Affairs (see Chap. XIV). The positions are usually under Civil Service, and staff salaries start at $3,100, but depend on the classification of the position.

PERSONAL QUALIFICATIONS

It is unnecessary to add to Miss Schwier's summing up of the personal qualities needed in successful tuberculosis nursing, except to stress three points:

1. *Health.* The employing agency has a very real responsibility for the health of its employees. You should expect an unusually thorough medical examination, including tuberculin tests and chest x-rays, upon entering your job; and continued, repeated examinations, both routine and whenever circumstances indicate the advisability for them—for example, after any unusual illness, respiratory infections, overfatigue, or strain. Some authorities recommend B.C.G. vaccination for those who do not react to the tuberculin test. Only by constant health supervision, checked by tuberculin testing, chest x-rays, and laboratory examinations, can you and your employer be sure that you are free from infection. You have a right to expect this sort of watchfulness and should request an examination if you do not receive it. Your part is to follow every rule of the hospital to the letter, get as much rest, fresh air, and change as you can, eat well and report at once every cold, unexplained weight loss, or any undue feeling of fatigue. Remember, for the few cases of tuberculosis among nurses that can be traced directly to tuberculosis hospitals, there are more that originated at home or in other types of hospitals. Many nurses feel safer in nursing all types of patients after their special training in the care of those with tuberculosis. Doctors feel that for nurses over thirty-five, in good health, and with a well-developed "aseptic conscience," there is nothing to fear. Close check on the younger group safeguards them.

2. *Keen Observation.* The successful nurse in the field of tuberculosis must develop and use all her powers of observation. In tuberculosis, more frequently than in many other diseases, little signs mean much. "The best tuberculosis nurse I ever knew," the head of a large tuberculosis hospital said to the writer, "was such a keen observer of symptoms that

I often told her the FBI would welcome her service. She never missed a
trick. She watched every patient in her unit unobtrusively, yet so carefully that her reports read like signposts to us doctors. We could almost
predict which patients would be found to be gaining, which losing, by
reading a summary of her notes. She knew everything about a patient,
his moods, appetite, sleep, interests, attitudes, as well as the usual physical
signs. She saw her patients through sympathetic but highly trained eyes.
She was sensitive to her patient's outlook on life." Probably it is this
ability to understand what being sick with tuberculosis does to a person
that makes the field a desirable one for nurses who have themselves been
victims of the disease. Doctors will usually point out that former patients
make successful and acceptable tuberculosis nurses.

3. *Breadth of Interests*. Miss Schwier's letter reveals clearly how nursing tuberculosis patients calls for a wide range of talents, interests, and
hobbies if the nurse is to keep pace with her patients' occupations. There
is considerable scope for one's imagination, and this variety compensates
in part at least for the occasional indifference on the part of an unre-
sponsive patient or the failure to get a patient under care in time.

Tuberculosis hospitals reflect very directly the spirit of the nurses,
doctors, and other personnel. If their attitude is cheerful, optimistic, and
imbued with a confident hopefulness, patients will be quick to sense this
and respond. These workers will have an understanding of each patient's
behavior and will know how to help each one no matter how difficult the
situation. The gloomy, self-centered, brooding nurse, who is, as psy-
chologists say, "an introvert," will be unhappy here or will learn to
change. Nowadays, tuberculosis is a hopeful disease. It deserves hopeful nurses.

Rehabilitation of the tuberculosis patient begins, in one sense, when
the definite diagnosis is made. From that moment, doctors, nurses, and
later the patient, begin to plan for a return to normal life. Both public
health and institutional nurses are assuming an important role in this adjustment and by interplay between hospital, rehabilitation services, and
home can greatly assist in preventing a breakdown. "Recrudescence of
active disease in arrested cases still occurs so frequently as to be a social
and medical disgrace. . . . Success depends on the 'carry through' in each
individual case." If a nurse can look ahead and work toward the goal of
returning an arrested, rehabilitated, and protected—because informed—
citizen to his home, she may know she has not only contributed to the

happiness of a human being, but safeguarded his community from infection and restored to his job a worker who will become a social and economic asset to the country and not a liability. Tuberculosis nursing is challenging—it deserves only well-prepared nurses. Here is a letter from one.

A Letter to Alice

Mt. Morris Tuberculosis Hospital
Mt. Morris, New York

Dear Alice:

Your letter informing me of your plan to join me in tuberculosis nursing made me very happy. Our discussions concerning the progress and future in this field have proved ever so true, as I believe you will agree after you've worked here.

Many of the nurses coming from general hospitals find the routine care boring at first, but if they are sincerely interested in tuberculosis, they soon discover that there is no limit to the good they can accomplish. Nursing groups are now stressing the patients' total needs, mental and physical, and I believe that here the nurse fulfills that role, completely. Perhaps if I tell you about our policies and types of treatment you will understand my enthusiasm.

Many of our new patients are contacts of patients now here and are sent to us through our own out-patient department. Others are referred by their own physicians after a diagnosis has been established. Discovery of new cases of tuberculosis through mass surveys has increased the size of our waiting list. During the interval between the diagnosis and the admission of the patient to the hospital, the public health nurse carries on a program of supervision and teaching in the home for both the patient and his family. After admission, this program is continued throughout the period of hospitalization. After discharge the public health nurse once more enters the picture, giving post-hospital supervision. Thus there is continuity of teaching and supervision during the entire course of the patient's disease until he is discharged from service.

Our aim is to teach and develop good health habits so thoroughly that they will be continued for the balance of the patient's life. He must understand that this is necessary for the protection of those around him, not only in the hospital, but also at home. Constant routine repetition is necessary to accomplish this end. We try to avoid antagonism by concentrating on the basic principles of good hygiene, which after all really covers the subject, rather than stressing his disease.

I could mention many obstacles that confront us, but I'll only give you a few so as not to discourage you. The greatest perhaps is language difficulty. A knowledge of Polish or Italian would be a great asset. However, I promise you that you will obtain a smattering of each eventually, as well as a thorough understanding of sign language in the meantime! It takes time to realize that patients don't understand our medical terms and one must speak in language a patient can understand. He should never be made to feel that he is being talked down to.

First impressions remain the longest, so it is necessary to establish a good rapport with our patients at once because we must teach immediately. The prolonged hospitalization affords us a better opportunity for teaching at a slower pace than is usual in a general hospital, but for some unknown reason, the initial instruction remains with them the longest. The mentally deficient cause us no end of difficulty. There isn't a great deal that can be done with this group except to use measures to protect ourselves and to keep their activity curbed to a point where they can do the least harm to others. For example, there is Benny—a sixty-year-old Italian, whose chief interest is the time of day. He is the proud owner of a cheap watch, but apparently he feels it is untrustworthy, as he is constantly making for each clock in the building to check it. Everyone in every department knows Benny and joins us in our efforts to restrict him at least to his ward. He has reached the point in his education where he has some idea of covering his mouth while coughing. He also has a saving nature and does not want to waste tissues, so he carefully folds one tissue into a 2-inch square. When he meets anyone, he very conscientiously holds the tissue 3 inches from his mouth and coughs a few times, whether necessary or not. Incidentally, unless these tissues are forcibly taken from him, he carries the same ones all day. Somehow we can't feel that much has been accomplished in this particular case! Yet he is safer here than he would be at home.

In addition to good hygiene, we teach the value of rest, both mental and physical, good eating habits, and living according to a routine pattern. This requires the vigilance of a prison warden, the love of a mother for her children, and the patience of a saint. Your sense of humor will aid you in keeping you from becoming discouraged. Although patients delight in "getting away" with something, a nurse can keep these slips at a minimum by tact and understanding. Many of these tricks are "attention getters." One soon discovers the time when it is best to ignore them and when it is time to be observant.

Absolute rest is a very important factor in curing tuberculosis. We encounter little difficulty with the strict bed patients, but as soon as they are permitted some activity, it's the same old story: Given an inch, they take a mile. They feel so good after their enforced rest that they think they can conquer anything. You can readily see our problem. While their activity is being increased, we feel like policemen. We often wish that like those worthy persons, we, too, were allowed the use of clubs in maintaining law and order.

Attempting to establish good eating habits is difficult and often impossible. Although the food is good and plentiful, it is not as palatable as home cooking. Like institutional food elsewhere, the menus vary little from week to week, and those whose appetites are good at the start soon become bored with the sameness. Surprisingly, most patients continue to gain weight, so apparently while they complain and fuss, they are not hungry. I am repeatedly astonished at the number of people who are averse to including fruits and vegetables in their diets. They will all agree that these valuable items are vital to health and should be eaten. But do they eat them? Usually not!

Hospital routine is accepted without question and usually enjoyed. It is strictly enforced. It runs like this:

7:00 A.M.	Hygiene—radio on	
8:00–8:30	Breakfast	
8:30–11:00	Baths	Treatments
	Bedmaking	
	Morning chores	
11:00–12:00	A.M. rest	
12:00–12:30 P.M.	Lunch	
12:30–1:00	Preparation for P.M. rest	
1:00–3:00	Rest period—radio off	
3:00–3:30	Hygiene—radio on	
3:30–5:00	Visiting period	
5:00–5:30	Dinner	
5:30–6:30	Rest period	
7:00–8:30	Visiting period	
8:30–9:30	Evening care	Lights out
10:00	Radios off	

The orthopedic cases—mostly spine at present—are, for reasons unknown, more cheerful and easier to manage than their pulmonary brothers. Maybe it is because they seldom have any real discomfort. Being flat in bed all the time seems to remind them that they are ill, a fact that ambulant patients forget. They are a grand group and we enjoy working with them. They do have hilarious moments, but work them off well with a minimum of damage. Recently, I walked into a ward that houses three intelligent men. Imagine my surprise to find the floor and beds soaked with water, the result of a water battle waged by the three! We nurses came swiftly to the rescue with dry linen and mops to remove the wreckage before the housekeeping department learned of it. The morale of these people is really wonderful, considering that they have so little diversion. Reading and listening to the radio are all that they are allowed. Some have their own radios, but for those who do not, there is a central system controlled at the switchboard with earphones at each bed. Individual sets are frowned upon because the temptation to listen to favorite programs during rest hour and after 10:00 P.M. is very great and so often yielded to. Radios are, however, permissible and are under the jurisdiction of the nurses.

Current movies are shown in the auditorium on Tuesday and Friday. Bed and stretcher patients with permission from the doctor are taken in the afternoon, ambulant patients go at night. From time to time additional entertainment is furnished—such as patient plays, high school plays, musicals, and readings. When enough talent is available among the patients, they usually set up a "broadcasting station" and go "on the air" for a half hour weekly. These programs are enjoyed by the bed patients as much as by the participants.

Religious services are held regularly for members of the various faiths. These, together with visits from the chaplains, do much for morale. Even the ones who are not religously inclined attend. At first, they probably go for a chance to dress and do something different. However, I'm sure this practice is firmly rooted in them while here and undoubtedly continued after discharge. The chaplains are very nice to work with and more than willing to assist us at any time. Very often they can get through to a patient when everyone else fails.

The hospital employs two teachers, one for the grade school and the other for high school and college students. This instruction is given at the bedside or in the classroom according to the needs of the individual.

Regent's examinations are given here and diplomas are granted by the home schools. Last June one of our patients was elected to the honor society, and we were as proud as though she had been our own sister. Occasionally, the patients seek our help with some arithmetic or algebra problems—and I have been forced to invent a very urgent mission elsewhere rather than to admit my inability to help.

Knowing your interests lie in teaching, I must give you a thumbnail sketch of our student program. Unfortunately, student nurses are only here for two months, although we have so much to offer them. The formal teaching consists of doctors' and nurses' lectures, movies, and demonstrations in a well-equipped classroom. They receive approximately 65 hours in this program. We also conduct an informal program—bedside conferences, ward conferences, and demonstrations—which consumes another 20 or more hours. The head nurses and staff duty nurses are responsible for most of these. Everyone enjoys the students because they bring us the reports of new ways of doing things from the general hospitals; and certainly they receive a completely new phase of nursing experience from us. The affiliating students help to keep all of us on our toes, because they want to know the "why and wherefore" of everything. We are using the team method at present and, although we've met with difficulties, it is proving successful. The staff duty nurse is assuming her share of responsibility and it amazes me how well she can, if given the opportunity.

Just a word about our occupational therapy department—even though I could talk about it for a long time. The personnel work with the nurses from the start. They visit each patient on his arrival and furnish him with a choice of reading material from a well-equipped library. This therapy is graded so that as his health improves and activity is increased he may learn to make many useful items. Some patients become so proficient that they are able, by selling their work, to provide themselves with spending money. However, our occupational therapy department is not maintained to provide an outlet for articles. While we cannot discourage selling entirely, we do try to keep it to a minimum. You can readily see why: a patient would forget that O.T. is for diversion and become so sale-conscious that he (or she) would work too hard, thus defeating its purpose. To appreciate O.T. in this branch of nursing, one must really see it in action. Many times, I believe, it has been the thing that has helped a patient to accept hospitalization when everything else has failed.

I don't want you to get the impression that tuberculosis nursing is the answer to a nurse's prayer for a perfect job. There are drawbacks, and in all fairness I'll give you a few. The hospital's location does not afford one the opportunities for entertainment offered by large cities. However, we are close to Rochester and Buffalo and if you own a car, this difficulty is conquered. On the other hand, we are not left completely destitute—we do have movies in town and the pictures are the current ones showing in the city. Mt. Morris's population is close to three thousand and there are several churches which offer card parties and other forms of diversion. Many of the nurses live in town, and through them we become acquainted and introduced to the town's activities. At present, we are all enthusiastic over the "Home Bureau." With all the items they teach, one surely can find at least one absorbing thing to do. We are planning to have a group right at the Nurses' Residence and I'm sure it will be fun. As in all small communities, we make our own entertainment, and as facilities are available we make good use of them. Summer takes care of itself. The place here is lovely and we have a swimming pool on the grounds, plus a cabin with outdoor fireplace for picnics. If you wish to try gardening, you may raise vegetables or flowers to your heart's content.

One thing I must prepare you for, knowing your leaning toward tidiness and orderliness. Any ideas you may harbor about neat, orderly rooms must be abandoned before you come to work in a tuberculosis unit. Upon entering a room, your eye, trained for years to observe disarray, may fall upon anything from hundreds of dollars' worth of leather in various stages of purse-making, to boxes skillfully designed to house moths in the cocoon stage! The best we can do is keep the rooms free from dirt and persevere in maintaining a semblance of order. The maids and porters must be pacified daily to keep them from throwing down their cleaning implements and walking out to a job where their efforts are appreciated. They, of course, are supervised by each patient while dusting his room, lest they destroy or mislay one of his prized possessions!

I hope this will give you sufficient information to help you feel at home on your arrival. I am looking forward to seeing you with impatience. Do hurry!

Sincerely,
LAURETTE C. SCHWIER, R.N.
Mt. Morris Tuberculosis Hospital
Mt. Morris, New York

Venereal Disease Nursing

Fifteen years ago the few nurses specializing in venereal disease were working mainly in clinics connected with hospitals and health departments and would have found it difficult to find specialized courses preparing for this one service. Today, as a result of the interest of the U.S. Public Health Service and the recent discoveries of new and effective drugs and methods of treatment in the control of syphilis and gonorrhea, the field has become a highly specialized one and the number of nurses employed in it has more than doubled. More attention is being given to the whole subject of social hygiene, and the public attitude toward these diseases has changed markedly.

In venereal disease nursing, as in all nursing, the demands on nurses in terms of time, degree of skill, and preparation, are continually affected by changes in medical treatment. Does the current schedule of medication call for penicillin every 2 hours or only four times a day? Do the doctors in the area prefer to send all patients to rapid-treatment centers, thus necessitating few clinic treatments, or are there other variations in the kinds of demands made on the nursing service? Currently, as Hazel Shortal,[7] Chief Nurse Consultant of the Division of Venereal Diseases (U.S. Public Health Service, Washington, D.C.) points out:

> Newer preparations in delaying absorptions media permit effective penicillin therapy to be given once daily for from four to ten days to complete a course of treatment. Thus we are now witnessing in many areas a return to out-patient therapy. This means that the local health department nurses will probably again be required to participate in the administration of treatments.
>
> Epidemiology service in venereal disease has also undergone changes within the past ten years which have affected policy and the extent to which nursing participates in the program.
>
> During the war years when local health services were experiencing critical shortages of nursing personnel, supplemental workers were added to many health department staffs to make contact investigations and to make post-treatment follow-up visits to patients who failed to report routinely for serologic study. . . . Now, it can be anticipated

[7] I am indebted to Miss Shortal and her assistant Rosalie Giacomo for much of the special information included in this section.

that the major responsibilities of case finding and case holding in venereal disease will again fall to the public health nurse carrying the family health services.

The field requires very well prepared nurses, alert to the constant changes in treatment and control policies. Much of the responsibility for case holding and follow-up rests with the nurse, whose tactful approach and understanding attitude can do much to keep patients returning for treatment and in a mood to provide confidential information regarding contacts. A tolerant and friendly acceptance of the situations revealed by patients and an effort to make their clinic visits painless—in every sense of the word—with due consideration for privacy, must be shown by the nurse. Here again, ability to explain things simply, to teach convincingly with tactful firmness, and to promote the doctor's plan of treatment, is essential. The nurse who is bored by repeating the same lesson again and again, who is discouraged or irritated by patients who fail to keep their promises or follow directions, or who has not the tenacity to follow up delinquent patients will discover that this field is a difficult one.

Adeptness and skill in interviewing is important to the success of all services in nursing, and it is vitally so in venereal disease. Ability to gain the patient's confidence regarding his sex intimacies, and an objective approach to a plausible solution of the problems in contact tracing resulting from these indulgences, is essential. The nurse who critically examines her own interviewing techniques, and is ready to utilize newer approaches, while at the same time helping the patient to maintain his dignity as a human being, makes the best contribution to the epidemiology of venereal disease.

Venereal disease control or, in its wider sense, social hygiene, calls for a good team worker. The "V.D. nurse" will find her work touches that of the medical social worker, the welfare worker, the public schools, the church, the law, the police department, and recreation groups—to name only a few. Sound knowledge, diplomacy, and the right psychological approach to all the aspects of these diseases must be combined in the successful worker in this field. These attributes do not come through reading or wishful thinking. They are the result of study and supervised practice in carefully selected situations. The control of venereal disease is still a community problem, and community attitudes are important.[8] For this reason, the nurse who is familiar with public health will be better prepared for the field, especially for the advanced positions.

The advanced positions may be in state or national agencies. Those on a state level are in the divisions of venereal disease control in state health departments or as consultants to state (or local) staffs of public health nurses. There are a few positions for specialists on the national level. Among the many interesting futures in this field are the positions for men nurses, which are increasing, especially with the Veterans Administration and the U.S. Public Health Service.

As Miss Shortal reports:

Education of nurses has progressed also in the last decade. The Rapid Treatment Centers have been used to give short, non-accredited courses in both the clinical and epidemiological phases of venereal disease for hospital and public health nursing groups. In a number of states, schools of nursing have arranged, with the approval of the State Board of Nurse Examiners, to provide one week of clinical experience for undergraduate nursing students at the Rapid Treatment Center. These experiences are given under the direction of nurses well-qualified in teaching and in venereal disease.

In the programs of study in public health nursing, venereal disease has been given increased emphasis during this era, and for nurses wishing to qualify as special consultants, three- and six-month courses are available at the University of Pennsylvania Institute for the Control of Venereal Disease.

Although there is some demand for nurses on the supervisory and consultant level in venereal disease work, it is the consensus of those responsible for program direction that the future will make many demands of *all nurses* in order that the gains of the past decade may be maintained. To this end, we as nurses are obliged to keep informed of changing schemes of treatments and to participate effectively in the epidemiology of veneral disease, as well as make adequate contribution to the education of students in nursing.

Courses in venereal disease nursing in institutions should be carefully checked with the NLNE, the National Organization for Public Health

[8] For information and literature regarding the social hygiene program, write to the American Social Hygiene Association (see Appendix A).

Nursing, or the U.S. Public Health Service. This is a field in which you can save yourself time and money by making the right selection of the course in view of your previous experience and future plans. The professional placement services will be glad to put you in touch with special consultants who will help you decide where to go and what your next steps should be. (For salaries in this field, see Chap. XI.)

SOURCES OF EMPLOYMENT

1. Counseling and placement services of state nurses associations, the American Nurses Association, and the New York State Employment Service
2. Local hospitals and schools of nursing
3. Federal services and U.S. Civil Service Commission
4. Local venereal disease clinics
5. Rapid-treatment centers

BIBLIOGRAPHY

General

1. ARNSTEIN, MARGARET G., and G. W. ANDERSON: "Communicable Disease Control," The Macmillan Company, New York, 1947.
2. ARNSTEIN, MARGARET G.: Communicable Disease Nursing—A Cooperative Venture, *Public Health Nursing*, p. 519, September, 1943.
3. "Communicable Disease Nursing (Bibliography)," National Organization for Public Health Nursing, 1950.
4. "Control of Communicable Diseases in Man," American Public Health Association, 1950.
5. MacCHESNEY, EMMA H.: What Is Communicable Disease Nursing? *American Journal of Nursing*, p. 266, March, 1940.
6. Program and Functions of the Public Health Nurse (Communicable Disease), *Public Health Nursing*, p. 280, June, 1944.
7. SHETLAND, MARGARET: Communicable Disease Nursing, *Public Health Nursing*, p. 543, November, 1948.
8. "State Programs for Care of Children with Rheumatic Fever," Children's Bureau, Social Security Administration, Federal Security Agency, Washington, D.C., 1943.
9. U.S. PUBLIC HEALTH SERVICE: Public Health Reports, Washington, D.C. (For current statistics on prevalence of communicable diseases.)

For references to nursing poliomyelitis, see Chap. VIII. Current numbers of the professional nursing journals offer accounts from time to time of the nursing qualifications needed in nursing specific communicable diseases. See index under name of disease.

Tuberculosis

1. CHADWICK, HENRY, and ALTON POPE: "The Modern Attack on Tuberculosis," Commonwealth Fund, Division of Publication, New York, 1942.
2. CODY, LOUISE L.: "Nursing in Tuberculosis," W. B. Saunders Company, Philadelphia, 1948.
3. CROWLEY, MARIE: "The Hospital Nurse in Tuberculosis Control," National Tuberculosis Association, 1951.
4. "Family Health Service in Tuberculosis," Guide 3A, Community Service Society, New York. (In pictures.)
5. FROST, HARRIET: "Nursing in Sickness and in Health," Chap. VIII, The Macmillan Company, New York, 1939.
6. Functions of the Public Health Nurse in a Tuberculosis Control Program, *Public Health Nursing*, p. 257, May, 1945; also pp. 175, 206, April, 1945.
7. "Guide for Advanced Clinical Course in Tuberculosis Nursing," National League of Nursing Education, 1947.
8. "A Guide to Work Conferences on Tuberculosis Nursing," Joint Tuberculosis Nursing Advisory Service, 1950.
9. HETHERINGTON, W. H., and FANNIE ESHELEMAN: "Nursing in Prevention and Control of Tuberculosis," rev. ed., G. P. Putnam's Sons, New York, 1950.
10. HINES, DOROTHY PALMER: "No Wind of Healing," Doubleday & Company, Inc., New York, 1946. (Novel about tuberculosis patients at Saranac Lake.)
11. HUDSON, HOLLAND: Placing the Discharged Patient, *Public Health Nursing*, p. 435, August, 1943.
12. JOINT TUBERCULOSIS NURSING ADVISORY SERVICE: "Instructional Plan for Basic Tuberculosis Nursing," 1949.
13. KIEFFER, NORVIN: "Present Concepts of Rehabilitation in Tuberculosis," National Tuberculosis Association, 1948.
14. KINGHORN, SARA M.: The Requisites of a Successful Tuberculosis Nurse, *New York State Nurse*, December, 1948.
15. LONGHURST, GRACE M.: "Tuberculosis Nursing," rev. ed., F. A. Davis Company, Philadelphia, 1949.
16. "Safer Ways in Nursing to Protect against Tuberculosis," 1950. Available from state and local tuberculosis associations.
17. SOUTH, JEAN: "Handbook on Tuberculosis Nursing," National Organization for Public Health Nursing, 1950.
18. SOUTH, JEAN: Tuberculosis Nursing Services, *Public Health Nursing*, March, 1949.
19. WALES, MARGUERITE A.: "The Public Health Nurse in Action," Chap. V, The Macmillan Company, New York, 1941.

Venereal Disease

1. AMERICAN SOCIAL HYGIENE ASSOCIATION: Publications, including the *Journal of Social Hygiene*.

2. BAUER, THEODORE J., and HAZEL SHORTAL: Prevention of Congenital Syphilis, *Public Health Nursing*, p. 81, February, 1950.
3. BAYLEY, H. LILLIAN: "An Interviewer's Aid for Venereal Diseases," V.D. Education Institute, Raleigh, N.C., 1948.
4. Bibliography, *American Journal of Nursing*, p. 740, August, 1944; also p. 548, June, 1944.
5. MORRIS, EVANGELINE HALL: "Public Health Nursing in Syphilis and Gonorrhea," W. B. Saunders Company, Philadelphia, 1946.
6. NELSON, NELS A.: Modern Venereal Disease Control, *American Journal of Nursing*, p. 75, February, 1950.
7. PICKENS, M. ELIZABETH: The Nurse in a Changing Venereal Disease Program, *Public Health Nursing*, p. 253, May, 1947.
8. SHORTAL, HAZEL: Nurse and Family in V.D. Control, *Public Health Nursing*, p. 56, February, 1946.
9. SMITH, C. P.: Community Action against Venereal Disease, *Public Health Nursing*, p. 368, July, 1944.
10. STOKES, JOHN H., and JANE B. TAYLOR: "Dermatology and Venereology for Nurses," W. B. Saunders Company, Philadelphia, 1948.
11. *Venereal Disease Information*, U.S. Public Health Service, Division of Venereal Disease Control, Washington, D.C. This is the most reliable and up-to-date source of information regarding the current developments in venereal disease control. Published monthly.

CHAPTER X

Private Practice

Private practice (private duty in homes and "specialing" in hospitals) is the oldest sphere of nursing service, and the nurse in this field is the "free-lance" member of the profession. In 1949, the inventory of professional nurses made by the American Nurses Association indicated that 21.6 per cent, or 65,032 nurses, were engaged in private duty.[1]

Although the nurse who "specials" in a hospital is subject to the rules and regulations of the hospital and owes loyalty to it, she is free to refuse a case if she wishes, may take a vacation when she "comes off" a case, and may state her preference as to the type of case and the shifts of duty. The nurse giving service in a home is equally free to plan her time between cases, and she, also, owes loyalty and must make adaptation to the needs of the patient and family for whom she is caring. The nurse registered with a professional or commercial agency is subject to the rules of that registry, but she has greater control over her time than the nurse in a salaried position. The nurse doing private duty who is not on the payroll of an institution, office, or other agency is classified as self-employed.

Those who have been successful in private practice in homes find great satisfaction in it. The secret, perhaps, lies in the fact that in the home the nurse feels she meets and masters the greatest challenge of all: adapting to ever-changing conditions surrounding one patient at home in the midst of his family.

The following account is the way one private practice nurse explains her enjoyment in this field of work to a senior student nurse.

[1] *Facts about Nursing,* p. 13, American Nurses Association, 1950. For the addresses of all organizations mentioned in this chapter, see Appendix A.

Private Nursing in the Home—An Adventure in Friendship

I can see you now, musing over and weighing all the aspects of the many fields open to you as you enter the nursing profession and leave your student days behind you. You are naturally giving thoughtful consideration to all the opportunities in an effort to learn just which is the one for you. Among the fields of nursing, private duty attracts you. You are ready for it, your qualifications are sufficient, and there is a special satisfaction in devoting all your skill and knowledge to nursing an individual through illness to complete recovery. It is your sincere wish to make your profession serve patients who are sick at home and, as you have seen the work of "special" or private duty nurses in the hospital, you feel familiar with the type of care and responsibility you will have to assume.

But do you have some questions about fitting into strange homes? Are you a little skeptical about being assigned to unfamiliar conditions, working for new doctors, meeting strangers, and working with different equipment? Of course, you have these doubts! Every private duty nurse asks herself, "Will I be able to please my patient, win the family's cooperation, find things with which to work, carry out the doctor's plan for the patient when I have never nursed for him before?" These are natural questions and every nurse feels uneasy when starting a new job, no matter where it is. But this is a condition of mind that disappears immediately when you begin the duties associated with the case. With continued practice, you learn to cope with any reluctance you may have in going into new surroundings in the home, and even though some nurses never lose that preliminary uneasiness when called on a case, they know that, once at work giving care to their patient, they will feel at home in every sense and be in command of the situation.

For, after all, you are not going into that home as a domestic or as a guest. You are going as a qualified nurse to be both companion and friend of a sick person. You need not think of the care you are going to give your patient as complicated or elaborate. You are fully prepared, if you have had sound nursing teaching and supervised practice, to meet every emergency. You can devote your entire energies to nursing at its best, remembering your instructions to exercise sympathy, conscientious attention to details, dignity, self-control, and self-forgetfulness. It is not necessary to remind you that while you are not a guest, you are a lady visiting in another's home and you will want to observe the rules of conduct of a thoughtful visitor.

One of your greatest contributions to your patient will be the sense of security and relief your presence brings. As a household is necessarily disquieted by illness, you can produce a calming effect by being as unobtrusive as possible. To invade the home, reorganize the mode of living for the entire family, insist on a special program for your own comfort, and request extra considerations for yourself only serve to add to the general disorder and will certainly not endear you to your patient or his family. By employing a little tact and good judgment, you will have everyone cooperating for the patient's comfort with little or no deviation from the daily routine of the houshold. You can be welcomed eagerly, regarded highly, and asked to return should need arise, or you can be tolerated only for the patient's sake and sent away as soon as possible. It is up to you.

It is important for you to remember that you are employed in the home with the patient as your charge. Your responsibility is second to that of the physician administering to the patient. As in every branch of the nursing profession, you will receive your orders from the physician, and these are the orders you follow as conscientiously as you have been taught. You are held solely responsible for seeing to it that these orders are carried out and for the constant nursing care of the patient while you are on duty. Possess a full knowledge of your nursing procedures and you will have no need to puzzle over your line of action in any instance concerning the care of your patient.

At one time it was found necessary to improvise a great deal of equipment in the home in order to keep a patient comfortable and to enable the nurse to perform necessary nursing tasks with the maximum skill and minimum discomfort to the patient. However, nowadays, equipment needed for a sick person and of standard hospital quality is found in most homes, or can be made available by concerns dealing in such supplies. There are, of course, some exceptions when you will find the need to improvise, but your instructions in your hospital plus your own imagination will be sufficient to meet these situations.

I know you have been wondering about the opportunities and the advantages for you as a private nurse in the home. I am glad to tell you about them. It is as common an occurrence for those endowed with intelligence and culture to suffer illness as it is for those who are uninformed. Frequently you will find your patient is of the former group. By your association with him your own knowledge is enriched. Perhaps he has traveled a great deal and enjoys recounting the highlights of his travels. Being the listener, you become familiar with far-off places and people. Perhaps he has a fondness for books and owns a fine library; possibly you will have access to this library. Your patient may be a collector, a linguist, a statesman, an educator. We all learn by contact; here is yours! Not infrequently, as your patient convalesces, he has a desire for a change in surroundings or the physician may prescribe such a change. You, as the nurse, may accompany the patient to another part of the country. Many nurses have traveled a great deal in this capacity. To enumerate all the advantages for a nurse as a result of these associations would be difficult, as they are as variable as are the patients and depend on the success with which the nurse fulfills her duties.

You are interested in the material, as well as the humane, aspects of nursing in the home. Your personal life and material gain are certainly to be considered, for to be satisfied in this regard is important so that you will not be carrying your disappointments and bitterness to a sickroom where serenity is desired. Nursing in the home frequently entails longer hours of duty than are customary in the hospital or in other branches of nursing. In the home, however, you are not constantly under pressure or bound by routine. Your day passes smoothly and at the tempo you would have it. At the close of the day your responsibility usually rests until the next day of duty. Your salary is that agreed upon by your state and district nursing associations. It is adequate to enable you to enjoy a few days of liberty between your cases, inasmuch as the private nurse is on duty 7 days a week while assigned to a case. There is also the great advantage of requesting an assignment only when you so desire. This tends to give you a feeling of independence which many of us covet.

When you have been engaged for a time as a private nurse in the home, you will find other compensations that you have gained beside those of a livelihood. You will find that your ability to converse, your speech itself, perhaps, have been greatly improved. You are more poised, more at ease, capable of holding your own in all sorts of situations. It may be that you have gained knowledge of a subject you were ignorant of hitherto. Your trust in your own judgment and ability has been proved and your sense of values heightened. You have made many friends, some of them friendships you will treasure throughout your life. These assets are not limited to the private nurse in the home, of course, but in the home the nurse is apt to be more aware of the possibilities of personal growth than is the case amid the distractions and routines of institutional nursing. Nor, be it said, does all the intangible personal return come from nursing in the homes of the well-to-do. Many of the most lasting, valuable, and important experiences are found among those who are not highly endowed with material things, but are rich in friendliness and appreciation of what you are trying to do. To them you are a member of the family. These are the most precious rewards of private duty nursing, not to be found outside of patients' homes.

MARGARET FUREY, R.N.
Buffalo, New York

Some of the advantages of engaging in private practice, say those enjoying it, are

1. It is a challenge to one's real nursing skill and adaptability.
2. It offers a variety of cases under a variety of conditions.
3. There is opportunity to meet interesting people.
4. There is frequently a chance to build up a desirable clientele among a group of doctors, thereby keeping rather steadily at work in congenial surroundings.
5. It offers occasional opportunities to travel.
6. Work is usually under pleasant conditions.
7. Patients may become lifelong friends. It is not unusual for a nurse to be retained many months, even years, in one family.
8. Work is usually under the direction of well-qualified doctors.
9. If private practice is in the hospital, there is opportunity to keep abreast of new developments in nursing and to see the latest treatments and procedures.
10. Experience in private practice for a year or two is good basic experience for every professional nurse, if only to accustom her to home situations, to getting along with families (quite a different proposition from care of a patient in the hospital environment), to developing her self-reliance and resourcefulness, and to nursing for private physicians.
11. The care of elderly, bedridden, or incapacitated persons who are not critically ill frequently makes an ideal occupation for professional nurses unable to carry the burden of acutely ill patients. The active professional life of nurses is proverbially short: in 1949 only 3.6 per cent of all employed nurses were over sixty years of age, and only 11

per cent were in the fifty to fifty-nine age group.[2] The fact that many nurses who are now reaching retirement age have not been able to provide for their old age makes private duty as a companion or guardian in a private home particularly attractive.

12. The nurse is free to take a rest between cases.

Private nursing in a home sounds very attractive, especially to young nurses who have been irked during training by fixed hours, close supervision, and rigid control of their freedom. It attracts more nurses than private duty in hospitals.[3] It is only fair to point out, however, that it has certain drawbacks, the first of which has already been referred to.

Irregularity of Employment. Time lost waiting for calls, during which personal expenses continue, makes income from this field uncertain. At best, no nurse will—or should—work 365 days in the year. On an 8-hour shift at $11 a day, the most she is likely to make in a year of steady work will be in the neighborhood of $2,600 and from this she must subtract nearly all living expenses, personal savings, insurance, and taxes. She bears her own cost of uniforms, meals, rent, telephone, laundry, and transportation when not on a case. Vacation and sick leave are taken at her own expense. Unless she lives in a club, at home, or with other nurses, she must have a telephone.

As the nurse who is not on salary is classified as self-employed, if she elects to go in under the Old Age and Survivors Insurance Act, she will pay $2\frac{1}{4}$ per cent of her earnings each month (1951–1953) toward a pension at age sixty-five (see Chap. XVI). She will be well-advised to make this slight sacrifice, but it must be realized that the tax is not shared by her private employer.

Lack of Promotional Opportunities. In private home practice there is no "future" in the sense of advanced supervisory and administrative positions with salaries in the upper brackets. Today's graduate on her first case receives the same compensation as the experienced nurse with 10 or 15 years of practice. Some private nurses point out with truth that there are chances of "lucky marriages" or long-time berths on salary under luxurious living conditions, and there is a future in the sense of a successful, steady career with an ever-increasing ability to give satisfactory skilled service. Also, there is some chance for specialization, especially if the nurse will prepare herself for the specialty through study and

[2] *Facts about Nursing,* p. 13, American Nurses Association, 1950.
[3] *Facts about Nursing,* pp. 13, 15, American Nurses Association, 1950.

practice. The special fields of psychiatric nursing, pediatrics, and communicable disease lend themselves to home practice. Nurse specialists may demand and receive slightly higher fees for the care of these patients.

Keeping Up to Date. It is difficult, but not impossible, for the nurse in home practice to keep up to date in new treatments and medications. She must make a real effort, at her own expense, to attend meetings, conventions, and institutes, read professional journals, and join professional organizations. In the future, the nurse with a specialty may have greater employability. The nurse in a home over a period of days has an unrivaled opportunity to teach health measures—both the prevention of illness and the positive promotion of well-being, home safety, and long life—if she is well prepared and her knowledge is up to date. A nurse who has been a convincing and tactful teacher in a family will be called again and again, and recommended to others.

Collection of Fees. Occasionally, questions of fee collecting arise when the nurse is being paid directly by the family. Nurses called to families on limited incomes cannot always collect, nor can they always bring themselves to ask for their regular charges. Yet they frequently remain on a case out of understanding sympathy with the patient so desperately in need of care. Until health insurance or prepayment plans cover the expense of illness in families of moderate means, the nurse working "on her own" will continue to face the decision as to whether to charge a part of her fee or leave the case. Few families today can afford $33 a day for continual home nursing except in dire emergencies. One of the reasons for the popularity of the Blue Cross plan, and the preference some patients express for practical nurses, is that the first provides hospital care including floor nursing, the second, nursing care at home and care of the home for less money than the professional nurse asks. In nearly all of our large cities, professional nursing on a part-time basis during the day can be secured from the Visiting Nurse Association. At present, unfortunately, visiting nurses do not cover night service,[4] nor will they remain more than 2 or 3 hours with one patient (see Hourly Appointment Service, below).

Lack of Supervision. As a student nurse, and perhaps as a graduate in the field of public health, you have been accustomed to supervision and have found how helpful such instruction and guidance can be. In private

---

[4] Except for delivery service in a few cities. Extension of evening service is being considered, however.

home practice, you will not receive supervision of this type. Two or three professional registries have offered supervision to private duty registrants, but there is nothing comparable to the assistance offered in other fields. The doctor on the case and the registrar in the professional registry will answer your questions and offer suggestions if specifically asked, but that is the most you can expect in home "supervision" in most cities. In the hospital, assistance of all kinds is at hand. If you are nursing in the hospital where you were a student, you will find your former instructors and supervisors more than willing to help you.

Lack of Growing Demand from Patients Sick at Home. The field of private practice in homes is definitely limited and not likely to expand rapidly. A trend away from home nursing was evident many years ago. A number of reasons for this have been cited: the increased use of hospitals for all conditions of illness; the availability of part-time home nursing from visiting nurse associations; the continued and probably increased use of licensed practical nurses; the reluctance of private physicians to carry large home practices when a good hospital is at hand; the development of highly technical diagnostic and treatment procedures requiring special equipment; the growth of prepayment and insurance plans providing hospitalization; dissatisfaction with professional nursing home care for long-time illness or subacute conditions.

Many of the nurses now giving service in homes are those who return with their patients from the hospital to tide over the early days of convalescence as long as full-time service is needed or wanted.

Irregular Hours of Private Practice. These make it difficult for nurses to count on freedom to pursue outside interests, hobbies, or courses of study. The 8-hour day has greatly improved this situation, however, and a much more normal life is possible.

PRIVATE PRACTICE IN HOSPITALS

Private practice in hospitals occupied about 34,000 of the nurses working in this field in 1949.[5] It is thought that the amount of "special" duty service needed by hospital patients in the future will depend greatly on the following:

1. Economic level of the patients, which is to say the nation's prosperity
2. Quality of nursing in hospitals given by salaried staff nurses

[5] *Journal of the American Medical Association,* p. 36, May 6, 1950.

3. Extent to which insurance and prepayment will provide nursing under the terms of their benefits to members
4. Extent of group nursing
5. Recommendations of physicians
6. Changes in the management and treatment of illness

Nevertheless, "specialing" in hospitals has definite conveniences and advantages to recommend it. The following is the gist of a conversation with a nurse with 10 years of experience as a private duty nurse in a large urban hospital. She prefers not to have her name used, but the author can vouch for her skill—having experienced it as a patient—and her enthusiasm and sincerity as reported by her coworkers and her supervisor.

MISS D.   Mrs. M., tell me why you like specialing in a large hospital like this? You must, or you wouldn't have stayed in it for 10 years!
MRS. M.   Yes, I love it. Why? Well, I'll be frank. First of all, this hospital has everything to work with. I guess I'm lazy or maybe just spoiled, but I like having the latest, best, and most effective things for my patients' safety and comfort—and that goes all the way from plenty of linen to the latest discoveries in medications and treatments. I like our private room facilities. I like seeing all sorts of diagnostic aids at work. I like nursing for top-notch doctors and I like the variety of my patients. I have surgical patients mostly, but all ages and all types.
MISS D.   And dispositions. Are most of your patients wealthy?
MRS. M.   Let's say comfortably off. Actually I might not know, because the hospital pays me, not the patient. It's different in some hospitals. Oh, another thing I like is being busy when I want to be and going off call when I feel like it. Only thing is I develop a conscience about that and am on call as soon as one patient leaves. While I am on a case I never leave unless I am sick. I try to see that I have 2 or 3 days between long, hard cases and I always take a summer vacation. The 8-hour shifts help a lot. I vary my shifts.
MISS D.   I'm taking notes! What else?
MRS. M.   We hear about and see the new developments in surgical care, we share in the hospital activities—lectures, parties, and so on— and we have use of the library. There isn't any excuse for getting in a rut. I have my own home; and my husband, luckily for me, is a musician so his hours are irregular, too, and we can usually plan our free time together.

MISS D.   You care for very prominent people—actors, generals, princes, —even kings!

MRS. M.   Often not so interesting as they sound! Quite often just like other patients—hard or easy to please, cross or pleasant—sickness is a great leveler! But often my patients become my friends. One old lady was my patient here for 3 days and she has sent me a Christmas card every year since for 8 years! Once she came back for a checkup and nothing would do but that I be present in the doctor's office throughout the whole examination! She is a dear.

MISS D.   I understand patients give nice presents when they go home.

MRS. M.   Yes, some do, some don't. I sort of wish they wouldn't. Some presents really mean something—you couldn't refuse them; but I never feel right about a cold-blooded check, even though the money is welcome. I hope that is not one of the reasons I like working here. Let me think—yes, I know another better reason: I like the feeling that I am not alone in the responsibility I take for my patients. Here there are always supervisors or doctors at the end of the telephone or corridor, and I can find solutions to my nursing problems by asking others what to do. Almost instantly, I can get aid—you know that doesn't often happen in homes. Yes, I like this job! Please don't quote me by name!

MISS D.   I won't, I promise, and thanks a lot. This may help other nurses decide to try specialing in a hospital. You make it sound very worth while.

ARRANGEMENTS FOR RECEIVING CALLS

PROFESSIONAL REGISTRIES

Professional registries are employment agencies, managed by professional nurses, which have been sponsored and approved by the local professional nurses association. They are supposed to meet the minimum standards recommended by the American Nurses Association. Many of the registries enroll both professional and auxiliary workers. A very few attain the status of true community centers for the distribution of all types of nursing service needed in the community.

The professional registry is nonprofit-making. It attempts to give its registrants employment. Investigation of the registrant's record is made before acceptance. It may refuse new applicants if there are fewer calls for nurses than there are registrants to be kept busy. An annual fee for service is charged to the registrant, who in turn agrees to abide by the rules of the registry. These rules may cover questions of "refused cases," and always fix the charge the registrant may ask the patient. The rates per hour are set by the local (district) nurses association.

Calls come to the registries from homes, hospitals, and doctors. Other agencies also use the professional registries and more and more attempt is being made to

1. Assist professional nurses to prepare for all types of cases (refresher courses, institutes, lending libraries, lectures)
2. Organize the registry with a view to filling community needs, thereby opening more avenues of employment to nurses
3. Provide services on a part-time basis
4. Supply practical nurses for appropriate cases
5. Interpret the registry's function to the public

Many reliable registries or bureaus are run by hospitals, but not designated as professional or official registries.

Young nurses are usually advised to start private practice by "specialing" in hospitals, becoming used to home service through accompanying their patients home after discharge from the hospital. They will receive more professional guidance from a professionally approved registry than from a commercial agency.

The U.S. Employment Service and state employment services have facilities in some of the large cities for the placement of private duty nurses. As this is a tax-supported activity, there is no charge for registration or placement.

"FREE-LANCE" WORK

As has been said, the nurse may be a completely "free-lance" worker and depend for her calls upon a group of physicians who use her service regularly. Under this arrangement she avoids paying registry or placement charges.

COMMERCIAL REGISTRIES

These may or may not be run by registered nurses. They try to respond to all demands from all services. They are run for profit. They charge a registration fee and a percentage of the nurse's earnings from each job to which the agency assigns her. Thus a series of many short cases may cost the registrant considerably more than she has to pay the professional registry in annual dues. On the other hand, the registrant is not restricted to the rules of the local district and in times of emergency or shortages may, unfortunately, feel free to charge what the traffic will bear if she is working in a private home. The more she charges, the more an unscrupulous commercial registry benefits. Such practices make for ill will toward the entire profession. Ethical commercial agencies operate under established rules.

Charges for Service

Nurses in private practice in homes are charging from $8 to $12 for an 8-hour duty. The lower charges are in small communities where the cost of living is less than in our large cities. Highest charges are on the West and East Coasts. In private practice in hospitals, charges range about the same. A higher rate is paid for night duty in many hospitals. To these rates may be added $1 to $2 or even $5 a day for care of mental illness, of communicable disease, or of more than one patient in the home.

Private patients very often wish to express their appreciation for care by a gift to the nurse at the close of her service. This may take the form of something rather simple, like a dainty handkerchief or a box of candy, or it may be a more substantial present such as an expensive watch or a generous check. Nurses use their own discretion about accepting these gratuities.

While on 8-hour duty in a home or hospital, it is usual for the nurse to receive one meal. In the hospital, the patient pays for that meal. On 20-hour duty in a home, all three meals are provided. This latter type of service is growing rarer in our large cities.

When nurses remain steadily in a home on a long-time case, employers sometimes ask for a monthly or weekly rate. When a nurse reduces her fee—an agreement which should be in writing—she usually receives other forms of compensation such as her room, meals, laundry, and use of the telephone. She may even be able to give up renting her own room, or she may sublet it. She should arrive at an understanding with her employer regarding tax deductions if she changes to a salaried basis.

Uniforms

It is the custom of nurses in private practice in hospitals and homes to wear the regulation white graduate nurse's uniform or the uniform of their school. It is especially necessary to present a spotless appearance in the hospital. In homes, when on a long-time case, or if the patient is convalescent and prefers to have the nurse appear in less formal garb, it is entirely appropriate to leave off the cap and wear colored washable dresses or simple tailored street clothes, depending on the situation. Nurses caring for private patients in hotels, summer resorts, or other more or less public places are often asked not to appear in uniform outside of the sickroom. This is a very reasonable request, for after all the white uniform suggests illness, is intended for use only in caring for the sick, and is both out of place and in poor taste in a general dining room, hotel lobby, or public gathering.

Hourly Appointment Service Center

If a community is not already supplied with an hourly appointment service from the professional registry or visiting nurse association, a nurse in private practice—or a group of nurses—may find this a lucrative field to develop. When it is undertaken by one nurse on a free-lance basis, she will need to have a telephone, with calls covered at all hours, and a car if travel to cases is difficult or time-consuming. She may have to build up her service through circular letters to physicians, cards for hospital patients, and an advertisement in the local newspaper and classified telephone directory. One satisfied customer usually tells another. The hourly nurse observes professional ethics very strictly; a licensed physician must be in charge of every case and treatments given only on his order.

A few nurses have developed their hourly service into a small organization with a paid staff. The advantage in this plan is a greater coverage and more flexibility in hours of service and therefore more regular hours for each nurse.

Charges for hourly appointment service range (1951) from $2.50 an hour (50 cents for additional hours) to $3 for the first hour and $1 for each additional hour. More than 4 or 5 hours at a stretch are seldom requested, as the cost would then approach that of the full-time (8-hour) private duty nurse. Special treatments are sometimes charged at a special rate, for example, $5 is the usual charge for colonic irrigations.

Nurses offering hourly service usually wear street clothes and slip into an over-all white apron or gown when giving nursing care on a case. A dark washable dress (worn under a tailored coat) is also serviceable, with a white "butcher" style apron to wear over it in the homes.

Hourly nursing fills a definite community need and is less expensive usually when under the auspices of public health nursing agencies. It is well to ascertain what the *community* plans for this service are before embarking on your own business. It may pay you to work through the already established program.

It is also wise to estimate the cost of setting up your "business," including extra laundry and your equipment. The hourly nurse must provide herself with a bag of supplies even more complete than that of the public health nurse. If possible, a period of observation or experience with a visiting nurse association should be arranged before venturing to take the responsibility of seeing several patients a day in their homes. Incidentally, these lessons in adjusting to home care and acquiring safe techniques mean greater speed and efficiency on your job, as well as safety for you, your patient, and his family.

OTHER OPPORTUNITIES FOR PRIVATE DUTY NURSES

Among the related opportunities for nurses in private practice are
1. The development of an employment service (registry)
2. The organization of an hourly appointment service
3. Perfecting a specialty and promoting calls for that service from a group of specialists
4. Part-time service in doctors' offices (see Chap. XIV)
5. A transfer to general duty on salary in the hospital (see Chap. II)
6. The addition of a special skill to the basic nursing preparation; for instance, an approved course in physical therapy

SOURCES OF EMPLOYMENT

1. Professional registries are probably the simplest and least expensive way for nurses in private practice to secure their calls. They offer the most ethical service.
2. Hospital registries
3. Alumnae associations or nurses' clubs
4. Developing one's own clientele of patients or group of doctors (frequently specialists) for whom a nurse serves regularly and rather exclusively
5. Contact with the Private Duty Nurses' Section of the American Nurses Association may prove helpful.
6. New York State Employment Service

7. Because private duty nurses are apt to change location fairly frequently, it is also suggested that contact be made with state and national professional placement services wherever they may be. Refer to the American Nurses Association for information, and to the Private Duty Nurses Section of the same Association for general information on personnel policies.
8. Commercial agencies

When changing to another state for employment, be sure to inquire regarding your legal right to practice under the state law.

BIBLIOGRAPHY

1. AMERICAN NURSES ASSOCIATION, CONFERENCE (NATIONWIDE) WITH GENERAL DUTY NURSES: Report, *American Journal of Nursing*, p. 255, June, 1949.
2. AMES, MIRIAM: Fifty Ways to Use an Hourly Nurse, *Hygeia*, p. 1115, December, 1931. (Still offers good suggestions.)
3. AMES, MIRIAM: Hourly Nursing Service, *American Journal of Nursing*, p. 113, February, 1933; p. 215, March, 1933.
4. BURGGREN, HANNAH: Part-time Nurses Can Be an Asset, *American Journal of Nursing*, p. 681, November, 1949.
5. CORRY, SARAH: "Notes on Nursing by a Nurse," Appleton-Century-Crofts, Inc., New York, 1944. (Procedures.)
6. DOTY, LORETTA M., and KATHERINE M. HOLFELTZ: Hourly Nursing Services Provided by Two Professional Registries, *American Journal of Nursing*, p. 113, Feburary, 1945.
7. Four Who Made Good (Hourly Nursing), *American Journal of Nursing*, p. 237, March, 1940.
8. Free-lance Hourly Nursing, *American Journal of Nursing*, p. 545, May, 1941.
9. GEISTER, JANET M.: A Long Road Turning, *R.N.*, p. 44, June, 1950.
10. GELINAS, AGNES: "Nursing and Nursing Education," pp. 58–59, Commonwealth Fund, Division of Publication, New York, 1946.
11. HANSEN, MARTHA: The Private Duty Nurse, *American Journal of Nursing*, p. 838, August, 1932.
12. HUGHES, LORA WOOD: "No Time for Tears," Houghton Mifflin Company, Boston, 1946. (Private duty in the early days.)
13. KOCH, FRANCES: A Case for Private Duty Nursing, *American Journal of Nursing*, p. 516, August, 1947.
14. LAURENTINE, Sister M.: Stepping Stones to Success in the Private Duty Field, *American Journal of Nursing*, p. 255, March, 1934.
15. *New York State Nurse*, p. 20, May, 1948. (Illustrations of private duty in a hospital.)

16. Private Duty Nurses: Independent Contractors, *American Journal of Nursing*, p. 172, February, 1937.
17. "Professional Nurses, The Outlook for Women in Occupations in the Medical Services," Women's Bureau, Department of Labor, Washington, D.C., Bulletin 203, No. 3, 1945. (See Index under Private Duty.)
18. QUIGLEY, GERTRUDE C.: Private Duty Nursing, *American Journal of Nursing*, p. 234, March, 1939.
19. SHELDON, NOLA SMITH: The Private Duty Nurse and Her Social Security Coverage, *American Journal of Nursing*, p. 235, April, 1951.
20. TATTERSHALL, LOUISE M., and MARION E. ALTENDERFER: Private Duty Nursing in General Hospitals—A Study, *American Journal of Nursing*, p. 651, July, 1944.
21. YOUNG, EDWARD L., JR.: What I Expect of a Private Duty Nurse, *American Journal of Nursing*, p. 761, July, 1937.

Some of the above are retained in this reading list because of historical interest and for their spirit of service.

CHAPTER XI

Public Health Nursing

Public health nursing, while one of the youngest children in the professional nursing family, has attained mature status in public acceptance, and future demand will undoubtedly require more and better qualified nurses. Estimates show that our country needs approximately 65,000 public health nurses; at present, there are 25,000. About 750 counties still have no public health nurses, while in 1950, 18 large cities were still without visiting nurse (bedside-care) services.[1]

"Firsts" in public health nursing are usually cited as: 1877, when a graduate nurse was employed by the Women's Board of the New York City Mission; 1885–1886, when visiting nurse associations started their services in Boston, Philadelphia, Buffalo, and Brooklyn; 1898, when the Los Angeles, California, first municipal nursing service began; and 1902–1903, when school nursing started in New York City.[2] Credit for the first rural nursing service goes to Westchester County, New York (about 1896); and Massachusetts claims the first nurse in a state health department (1915).[3]

Public health, defined as the art and science of preventing disease, prolonging life, and increasing physical and mental happiness through organized community effort,[4] is not only a steadily expanding field within the United States, but is calling for experienced public health nurses to

---

[1] *Facts about Nursing*, pp. 19, 21, American Nurses Association, 1950.

[2] For industrial nursing, see Chap. XIII.

[3] CHAMPION, MERRELL E.: Seventy-two Years of Public Health in Massachusetts (reprint), *New England Journal of Medicine*, pp. 241–247, March, 1945. Also HUBBARD, RUTH W., Public Health Nursing, 1900–1950, *American Journal of Nursing*, p. 608, October, 1950.

[4] Adaptation of definition originally phrased by Dr. C.-E. A. Winslow.

work beyond our boundaries—in Mexico, South America, Europe, the Near East, and the Far East.

Public health nurses work in two types of agencies: those publicly (tax-) supported and those supported by private funds (such as individual gifts, patients' fees, community-chest or foundation appropriations, and income from business contracts). Occasionally, agencies draw their income from both sources and are called "combined" services. The expansion of rural hospital and clinic services will strengthen the place of the voluntary agency. Health departments now spend about half of their budgets on salaries for public health nurses, and with boards of education are employing about three-fourths of the total number of public health nurses in the United States. The remaining one-fourth serve in privately supported health agencies, the majority of them in visiting nurse associations.

The positions in both types of agency—official and voluntary—are much the same in title and general duties. They are staff or field nurse, assistant supervisor, supervisor, specialized consultant, educational director, assistant director, and director. In small agencies—three to six nurses—there may be only the staff nurses and their director who combines supervisory duties. In very large agencies (the largest public health nursing staff numbers approximately a thousand when fully staffed), there may be subdivisions of these positions, such as junior and senior staff nurses, district or regional supervisors, and an associate director. A few agencies employ a "graduate" or "clinic" nurse without special preparation in public health nursing. However, promotion of these nurses is dependent on their qualifying as public health nurses.

Public health nursing agencies function on a city (or town), county, state, and national basis. Federal, state, and county agencies are nearly always tax-supported. Many of the positions are classified under Civil Service (Chap. XV). Private agencies flourish in cities and towns, with the large voluntary organization, the National Organization for Public Health Nursing, covering the nation with advisory and consultant services.[5]

The public health nurses, like their sisters[6] in the institutional field, are developing clinical specialties. Those with advanced public health preparation in a specialty—for example, orthopedic, tuberculosis, or

[5] For addresses of organizations mentioned in this chapter, see Appendix A.

[6] See also TRUDEAU, REMI ALCIDE: Men Nurses in Public Health Nursing, *Public Health Nursing*, p. 432, August, 1949.

venereal disease nursing—may receive consultant appointments or qualify as teachers.

The functions of public health nurses are pretty much the same everywhere, with the following exceptions:

Bedside nursing may not be included in the service expected from the nurse in the tax-supported agency. This situation is changing, however, the trend being toward its inclusion. Visiting nurse associations always include it.

School nursing (see Chap. XII) may or may not be a separate service. Except in parochial and private schools, it is tax-supported.

The public health nurses serving in rural areas work under different conditions from those in a city, but what they teach and do are based on the same general principles.

Public health nursing is carried on by some 181 local chapters of the Red Cross. The objective of such service is usually to concentrate on a demonstration of the value of bedside nursing service as an essential part of a community health program. The chapter services are especially needed and active in areas otherwise unprovided with public health nurses. Qualified nurses are desired for these positions.

The following sketches from public health nurses on the job represent three types of service: an urban health department, a rural county health department, and a large urban visiting nurse association. The first is presented here.

Hi, Nurse!

Your nursing school is certainly progressive, Mary, to include community nursing in its curriculum. We, who find real satisfaction in this type of work, hope to see the new graduates coming into our field of nursing. I am going to take you with me into the district just for a day. It really takes a year to know your families and to find out whether you have made progress in your work, because in public health nursing your patients aren't here for a day or a week, but all the year round; and it takes longer to realize results in working with them. Your rewards are real and lasting, however.

We in the official agency do not perform bedside nursing routinely as do the visiting nurses, but our principles are the same: to promote health and prevent disease through practice, demonstration, and instruction among families and individuals. You have asked how we work, and what we do, and what is meant by the phrases: "community aspects," "referral systems," "family health service," and "a generalized service." Let me explain.

First of all you must enjoy people, for public health nursing is for all persons—from the happy school child who calls, "Hi, Nurse! are you coming to my home?" and the young and insecure mother caring for her new baby, to the elderly lady who looks forward to the cheerful "Hello" of the nurse who calls on her. The people we meet are all part of a family living together with other families, forming a town or a city or, in rural areas, a country village. But the people we work with are humans with feelings and attitudes and sensibilities. They are the people who make up America—people of different colors, religions, and personality types—and they all have problems! Sometimes the problems are economic or social or medical, but as Emerson has said: "Health is our first wealth." As nurses we can spend special effort in teaching others to be healthier citizens through our help.

But you have asked specifically, "Just what do you do in public health nursing?" Let's begin with an example. As you know, there isn't anything more thrilling in life than the arrival of a new baby. Somehow, they just wind their fingers around your heart. If you love babies, you have a place in community nursing, because so many babies have mothers who need just a little of the help that a nurse has to offer in the care of this new creature who suddenly upsets the whole routine of the household. New mothers become alarmed at the strangest things. The baby's noises, hiccoughs, or sneezes send the mother into a panic; and when her baby cries, how she wishes he could say why!

We like to meet the mother long before the baby's arrival because we know that a healthy mother needs medical supervision during her pregnancy, and often she needs instruction in the preparation of foods and in selecting foods for a well-balanced diet for herself and the coming baby. She may need a bit of encouraging to secure the dental appointment she has postponed. We can be of special aid in answering questions about the growth and development of the baby, about his emotional needs and about his clothes, his crib, and other supplies. We help prepare the mother to breast-feed her baby if possible. We aid in formulating plans for the care of the children when she is away at the hospital, and we help her to develop receptive attitudes in the other children toward the new baby.

When mother and baby return from the hospital there are so many

things with which even the most confident mother needs help and assurance! Here we play a really helpful role by urging medical care and
supervision, giving information about the preparation of the baby's
food, explaining about the value of immunization, and being of service
should the child be ill by teaching her how to give nursing care under
the supervision of the family physician. The biggest thrill comes when
you demonstrate the first tub bath. Showing the mother a simple, safe,
and easy method of giving the baby a bath will help her in making the
bath a safe and happy occasion. We try to impress the new mother with
the basic need of all mankind: to be loved; and how this love will aid
her boy in life's development. I would so enjoy taking you to see a
blind couple in my district who have a fine young son. So much of
what we know we learn through seeing, but Mrs. Hampel has to learn
through hearing or feeling. She was blinded in an accident when she
was five. She was a most attentive listener when I gave Harry his first
bath and then she demonstrated his bath to me. I wish you had been
with me! It was a pleasure to see how well she bathed the baby. He is
five months old now and she is feeding him cereal, vegetables, and fruits
and he has already doubled his birth weight. He is just about the finest
specimen of babyhood you can imagine. Even though both mother and
father are blind, they are so self-reliant that the only service I give to
Harry is to cut his fingernails!

Some mornings I begin my day in one of our elementary schools. One
of our important school health services is to work with parents of the
children who need medical care—for instance, the boy who does badly
in school because of poor vision. Other services deal with children with
deafness, cardiac disease, or crippling conditions. Then there are the
epileptic and the spastic children. You might ask, what has the nurse
to do with these children: don't the teachers teach health and notify the
parents when the child is ill? Yes, but the nurse in school aims to see that
the children's physical defects are corrected as far as possible. We interview the parent to secure information about the medical care already
arranged—perhaps the mother is new in the city and does not have a
family doctor, or she may be unable to pay for the needed care because her husband has been on strike, or he may be ill, and the money
saved for a rainy day has been used for food. We have at our disposal
the names of hospitals and clinics where people in unfortunate circumstances may secure medical care, or eye examination and glasses, or
hearing aids at a reduced rate. Some communities, which have through

the years become conscious of health needs, have established schools for crippled children, the hard of hearing, the blind, the epileptic, and the unfortunate child who is mentally defective or a slow learner. We have knowledge of these schools, and when we find a child who has a disability, we explain to the parents the services available so that they in turn may enroll their child in a special school or secure special care for him. We aid the teachers by giving them information about the home situation, which may help them to a better understanding of the child.

For example, Kenneth was a problem to his teacher, as he feigned deafness, and when the audiometer readings were normal, he developed a visual defect. Luckily, he had an understanding mother. She stated that Kenneth's father died when he was four and that he still mourned him although he is now ten years old. His teacher has given him extra responsibilities. The visiting teacher has persuaded him to talk about his father and has advised his mother about her reactions toward him. Kenneth no longer weeps when he talks about his "Dad."

By law, the department of health is responsible for the control of communicable diseases. The nurse in the school has her responsibility as a member of the team in this control program. The teacher has a morning inspection of the children. Those who show symptoms of illness or of suspicious communicable disease are referred to the nurse. We inform the parents of the symptoms and urge medical care. In the more serious communicable diseases, we play a special role. After the diagnosis of disease is secured, we instruct the mother in setting up satisfactory home isolation of her ill child. We try to pattern our isolation at home on that of the hospital, hoping to break the chain of infection from the patient to those about him and to protect him from other illness until he is well.

We share in promoting protective measures against whooping cough, tetanus, smallpox, and diphtheria. We teach that gamma globulin is helpful in making measles less serious in the child already exposed to the disease, and that gonorrheal ophthalmia can be prevented by the administration of silver nitrate drops. We worry when a newborn baby has an infected eye, being suspicious of gonorrheal ophthalmia. Then it is our duty to obtain an eye smear and to see that the baby is under a doctor's care. It does not happen often—perhaps once in a year—but should the baby have gonorrhea, then we must see that the baby is placed immediately under medical care, that the mother and father have a doctor's examination, and that treatment is given if either is infected. Immunization is an important phase of our total health program.

Perhaps you may not have realized that one disease which handicaps many school children is rheumatic fever. We aid the young rheumatic fever patient by helping his mother prepare for home care and by suggesting pastimes for the child who may have to spend long hours in bed at home.

Tuberculosis is one communicable disease which is still a serious problem in many of our families because of its long period of hospitalization and follw-up, but many people recover from the disease if it is discovered early and properly treated. Here is one of my families where there is tuberculosis. Mary Saunders is a very pretty young mother of three children. She has had so many problems to face in the past few years that she had a nervous breakdown, along with tuberculosis. First her husband was called to service when Johnny and Susy were two and four; and then when he returned from overseas, Dennis came; and then Mrs. Saunders became very tired. A chest x-ray showed tuberculosis and she had to face a long hospitalization. In answer to my questions, she recalled that when she was a small girl her grandmother had been very ill, but her illness was never discussed. With her new understanding of tuberculosis, Mrs. Saunders felt that her grandmother had been the one in the family from whom she had received the primary infection. During Mrs. Saunders's hospitalization, the children were placed in boarding homes. Coming home was a bigger problem: she had three children to care for, she had to maintain rest periods for herself, and she had to keep her home. It took about a year before she felt she was well enough to have Dennis with her, as he required more care than the two older children now in school. Mrs. Saunders has been faithful in keeping the children under doctor's care and she has secured her needed rest and goes periodically for her chest x-ray and physical examination. We have felt that through our visits with her she has developed a healthy outlook toward her illness and that she realizes the need for regular rest and a well-balanced diet for herself and her family. We feel that we have helped her to accept the care of Dennis and have aided her in understanding his behavior when he first returned home. She is interested in her children's welfare and realizes the need of caring for herself for their sake. This is one example of the complications in family living which comes with a diagnosis of tuberculosis. We, as public health nurses, know the hospital facilities for the care of tuberculosis, we know the social agencies provided by our government and the people of our city for the care of those less fortunate, who, through no fault of their own, have developed this disease, and we know what measures can be taken to control and prevent it to an even greater extent than at present.

During our follow-up visits to recovered tuberculosis patients, it is sometimes our task to tell the patient that he must return to the hospital because of a series of positive sputum examinations or for a repeated chest x-ray and hospitalization. It is then that your heart aches and you wish harder than ever for better protection against tuberculosis and for a more specific drug than streptomycin.

Should we find a child or an adult with a suspicious-looking throat that might mean diphtheria, it is our responsibility to take a throat swab and send it to our hospital laboratories for culture and examination. In all cases of diagnosed diphtheria, we take throat cultures of all persons who have been in close association with the patient. We are trying to prevent disease and, by taking precautions when a specific communicable disease is known, we are able to prevent others from getting that disease. In our instructions to parents who have children with whooping cough, we teach the care of the children, and we instruct the mother to keep her children at home; not allowing others to come to her home until the children are recovered. When people know the facts about a disease, they respond to our instructions and do their part in the control of disease.

There are many health problems in our daily work that I have not told you about. There is the problem of minor contagion, which includes impetigo, scabies, ringworm, and pediculosis. If we find people who have symptoms of cancer, we urge them to seek immediate medical attention, as we know that early care for cancer means possible cure, and because we know the seriousness of delay, we return to the home to assure ourselves that the family has secured medical care and that the physician did not find the symptoms serious. I am sure you know from your sociology classes all about our aging population. We, in the district, know this group well. We try to give grandfather a little attention, urging him to take life easier. Or we help the older woman with diabetes, teaching her to give herself insulin or helping her to plan her diet. Sometimes we find a grandmother, in a motherless home, who knows all the answers for raising children. Then we try to win her confidence and persuade her to follow the new methods and new ideas of care. Young and old have many superstitions about illness and about themselves— very distorted notions about the normal functions of the human body.

We try to bring the truths that we have learned about disease and its prevention, about the care of the sick and the promotion of health, to the people whom we serve in our districts.

Should you consider making public health nursing your specialty, I am sure you would enjoy it. You would certainly feel a warm thrill of elation when some youngster, whom you have known in school or at home, calls, "Hi, Nurse! Are you going to MY home?"

MRS. MARION E. BECKER, R.N.
Staff Public Health Nurse
Detroit Department of Health
Detroit, Michigan

PERSONAL QUALIFICATIONS

Sound health is an almost indispensable asset in public health nursing. Anything less would be a contradiction in terms and would be a real hindrance to successful health teaching, of which the job so largely consists. Through her appearance, posture, energy, and alertness, the public health nurse should be able to give the impression of having surplus reserves of health. In a sense the nurse in public health is always before the eyes of the public; the impression she makes, especially when she is in uniform, is of importance in selling her service and impressing her lessons in health. One recalls the mother of an undernourished child who looked sternly at a thin and drooping school nurse and asked, "Nurse, do you eat these green vegetables you say I should cook for my Johnnie?"

"Oh, surely. I eat them every day."

The mother shook her head. "Then they would surely make Johnnie worse."

Many nurses find their health improving after a few months in this field. They are in the open air daily, get more exercise than is usual on the wards, have better meals, and are actually practicing what they preach in observing regularity of habits. A constant variety of patients, circumstances, and experiences keeps their interest at high pitch, while the happy spirit of informality among the members of the professional staffs is a pleasant contrast to the necessarily more formal staff relationships in hospital and clinic situations.

A public health nurse writing from Michigan gives a quick glance at the rural situation:

So rural it was, in the Upper Peninsula of Michigan, across the Straits of Mackinac. This part of the country is rich in early American history; the winters are long and the snow is deep. Learning how people lived on the farms, in the villages and in the log cabins of the lumber camp was exciting though rugged. I found that the county public health nurse was an important person in sickness and in health. The county had two doctors, and one 15-bed hospital located above the one village drugstore. A journey of several hundred miles was necessary for patients referred for consultant medical care. The first winter brought a severe scarlet fever outbreak and reaching some of the homes was impossible by car, so that snow shoes and a ski suit were in order. Helping the doctors at deliveries, instructing mothers in infant care, assisting in a new tuberculosis control program and visiting the 19 one-room rural schools were all a part of service to the community.

This and subsequent experience pointed out the uneven distribution and quality of medical, nursing, and hospital services which exist in rural areas, and the need for many more qualified workers.[7]

It is customary to require fairly rigid medical examinations before acceptance in public health positions, and yearly examinations thereafter, including chest x-ray and blood tests. Immunizations are also kept up to date.

The public health nurse must like to teach. If she loves teaching, she will learn how to do so correctly and get results from her pupils—the patients and families with whom she works. If she does not like to show others how to do things, does not like to explain and share her knowledge, then she will be unhappy and indeed out of place in public health nursing. Someone has said, "Public health nurses are always trying to work themselves out of their jobs by teaching people how to keep well." So thoroughly is this desire to make use of every opportunity to teach health inculcated in public health nurses, that one, visiting a hospital ward while temperatures were being taken, exclaimed in surprise, "Haven't you taught the convalescent patients to take their own temperatures? Why not?" This ardor to teach others is evident in the reports of public health nurses in this chapter.

A public health nurse must be adaptable. A contributing quality is that of imagination. How else can she give safe nursing care in a home

[7] *New York State Nurse*, p. 9, April, 1947.

without running water? How else can she make lessons in balanced diet acceptable to a Greek family of six living on $35 a week?

Public health work calls for considerable assumption of individual responsibility. Good though the supervision may be—and it is usually excellent—a supervisor is not with the nurse in every home. Quick decisions must be made, sound judgment evidenced in the advice given to families. A nurse must stand on her own two feet and know why she takes certain action—which may not be on the subject of health at all, but perhaps concerns the rent! Self-reliance and good judgment are important. Maturity of judgment must be attained fairly rapidly for work in this field, and decisions have to be practicable and based on principles of sound psychology.

Another quality desirable in a public health nurse is initiative. Records will show a nurse who has worked for years in a district, with the case load remaining about the same. A new nurse takes over and the case load doubles in 6 months. The second nurse had initiative and *looked* for patients. She was, perhaps, quicker to grasp opportunities.

"I am several kinds of person every day in my county," wrote a county nurse. "With Mrs. Jones I am stern and formal and insistent, for Jerry Wayne I play the role of sympathetic big sister, I joke with old Mr. Woods, and I am an expert consultant in chicken raising when I visit Farmer Hale."

You will need an unquenchable flame of courage—a refusal to be downed by repeated disappointments—if you are to become a public health nurse. People seldom learn new habits in one lesson, and it takes more than one visit to convince a family that a recommended line of action is the one they wish to adopt. The best-laid plans fall apart at the last minute. There are times in public health, as in other fields of nursing, when conditions seen and shared nearly break a nurse's heart. Sentiment, Miss Wald once said to her staff, has its place in public health nursing, but not sentimentality, and sentiment must always be directed toward a practical plan of service and not allowed to become morbid or develop into a passive acceptance of conditions. Herself so sensitive to people's needs, Miss Wald practiced this precept every day of her life. "Let's do something about it!" is the public health nurse's response to those overwhelming situations which spell futility and frustration to others.

The public health nurse meets a very wide variety of people in every walk of life. Families, lonely patients, groups of all ages, doctors, social workers, "lady bountifuls," public officials, teachers, politicians, business-men, lawyers, editors—there is literally no limit to her acquaintances. More than most workers, this nurse must know how to get along with everyone. Tact and friendliness are basic to her success. No one knows this better than the rural nurse.

The rural nurse, Eva Mae Hardin, who wrote the account of rural nursing for the first edition of this book, died the following year. Out of appreciation for her contribution, and because she expresses a desir-able attitude for the nurse who expects to go into public health nursing, a part of Miss Hardin's story is quoted:

Make the most of your student days. Ask yourself why this patient is here. Would not an ounce of prevention earlier have obviated this trip to the hospital and possibly a long-drawn-out stay? Why didn't the patient seek medical advice? What are the home conditions? Why is the mother so anxious to return to her home and children? Could health teaching in the home have helped this patient in some way? In the children's ward, check the case histories and discover, possibly to your amazement, how many of these conditions could have been pre-vented by proper health teaching and early medical care. While work-ing in the out-patient department, consider how many need the care and help that public health nurses can give. Look about you and see what kind of family, home, and community these people come from. Yes, here are the first lessons in training for public health nursing. Develop a sense of obligation to help these people; try to understand their problems, physical, mental, social, and financial. You will not be so quick to judge them, and you will start the foundation of your ap-proach to public health nursing—service to others.

When you graduate, if you have had the affiliation in public health nursing, you will perhaps want to enter the field directly. I am a firm believer in in-service training. I believe that several months of well-supervised in-service training will be of great help to you. Then, by all means, continue your course of study. After a few months of experience in the field, you will have more than a speaking acquaint-ance with public health nursing; you will have a working knowledge. Then enter your course of study with enthusiasm and learn from books.

A report from another Texan nurse working in a county health de-partment carries out the picture.

A County Nurse Speaks from Texas

When I finished my nursing training I went to work for a large hospital as operating-room supervisor. The hours were long and hard and the pay not too good. I soon realized this was not the phase of nursing that I wanted. So I did private duty for a while; this was not what I wanted either. A friend of mine was doing public health nursing. I asked her to let me go with her one day and see what public health nursing was like.[8] I also inquired into the training needed and its cost. I knew that I could not take up any phase of nursing that would involve expense and time without some salary, as I had two children at home to support.

I learned that the public health nurse's hours were such that I would have more time at home with my children; I would be able to be a part of the community in which I lived; I would have time to go to church and do some church work—things I had not been able to do in the other nursing positions. After spending a day in the field with my friend, I *knew* this was the phase of nursing that I was interested in! I immediately wrote the state department of health for an application blank and to ask if I would be accepted for a scholarship for my needed training in public health nursing. I had graduated from a well-recognized school of nursing so I knew I could qualify as far as basic nursing preparation was concerned.

Among the questions asked me when I went for my personal interview was: did I think that I could sit on a box in a little store and sell my work to the rural people in a backwoods part of the state? At the time I thought this just a casual question thrown in to relieve the tension of the interview. But how many times since entering the field of public health I have done this very thing! I have even made home visits with nothing to sit on except an apple box—and this about ready to fall down.

I was accepted and I prepared for my training. I spent a month in a well-organized health unit, visiting with the unit nurses, meeting the doctors, visiting in the schools, and meeting the people of the community. This month of orientation gives a nurse a general idea of all the things she will do as a public health nurse. I then spent three months in an approved school for public health nursing, starting the program of study which would lead to a degree in this field. This period of work represented about a third of my training. (I finished the year's program of study several years later after having worked in the field.)

[8] This is one of the best ways to become acquainted with a new type of work.—Editor

After the 3 months in college, I was assigned to a county unit with two other nurses. The county and city were divided into thirds and each nurse was expected to carry the load in her third of the county. I am senior nurse now in a county health unit with a population of about fifty thousand. There is one large town of about twenty-two thousand people and several small towns in the county. I now cover one-half of the county and one-half of the city. We have only two nurses in the unit—not nearly enough. We are able to do only a small part of what we would like to do.

Here is my day.

I report to the office of the County Health Unit at 8 A.M. and review my records for the families I plan to see today. My first visit is to Mrs. Smith. Mrs. Smith is a very young woman who is pregnant for the first time. She is glad to welcome me into her home because I am a nurse. She knows nothing about the work of the public health nurse or what the health department is for, except that she has heard that it is where people go to get blood tests and be treated for a "bad disease." I try to explain to her a little about what the health department does and especially how the nursing division can be of help to her. I find Mrs. Smith is frightened about her pregnancy, as her own mother died when she was born and her neighbors and friends have been telling her of many sad experiences during delivery. I try to explain to her that pregnancy is a normal condition and with proper care she need have no fear of the outcome. The first thing she must do is decide on her doctor and listen to him and pay no attention to what the neighbors or friends have to say. I explain that she should expect a blood test, urinalysis, blood pressure test, and pelvic measurements when she visits the doctor. If he does not do these things, she should ask to have them done. She should also have a dental check.

I open a record for the family and write down the things we have discussed together. Keeping this record makes the patient feel that what you tell her is of importance and shows that you are interested in her. I tell her when I will be back and suggest that she jot down any questions she may have. These we will discuss on my next visit. Often a young woman will be hesitant in asking her doctor some of the personal questions that bother her.

The amount of teaching done on the first visit to an expectant mother depends on several things, among others the attitude of the family, their intelligence, and whether the patient is under a doctor's care. This first visit in the home is of vital importance because you can either build a good rapport with the family or put them on the defensive so that you will not be very welcome on the next visit.

Next, let's visit Mrs. Jones, a newly delivered mother, and her baby. This family has been seen periodically during most of Mrs. Jones's pregnancy. She was delivered by a midwife. The card from the midwife came to the office just before I left for the day.

Mrs. Jones is expecting me and has many questions that she asks too fast to be answered! She had thought she was all prepared for this new arrival as she had been shown how to bathe the baby and care for his eyes and genitalia, but after the baby's arrival, she found she had to explain to a neighbor how to do things and she "got all mixed up." So once again I bathe the baby showing the neighbor how to care for the eyes, cord, genitalia, etc. I examine Mrs. Jones's breasts, check her blood pressure, take her temperature, and note her flow. She has been told what symptoms to watch for after delivery and has remembered them. The feeding schedule is carefully gone over and the mother's diet discussed. Once again I explain why she should eat a well-balanced diet and drink plenty of milk and other fluids.

This is a very gratifying visit. I feel the nursing is welcomed by the family, they were looking for me and the father was home to see that everything needed was done for his wife and baby. They are a very poor family measured in dollars and cents but a very rich one in many other ways. They did not have the money to pay for the medical care that is most desirable at this time, but they had the wisdom to take advantage of the services available from the health department and to try to follow our instructions.

The midwife who delivered Mrs. Jones's baby is under the supervision of the health department. She is visited regularly by us and is furnished silver nitrate to instill in the babies' eyes, given sterile cord dressings, and taught to recognize danger signals and to get a doctor immediately. She is also taught how to fill out the birth certificates. She is required to have a physical examination each year. She refers all prenatals to the health department as soon as she knows about them. She encourages her patients to get a blood test.

It is time now for lunch. I eat it leisurely, sitting at the side of the road under a shade tree. I review the two visits, making plans for my return and checking to see if anything was omitted that should have been explained.

You might suppose, at this point, that all public health work is as pleasant and satisfying as these two visits. That there are many discouraging experiences, will be evident during my afternoon rounds.

After lunch, I stop to see Mrs. Davis, mother of Don, who had infantile paralysis when he was three years of age. Don is now nine years old. He is developing a scoliosis of the spine, weakness of the right ankle, and shortening of the left leg. His mother is not willing to have the child see an orthopedist as she is afraid he will want to operate and she has had an unpleasant experience in the hospital and does not want her boy to go to a hospital. I try to show her how his condition will gradually become worse and that she will be to blame for this crippling condition if she continues to keep the boy from proper care. I have already made several visits in this home. The family has been referred to the school for exceptional children and the fieldman from the school has visited in the home trying to interest the parents in letting the boy have a corrective operation—so far to no avail. Such visits are very discouraging. You feel you are not doing all you should. But I'll keep right on visiting, each time hopeful.

I next stop at the little country store for a cold drink and to have a brief chat with the owner. The public health nurse should be known by the storekeepers and by all the key people in her community, so they can refer families to her when they are in need of her help. Today Mr. Goodwin tells me about a new family which has recently moved into the community; the father is ill and rumor has it that he has tuberculosis. Mr. Goodwin feels that I will be welcome in the home and he will appreciate it if I can go over this afternoon. So I change my schedule and go at once to see the new family.

Mr. Jordan is in bed with his clothes on and his wife is nursing the baby when I arrive. The house is clean and the children are clean. You can tell the family is trying to do the best they can under the conditions. I introduce myself and my organization and I am welcomed gladly.

Mr. Jordan went to see his doctor a few days ago and was told that he has tuberculosis. He must stop work for at least a year and go to the sanatorium for treatment. Naturally, he does not see how he can stop work and leave his family with no income at all. Mrs. Jordan is not too willing to accept the doctor's diagnosis, as her husband has not lost any weight and he still has a fair appetite. He is tired all the time and is having night sweats, however. I explain all I can about the disease. I select some leaflets for her to read so she can know more about it and be more sympathetic with her husband's plight. The application has already been filled

out for the hospital. The doctor has urged that the family be tuberculin-
tested and x-rayed if positive. But they do not know how they can afford
these services and have been too proud to ask for help. I explain about the
work of the Active Tuberculosis Association in the county and that they
can get the tuberculin tests at the health department without charge upon
referral from their doctor. This explanation helps the tense situation
considerably.

Next I begin to plan with the mother how she can best care for her
husband with the least exposure to herself and the children. We select a
nice sunny room for Mr. Jordan's bedroom. It is convenient for him and
not too inconvenient for the rest of the family, with relation to the
kitchen and the other bedrooms. Then I show her about boiling her
husband's dishes, burning any waste food on his tray, the care of nose
and throat discharges, and the care of his linens. I explain why dry
sweeping should not be done and show Mrs. Jordan about wet-mopping
and dusting. I know from observation and listening to the Jordans talk
that they will be in need of financial help while he is in the hospital. I
explain to Mrs. Jordan about the State Department of Public Welfare
and give her a referral note to the case worker in this district.

When I leave, Mrs. Jordan's attitude is much better. She wants to
know when I will be back to see if she is doing all the things I have suggested. I promise to be back in a week and give her further help, and
answer any questions.

Perhaps some of you are asking: Why are you so concerned with the
entire family?—nurses are trained to care for the sick. That is one of the
biggest joys and satisfactions experienced in public health nursing. You
do not see just the sick member of the family—Don, the crippled child,
or Mr. Jordan—you see the entire family as a family unit and you become interested in each member of the family and try to help work out
their problems together.

It is growing late—time to turn the car toward home. This unexpected
visit has taken more time than I had planned. The sun is already setting,
but perhaps it was my most important visit of the day!

These are but a very few of the many conditions a public health nurse
meets in her line of duty. She helps at well-child conferences, maternity
clinics, immunization clinics, venereal disease clinics; and is ready to talk
to any civic group that calls on her to tell of her work or some special
phase of her work.

To young graduates planning to take up public health nursing I would
like to say: Do not consider going into public health work unless you

have the ability and desire to meet people on any level of life, like to teach, have skill in teaching, and are able to improvise material and to think out ways of getting things done by other methods than just the everyday obvious one. The hours and salary are good, and you are more or less on your own, but the greatest satisfaction, believe me, comes from helping families adjust to their lot—or improve their lot by better planning and managing.

MARY L. PROCK, R.N.
Senior Public Health Nurse
Paris-Lamar County Health Unit
Paris, Texas

PREPARATION FOR PUBLIC HEALTH NURSING

Preparation for this field consists of 1 year of study and practice in public health nursing at a college or university approved by the National Organization for Public Health Nursing.[9] The advanced positions call for additional postgraduate study and experience. The supervisor of staff nurses, for example, should have a baccalaureate degree, a course in principles of supervision, and at least 2 years of experience under direct supervision. [10] A master's degree is desirable for the higher level positions.

Nurses who are planning to accept public health nursing positions where there is no continuous supervision, as in rural areas, should have at least 1 year of experience, preferably 2, on a staff that provides qualified supervisors and offers a generalized[11] family service.

PERSONNEL POLICIES

In public health nursing agencies, 3 to 4 weeks' vacation on pay, 2 weeks' sick leave, and the usual legal holidays are allowed a regular member of the staff. The working week is usually 40 hours, and only emer-

[9] There are an increasing number of collegiate schools of nursing where approved preparation for staff positions in public health nursing is combined with the basic nursing curriculum—approved by the National Nursing Accrediting Service.

[10] For a list of approved programs of study, loans, or scholarships to assist in preparing for this field, write for information to the National Organization for Public Health Nursing (see Appendix A). See also special training courses, such as are offered by the New York State Department of Health, Albany, N.Y.

[11] By "generalized" is meant a program of nursing and health supervision in homes, and clinics or conferences in which all types of service are offered by the staff nurse —not just a specialty, as in tuberculosis care or child welfare.

gency work is carried on Saturday afternoons and Sundays. Staff nurses usually take turns, or are on call, for holiday and week-end work; compensating time off duty is given on some other day.[12]

In public health service, not all nurses are required to wear a uniform. An effort is made to suit the clothing to the demands of the job. For example, nearly all public health nurses giving bedside nursing care routinely in homes wear a washable uniform, usually blue. Those nursing only occasionally may carry an allover apron or smock; in clinics, a washable smock, hoover apron, or slip-on gown may be worn. Public health nurses who travel a great deal or who have less direct contact with patients wear tailored suits, often with identifying insignia. The cost of cleaning or laundering uniforms is usually borne by the nurse, except in clinics. Aprons for wear over uniforms are supplied and laundered by the employer. Exclusive of wartime requirements, the most *uniform* uniforms, including outdoor garments, are worn by nurses on the staffs of visiting nurse associations and the Red Cross.

The following account tells of the typical program of that oldest phase of public health nursing—visiting nursing—this time in San Francisco.

Nurse, the Door Is Open

Pinned to the outside of a curtain in a kitchen window in San Francisco is a piece of paper. On that piece of paper these words are written: "Nurse, the door is open!"

It is early morning. Cars move toward the Bay Bridge, which spans the harbor like a giant fork. These cars are moving toward the city of San Francisco. In one of the cars driving toward the city are two women. Both are visiting nurses. This morning one of these women will pass the kitchen window where the penciled note is pinned . . . she will read the words . . . she will open that door and enter. . . .

At approximately the same time there will be 30 other visiting nurses opening and entering 30 other doors throughout the city. They will close these doors when their work is finished and go on to enter 30 other doors. At the end of the day each individual nurse will have passed through the doors of six to eight homes in the city of San Francisco.

Working with the regular staff nurses in the field are eight to ten student nurses. These student nurses come from Stanford University and

[12] See also the personnel policies recommended by the National Organization for Public Health Nursing. (Revised, 1950.)

the University of California Nursing Schools. Both institutions are located in San Francisco. These schools rotate their students through the Visiting Nurse Association of San Francisco at 2-month intervals for their affiliation with a public health nursing agency. After being coached and briefed by the Association in the technicalities and philosophy characteristic of public health nursing in this area, they too will simultaneously be opening and entering the doors of additional homes.

A rough estimate of the number of home visits made by this combined graduate and student field staff falls somewhere between 240 and 320 visits per day. It is a big job in a big city. This tempo is maintained 5 days a week, with a slight slowing down over the week ends, as about one-fourth of the graduate and student field staff carry the week-end work. This skeleton staff stands by for all essential and emergency home calls—giving a sort of blanket protection throughout the city. Holidays fall under these week-end regulations.

Circulating out of the office into the field with this combined nursing staff are two occupational therapists. They are on call in all districts in the city. They carry a heavy load of patients referred to them by the whole nursing staff.

The two nurses in the car moving with the traffic across the Bay Bridge toward San Francisco this morning are members of the graduate field staff of the Visiting Nurse Association. Both women happen to be new to San Francisco—new, in fact, to California. But the idea of becoming visiting nurses is not new to them. Their student exposure to this phase of public health, in faraway Connecticut, set their course of action. Two decisive events occurred for them in the summer of 1950: graduation and employment—their careers as graduate visiting nurses began here 3 months ago. Each morning they cross the Bay Bridge on their way to the office in San Francisco. The fog that sometimes clings to San Francisco and the East Bay area has burned off early today. M.A. speaks:

M.A. Look, the formation of the ships in the harbor has changed. They have weighed anchor. They're moving.

J.V. There's one under the Golden Gate now, going out to sea. I wonder where she's going?

M.A. The Embarcadero—the street that snakes the waterfront— is rightly named. It starts at Fisherman's Wharf and winds around to the China Basin. It's the eastern border of my district.

J.V. What about Russian Hill, is that part of North Beach district too?

M.A.   Yes. I had quite a time when I was first assigned to North Beach. I kept running into Telegraph and Russian Hills. I'd be driving along a street and suddenly it would dissolve in front of me with nothing but atmosphere beyond. Climbing out of my car, I could spot my street, at what seemed a thousand feet below me. Actually, the elevation is not over 302 feet at any point.

J.V.   San Francisco is a cosmopolitan city, but there seem to be areas of racial concentration. Who lives in North Beach?

M.A.   It is cosmopolitan indeed! All types of people at all economic levels live and work in this section. It's known as the Latin Quarter, because of the high concentration of Italians and Spanish. But there are Irish, Germans, and people of many other origins. The Chinese are now crowding the edges and are spilling over into North Beach.

J.V.   There is an International Settlement down there, isn't there?

M.A.   Yes, at the foot of Pacific Avenue. But, I think it's more international along Broadway, where there are blocks of foreign restaurants, night clubs, and family hotels. We often get calls to these family hotels. The Italians seem to enjoy this type of group living. What are those hills in the far west?

J.V.   Those two hills are called Twin Peaks, the highest elevation of the city. They are also in my district. One of the buildings you see is part of the University of California Medical Center. The famous Langley-Porter Clinic, where some of our patients go for psychiatric treatment, is right there.

M.A.   Do you climb any of those hills?

J.V.   I'll say I do! I climb up and down them every day. You can't escape the hills in San Francisco. But where there's a hill, there's a view. I learned early to ride the buses or streetcars to the top of the hills and walk down as I cover my district.

M.A.   Some of the nurses who have walking districts use the cable cars.

J.V.   Here's Grant Avenue.

M.A.   The beginning of Chinatown.

J.V.   It's unbelievable that approximately twenty thousand people are living in 12 blocks. Isn't that what one of the supervisors told us?

M.A.   Yes, they're really packed in. I think the nurse who has Chinatown has a choice district. Have you taken a call down there yet?

J.V.   No, have you?

M.A.   Yes, the north part of Chinatown skirts my district. I was sent in to give nursing care to a patient who had had recent surgery. She was still in traction but was able to be sent home from the hospital to complete her recovery. As I approached the assigned address I noticed it was a jewelry store. I double-checked the address before entering; then I stepped into the store. A Chinese woman behind the counter looked up and announced in a loud voice, "Nursie!" A man arose from a table in the back of the store and came forward holding some keys in his hand. He nodded to me and motioned for me to follow. We walked out of the store and down the busy narrow street. He suddenly turned into a doorway, and opened the door with the key. We climbed some stairs leading up to the third floor of the building, which was cold and dimly lit. I followed him into one of the rooms off the hallway. There was my patient in bed.

"Hello," she said. I would have guessed her age to be twenty-four, but discovered that she was actually forty-three. She had been home from the hospital for several days. Being in traction, her activities were restricted. She needed full general care. A friend had told her about the visiting nurses, and she had contacted her doctor and requested that he call us. She spoke enough English for us to understand one another. When words failed, we got along with gestures. She was admitted as an acute case.

I went to give her care three times a week for several weeks. She's well now. The man I followed the first day is her uncle. The place where the patient is living is a community rooming house. In making return visits, I noticed that whole families lived in one room. There were common bath and kitchen facilities at the end of each hallway on each floor.

That's the explanation as to how 20,000 people can be packed into 12 city blocks. We get many calls throughout Chinatown. The reason is obvious.

J.V.   Are they friendly in Chinatown?

M.A.   They are shy, but their friendliness is unmistakable. If you wear a blue topcoat and carry a black bag, you are "Number One Nurse" in Chinatown.

J.V.   This is Gough Street. We turn here.

M.A.   So we do.

The two nurses park the car on Gough Street and walk around the corner to the office at 1636 Bush Street. It's almost 8 A.M. and some of the nurses who live in the city have already arrived at the office. When you work as a visiting nurse you hold a combination office and field position. In the office the staff nurses plan their day's itinerary and chart yesterday's visits. New calls coming into the office are screened and distributed by the divisional supervisors. All calls are checked for doctors' orders before being assigned to staff nurses, but it's up to the individual staff nurse to keep these doctors' orders current. This is an absolute *must* as The Visiting Nurse Association does not give nursing care without orders from a physician. The divisional supervisors aid the staff nurses in planning the day's work. They are more or less referees in equalizing the work throughout the city—guarding against the overloading of any one nurse. They are experienced nurses and are always ready to answer questions pertaining to the nursing care of any patient in their district. They are stationed at the office throughout the day and are only a telephone call away from any of their nurses who want on-the-spot advice. The educational director at the office is also available to give information at any time. Up-to-date reading material is supplied for the staff at the office.

It takes about an hour for the charting of yesterday's visits and the organization of the current day's work. Reequipped with supplies, the staff nurses take off for the field. This mobile nursing unit fans out from the office and moves like a large infiltrating force throughout the city. The field nurses report back to the office via the telephone twice during the day. In this way, the supervisors have contact with their nursing force at all times.

There is a time of day when the visiting nurse closes her last door. Officially, the day ends at 4:30 P.M. Unless it is a Friday, when the staff must return to the office to turn in their week-end calls, the nurses leave from their districts and go home.

Again, the two new nurses are crossing the Bay Bridge, this time headed east for home.

M.A. Busy day?

J.V. Quite. Diversified too. I went from a tub bath demonstration on a new baby to a tub bath on a ninety-five-year-old grandpa.

M.A. For the visiting nurse patients are neither too young nor too old!

J.V. Right you are. Our work may swing from pediatrics to geriatrics with a mere turn of the record card!

M.A. Or fall into any age group between these extremes.

J.V. When you get right down to it, figuratively speaking, the visiting nurse is actually the general practitioner in nursing.

M.A. Did you get into any health supervisions?

J.V. Yes, I went in to see an antepartum case referred to us by the John

Hancock Mutual Life Insurance agent. I also saw a cardiac patient, a diabetic woman, and a baby eleven months old.

M.A. How about the twelve-year-old boy who has tuberculosis of the spine? Gerald?

J.V. Oh, yes, I give him 2 cc. of streptomycin every day.

M.A. How is his mother taking the confirmed diagnosis?

J.V. She is still not accepting it. She won't admit that Gerald has tuberculosis.

M.A. Is she following the doctor's orders? Does she accept your teaching concerning the boy's care at home?

J.V. Very well. She gives excellent physical care. She is not mentally morose. She simply refuses to believe her boy has tuberculosis of the spine. I have trained her to the point where she is giving full general care every day. This is really a big job, as he has been in a bivalved body cast after his bone-graft operation on the spine. I have not approached her yet with the idea of learning how to give him the streptomycin injection. She still has a high degree of nervousness and apprehension.

M.A. It will probably take time. The nervousness and apprehension are most likely due to her unwillingness to accept the diagnosis. How long will Gerald be in bed?

J.V. The doctor thinks for 9 months at least.

M.A. That's a long time—especially, if you are twelve years old!

J.V. Yes, it is. I have called the Board of Education and a homebound teacher goes in for an hour three times a week. So he will not fall behind in his education.

M.A. What about our occupational therapists? Have you referred Gerald to them?

J.V. Yes, indeed, he is on their waiting list. When I went in to talk to one of the occupational therapists about Gerald, I asked her about some other patients. She told me about her youngest patient—an eighteen-month-old child with Erb's palsy. One of our nurses referred the patient. The mother was allowing the child to shelter the arm instead of encouraging its full limited use. The occupational therapist suggested some toys for the child which would bring the affected arm into play unconsciously.

M.A. What sort of toys, for example?

J.V. Well, for instance, a set of boxes which fit inside of one another, As the child lifts these successive boxes out, he uses an upward motion of his arms. The boxes are cut to definite size necessitating the definite upward swing of his arms. He gets so engrossed in successively pulling the boxes apart that he unconsciously uses the affected arm.

These toys are used at definite times during the day so that his arm is exercised in a routine and scheduled fashion. The mother had to be instructed and encouraged to play certain types of games with the child which will bring the affected arm into action. The occupational therapist goes in and has a "play period" with the child several times a week.

M.A.   Have you ever watched one of the occupational therapists at work?

J. V.   No, I haven't, have you?

M.A.   I was in a home the other day caring for a patient when one of the occupational therapists arrived.

J.V.   What's the patient's diagnosis?

M.A.   A chronic condition—she had a cerebral accident several months ago and her right arm was paralyzed. "It's lazy now," she said; and did nothing about it except to spend most of her time brooding over her misfortune. Consequently, her arm hung limply at her side, and her hand was closing into a fixed fist. One of the nurses sent the occupational therapist in to work with the patient.

J.V.   What are her hopes for this patient?

M.A.   Well, I asked her that question after we left the house. She said that a large part of their time is spent with cerebral-accident patients, and that their hopes are twofold—first, ultimately to help the patients to see that they can be useful individuals in spite of their handicaps; and second, to prevent grotesque deformities incurred from disuse of the parts.

J.V.   They don't hope to restore full physical normalcy to an affected part?

M.A.   That's right. Their eyes are focused on the whole and not on any one part. It is the physical therapist who has hope of bringing about a degree of normalcy.

J.V.   The occupational therapist hopes to weave the affected part into a generally useful pattern of living?

M.A.   Yes. They establish new attitudes by giving the patient something to do. They deal with what is left and are not concerned with what has been knocked out. They hope to change the attitude of, "Well, what can I do?" of so many of our patients to, "Look, I'm doing something!"

J.V.   The occupational therapist carries these same hopes to cardiac or arthritic cases, amputees, or any other patient we refer?

M.A.   Yes.

J.V.   I think it is our work with the chronic patients that makes it so very clear to us, as nurses, that we cannot meet all of the patient's needs alone. There must be a sharing of responsibility.

M.A. But isn't it up to us to recognize our patients' needs and to be informed concerning other resources in the community that are available for effective dispersing of the total responsibility.

J.V. Sometimes the needed resource is available in the community and sometimes not. I went into a home today and found that it was housekeeping service that was chiefly needed and not nursing care. The family finances cannot possibly stand this extra drain for any prolonged period of time.

M.A. Whom are you planning to contact to inquire if a housekeeping service is available in the community?

J.V. I shall call the Social Service Exchange tomorrow to see if there are any registrations on the family. There may be or may have been a social agency assisting the family. If not, I shall discuss with my supervisor the possibility of referring the family to one of the social agencies which may be able to meet this family's need.

M.A. It certainly is becoming more and more apparent, with the increasing number of chronic patients, that a housekeeping service in a community will have to be a necessity and not a possibility.

J.V. Yes.

M.A. Look, it's dusk already—better turn on the lights.

J.V. Have you noticed how suddenly darkness falls? There's no ifs or ands about it out here at this time of year. It's either night or day. There are no twilight periods.

M.A. I was talking to a doctor today. He asked me if I liked what I was doing.

J.V. What did you say to that?

M.A. I said I loved what I was doing! What about you? If you were a student nurse again facing graduation and subsequent employment, would you still choose to be a visiting nurse?

J.V. *Absolutely*. To me it is the ground floor in public health nursing—a firm foundation.

M.A. And an open door to many other doors! Well, here we are—and am I hungry!

JANICE VORDALE, R.N.
MARY ALTER, R.N.
Staff Nurses, The Visiting
Nurse Association of
San Francisco, California

Administrative Positions in Public Health Nursing

In large public health nursing agencies the administrative positions are

Director and assistant director
Consultants (representing specialized fields)
Educational director
Supervisor and assistant supervisor

Occasionally senior staff nurses will have some administrative responsibilities, as, for instance, when in charge of a small office or desk space in an outlying urban area, or when relieving in any one of the positions listed above.

In rural agencies or very small suburban offices where there is just a one-nurse staff, the public health nurse combines administrative, executive, and field-service duties.

In medium-sized agencies (10 to 50 nurses) the responsibilities of supervisors, consultants,[13] and educational directors may be distributed among only two or three assistants to the director, or one assistant may combine several duties, those of a consultant and educational director being frequently found together.

The positions in supervision require both theoretical and practical preparation. Every nurse considering the field of public health nursing should look ahead to the time when, after her basic year's training and a few years of experience, she will want to develop special skills. Besides the approved program of study, supervisors will need 2 years of experience in generalized service under qualified supervision. A few months serving as assistant supervisor are helpful. They should have completed courses in the principles of supervision, educational psychology, and guidance.

Consultants and educational directors are increasingly expected to have completed advanced study in their specialty and to hold a master's degree. At least 2 years—and preferably 5—of supervised general field experience are necessary to provide sufficient knowledge of staff and community problems to enable these nurses to fill their positions successfully. Courses that will assist in making studies, surveys, and evaluating the work of staff nurses and students are of special importance to these employees.

[13] For interest, see STOKES, JOHN H.: What Is a Consultant? *Public Health Nursing,* p. 239, May, 1947.

Examples of the currently classified consultant positions in state health departments include public health nursing consultants in orthopedic nursing and physical therapy, cancer, tuberculosis, venereal disease, communicable diseases, maternity and child health, mental health, education, nurse midwifery, home safety, industrial hygiene, and rheumatic fever.

Besides basic preparation as public health nurses, most of the consultant positions call for a year of experience at least and an advanced course of study in the specialty. Consultants must offer at least 6 years' experience in nursing, two of which should have been in supervisory, teaching, or administrative positions—this is based on or follows the usual year of basic theory in public health nursing. Some states offer "equivalents."[14]

Administrators—directors of public health nurses—should hold an advanced college degree, and offer at least 3 years—preferably 5—of experience in more than one type of agency, including experience in supervision. In the large organizations, administrators are expected both to be very well qualified educationally and to have had wide experience in supervising and directing smaller staffs of various types. Courses in public administration, statistics, personnel management, and business will be found helpful, although not specifically required at the present time. (For positions in national and Federal agencies see Chaps. XV and XVII.)

As the qualifications for public health nurses are growing more clearly defined and are constantly under revision, it would be wise to write to the National Organization for Public Health Nursing for the latest recommended requirements for this field.

SALARIES[15]

Salaries range (1950) from $1,800 to $2,800 in staff positions for qualified public health nurses; $2,200 to $3,800 for supervisors; $3,800 to $5,500 for consultants, educational directors and assistant directors; and $3,500 to $8,500 for directors. The lower salaries for directors are in small agencies; the top salaries are paid in positions carrying very heavy administrative responsibilities and calling for 8 years' experience or more. Salaries in public health nursing vary greatly with the area and the country. The New England and Southern states pay less than the rest of the country.

[14] It is always possible to secure the requirements for state Civil Service positions from the state Civil Service Commission or merit system agency at the state capital.

[15] See also salaries recommended by the National Organization for Public Health Nursing, *Public Health Nursing*, p. 203, April, 1949.

SOURCES OF EMPLOYMENT

1. Professional placement bureaus
2. For Civil Service appointments on a Federal level (U.S. Public Health Service, Children's Bureau, Bureau of Indian Affairs, District of Columbia Health Department, Panama Canal Zone, and others, see Chap. XVI), U.S. Civil Service Commission. For positions on a state or local level, the Civil Service (or merit system) Commission at the state capitol or listed in your local telephone directory under county and city departments.
3. State, county, and local health departments—direct application
4. Visiting nurse associations (see local telephone directory—may be under District or Public Health)
5. New York State Employment Service, New York, N.Y.
6. American Red Cross, Washington, D.C.
7. Out-patient departments of hospitals, clinics, dispensaries, and local agencies engaged in public health projects, such as care of crippled children
8. Schools of nursing (collegiate)
9. A few industries with home visiting services employ public health nurses (see Chap. XIII).
10. National Organization for Public Health Nursing
11. American Public Health Association
12. Advertising sections of nursing journals
13. Professional nurses', hospital, and commercial registries. These are less likely sources of employment information for public health nurses.

See also Sources of Employment, Chaps. XII, XIII, and XVII.

For national voluntary agencies employing public health nurses, see Chap. XVII; for Federal opportunities, see Chap. XVI.

BIBLIOGRAPHY

1. BOGGS, LYDIA B.: Going My Way? *Public Health Nursing*, p. 606, December, 1947.
2. BRAINARD, ANNIE M.: "Evolution of Public Health Nursing," pp. 200, 297, W. B. Saunders Company, Philadelphia, 1922.
3. COLCORD, JOANNA C.: "Your Community," 2d ed., Russell Sage Foundation, New York, 1941.

4. DEMING, DOROTHY: "Penny Marsh Finds Adventure in Rural Nursing," Dodd, Mead & Company, Inc., New York, 1940.

5. DEMING, DOROTHY: "Penny Marsh, Public Health Nurse," Dodd, Mead & Company, Inc., New York, 1938.

6. DEMING, DOROTHY: "Penny Marsh, Supervisor of Public Health Nurses," Dodd, Mead & Company, Inc., New York, 1939.

7. DUFFUS, R. L.: "Lillian Wald, Neighbor and Crusader," The Macmillan Company, New York, 1938.

8. EMERSON, HAVEN, and MARTHA LUGINBUHL: Local Health Units, *American Journal of Public Health,* pp. 898–904, September, 1945.

9. FREEMAN, RUTH B.: Red Cross Nurses Serve the Community, *American Journal of Nursing,* p. 144, March, 1950.

10. FREEMAN, RUTH B.: "Supervision in Public Health Nursing," W. B. Saunders Company, Philadelphia, 1949. Also "Public Health Nursing Practice," 1950.

11. FROST, HARRIET: "Nursing in Sickness and in Health," The Macmillan Company, New York, 1939.

12. GARDNER, MARY S.: "Public Health Nursing," The Macmillan Company, New York, 1936.

13. GARDNER, MARY S.: "So Build We," The Macmillan Company, New York, 1942. Also "Katharine Kent," The Macmillan Company, New York, 1946.

14. HAMM, ELSIE MAXWELL: Boom-Town Nursing, *Public Health Nursing,* p. 521, October, 1945.

15. HEISLER, ANN: 1950 Census of Nurses in Public Health Work, *Public Health Nursing,* p. 558, October, 1950.

16. HUBBARD, RUTH W.: Public Health Nursing, 1900–1950, *American Journal of Nursing,* p. 608, October, 1950.

17. KANEKO, MITSU: Public Health Nursing in Japan, *Public Health Nursing,* p. 97, January, 1950.

18. KIDDER, CAROLINE E.: Way Down East in North Carolina, *Public Health Nursing,* p. 93, February, 1945.

19. KNIGHT, CORNELIA: I'm Glad I Affiliated in Public Health Nursing, *American Journal of Nursing,* p. 286, May, 1949.

20. MILLER, MRS. D. G.: What Does the Rural Area Offer the Public Health Nurse? *Public Health Nursing,* p. 350, July, 1947. See also The Rural Nurse, p. 331.

21. O'HARA, HAZEL: Public Health Nursing in Latin America, *Public Health Nursing,* p. 73, February, 1950.

22. "Personnel Policies in Public Health Nursing Agencies," National Organization for Public Health Nursing, 1949.

23. Plan for Observation in Public Health Nursing, *American Journal of Nursing,* p. 117, February, 1951.

24. "Public Health Nursing," p. 376, and "School Health Services," p. 438, in the Social Work Year Book, American Association of Social Workers, New York, 1951.

25. "Qualifications of Public Health Nurses," National Organization for Public Health Nursing, New York.

26. Retirement Plans in Public Health Nursing Agencies, *Public Health Nursing*, p. 158, March, 1947.

27. SMULLING, CATHERINE: *M. S. Hygiene*, Alaska's Floating Health Unit, *Public Health Nursing*, p. 258, May, 1947.

28. WALD, LILLIAN D.: "The House on Henry Street," Henry Holt and Company, Inc., New York, 1915.

29. WALD, LILLIAN D.: "Windows on Henry Street," Little, Brown & Company, Boston, 1934.

30. WALES, MARGUERITE A.: "The Public Health Nurse in Action," The Macmillan Company, New York, 1941.

31. WATT, Dame KATHERINE: The Public Health Nursing Services in England, *Public Health Nursing*, p. 433, September, 1947.

32. WILCOX, BARBARA: Where Will You Work—City or Country? *Public Health Nursing*, p. 409, August, 1948.

Public Health Nursing, a monthly magazine published by the National Organization for Public Health Nursing, contains job descriptions of public health nursing from time to time, as well as salary studies.

CHAPTER XII

School and Camp Nursing

SCHOOL NURSING

School nursing as we know it in the United States was begun in New York City in 1902–1903 at the instigation of Lillian D. Wald. After visiting the schools in England in 1902, Miss Wald returned to offer the services of one of the nurses (Lina Rogers Struthers) from the Henry Street Settlement to the New York City schools. A demonstration of school health service carried out in four schools was so successful that the health department took over the service, which was gradually copied by other cities.[1] Today there are approximately 5,852 school nurses employed full time by boards of education and many public health nurses giving part time to schools as an activity in their generalized community services. They are scattered all over the United States and its possessions. In addition to work in the public schools, which may cover all ages from nursery school to college, many nurses serve in parochial and private schools, day nurseries, boarding schools, schools for the handicapped, teachers' colleges, colleges, and universities.

As you read Mrs. White's enthusiastic account of "Jane Wilson's" day with the student nurse who is observing school nursing, one fact is evident: You have to like to be with children to be a successful school nurse. You already know whether you like *sick* children—but do you like noisy, restless, giggling, excitable, and ever-curious boys and girls around you—not in twos and threes, but by the dozens? If you do—most nurses do!—here is your chance to grow close to them, to win their priceless confidence, and to influence their lives at, as Mrs. White says, the "hub": their health in schools and homes. The child who is not

[1] Annual Count, U.S. Public Health Service, 1950.

full of boundless energy, good spirits, and lively interest in what goes on around him is usually not a well child. Perhaps he is just overtired, he may be hungry, or something far more serious may be the cause of his behavior. The teacher, with the help of the school nurse, the school physician, the family doctor, and the parents, learns to know her pupils, to be sensitive to their physical and mental condition, and to understand when to call for expert health advice. Teachers rely greatly on the school nurse. A breadth of sound knowledge in health education, unfailing tact, and understanding of people are needed by the school nurse if she is to respond to all the demands made upon her. From the variety of duties carried by "Miss Wilson," one can see that she must be ready to answer the simple questions of the children, the searching questions of the teachers, and the worried queries from troubled parents —all more or less unpredictable in their nature.

"Nurse, if I use Gardine drops in my eyes, will they be large and sparkling like this bottle says?" asks the fourteen-year-old girl. "Miss Wilson, what does penicillin come from?" the music teacher asks at lunch. "What can I do to stop my husband's hiccups?" Helen's mother wants to know. Then, of course, there is always that staggering request from a prominent ·citizen to "speak to my group" on any subject from compulsory health insurance to sex education! For the school nurse is a respected member of the community and her opinion carries weight.

In addition to teaching, counseling, and guiding, there are the occasional real emergencies for the school nurse to handle: the accident on the playground, the fire in the chemistry lab, the teacher with a fainting spell. An outbreak of sore throats may mean almost anything, from too many parties over the holidays to scarlet fever. A school nurse needs a thorough knowledge of first aid, close acquaintance with the early symptoms of communicable disease, and calm judgment in emergencies.

As Mrs. White's description so plainly reveals, the school nurse is a member of a team. The principal, the teachers—especially the director of physical education and the home-economics instructor—the school physicians, and the parents are members of this team, all directly concerned with the health and welfare of the children and the safety of their environment. The school nurse is as much an interpreter and coordinator as she is a nurse; indeed, she does very little actual nursing. Through teamwork the school nurse meets the health needs of the children and school personnel and, indirectly, thus contributes to community health. In all she does, she is trying to lay a firm foundation of good health habits which will last the individual a lifetime. More and more emphasis is being placed on the home visit and the contact with parents.

The school job is particularly desirable for nurses who prefer "living health" in the school atmosphere to bedside nursing in a hospital, who love children, who enjoy contact with adults of widely varying interests, and who want the long holidays of the school year for additional preparation and self-development. In rural areas and in many small cities, it will be necessary for the nurse to drive a car. It perhaps goes without saying that a school nurse should be herself an example of good health, good posture, and good grooming. Teachers, parents, and children are quick to notice if their nurse fails to practice what she preaches to them so earnestly!

QUALIFICATIONS

Qualifications for school nurses vary, but in the elementary and secondary schools, nurses are, like Mrs. White, well-qualified public health nurses with special preparation in the health problems of the school-age child. Mrs. White has a B.S. degree as well as her formal preparation in public health nursing. In high schools and colleges nurses may serve in the capacity of teachers, in which case they must hold a teacher's certificate. If they are employed by large private boarding schools and colleges, they are more likely to serve in the "infirmaries" or hospitals as general duty and supervising nurses or as clinic nurses. In the latter positions, a knowledge of public health and teaching methods is an advantage but not a prerequisite. Positions for public health nurses with school experience and academic degrees who can meet the qualifications of college faculties and serve as health educators, consultants, and instructors in colleges have been slow in developing, but are among the many interesting jobs of the future. Qualifications for the position of health educator are even higher and call for additional special preparation.[2]

There are a few supervisory positions in school nursing, chiefly in large city school systems, and a few positions with administrative and consultant responsibilities on the state level. Qualifications for these are the same as for supervisors and directors in public health nursing (see Chap. XI). Usually, the incumbents of these advanced positions have

[2] For qualifications and information, write to the American Public Health Association. Addresses of organizations mentioned in this chapter are given in Appendix A.

had education beyond the bachelor's degree and hold teacher's certificates.

Forward-looking school nurses try to secure the same preparation as for public health nursing: study in public health nursing, including supervised field practice with emphasis on the health of the school-age child.

There are no men nurses in this field. It would seem that there might be positions for men nurses in men's colleges and vocational schools.

SALARIES

Salaries for full-time qualified school nurses range from $2,000 to $3,000 a year, with $3,000 to $6,000 paid in the administrative and executive positions. Supervisors' salaries fall between these two levels— approximately $2,500 to $4,000, depending on the amount of responsibility, size of staff, and area of the country. These are cash salaries, subject to certain deductions depending on state and Federal tax rates, pension benefits, and insurance plans.[3] Salaries may be paid on a 10 months' basis, or for the year with a month's paid vacation.

The school nurse (unless a resident in a teachers college, private school, or college) lives in her own home, receives an allowance for or the use of a car, and is in all respects treated as one of the school faculty.

Sick leave is usually the same as that allowed the teachers.

The school nurse usually wears the public health nurse's uniform or strictly tailored business clothes. When assisting the school physician, taking active part in or demonstrating nursing procedures, she may wear an intern's white coat, a washable smock, cover-all apron, or other simple washable dress. As this is a health service, reminders of sickness are out of place and the all-white uniform and cap quite unnecessary.

The following account of a school nurse's day is written by a school nurse employed by the board of education in a town of less than 10,000 population.

Ruth's Day with a School Nurse

"Our students have each a chance to spend some time with a school nurse, Miss Evans," the educational director of the Springside School

---

[3] Your state health department or state board of education can give you current salaries being paid school nurses within your state. If you wish to know salary scales on a nationwide basis, write to the National Organization of Public Health Nursing (for address, see Appendix A).

of Nursing had said to Ruth Evans, senior student nurse, the day before sending her to visit with Jane Wilson, school nurse in the town of Springside. "School nursing is the hub of public health. We believe every student nurse should have some acquaintance with it to increase her understanding of the family and the community aspects of health in a democracy. I think you will enjoy your visit with Miss Wilson."

Ruth Evans was not too enthusiastic over the prospect of this visit. She had just about decided to specialize as an instructor of nursing arts in her own hospital. School nursing seemed rather irrelevant. However, she reported promptly at 8:30 on a bright April morning at the Springside Public High School.

The secretary to the principal directed her to the health office. Ruth was surprised to find the pleasant room located just opposite the door marked: Supervising Principal. She remembered that the nurse's room in her own high school had not been so close to the administrative offices nor so convenient to the main entrance. The advantages of this arrangement in easy access to records and personnel were immediately apparent.

Miss Wilson welcomed Ruth cordially with the reminder that they were already acquainted because she was a graduate of the school of nursing Ruth was attending. After the visitor's outer clothing had been placed in the nurse's locker closet, the nurses sat down facing each other across the wide desk near the window.

"Well, Miss Evans, this is where my day's work begins. Each school nurse must adapt her daily routine to the needs of her school family. I must always be prepared for interruptions, for emergencies, or to join in special health surveys. Here in Springside we have two elementary schools and the high school served by one nurse. Health and educational authorities have estimated that a well-qualified public health nurse can give satisfactory service to 1,500 pupils of elementary school age or 2,000 to 2,500 secondary school pupils, unless travel between schools requires a great deal of time. School nurses may be working in large cities, suburban or rural districts, in colleges or special schools. Sometimes there will be 1,500 pupils in only one school, or a nurse will have as many as 10 schools to serve. Do you see what a variety of opportunities for individual preference exists in school nursing positions?"

Ruth Evans nodded. "I never thought of that! I've always thought of a nurse for each school, because I lived in a large city."

"Our nurse educators and vocational guidance consultants have found that most young nurses do not realize these wide differences of opportunity and need for special preparation in nursing positions. That is one reason our school of nursing arranges these field visits." The phone interrupted Miss Wilson.

"Miss Wilson speaking. Yes, Miss Reed, we'll be ready to receive the admissions at the usual time."

Turning to her visitor, Miss Wilson explained that the attendance clerk had several pupils awaiting an interview with the nurse. All pupils who returned to school after a brief illness without a doctor's certificate were seen by the nurse. This procedure had been instituted in this high school because many parents did not call the family doctor for minor ailments. Early symptoms of communicable diseases were frequently overlooked in the older children. These interviews provided a brief contact with the nurse and an opportunity to offer some health education to the pupil.

Each pupil arrived with a referral form for the nurse. A visible index file made it possible for Miss Wilson to pick out quickly the complete health record for each pupil. Ruth was surprised at the amount of information the school nurse had accumulated about the students and the interesting leads she had gathered in the brief, friendly talks with them.

After the group had been sent to their classrooms, several messages arrived by student messenger from the main office. While these occupied Miss Wilson's attention, Ruth used the time to observe her surroundings. The fine murals portraying health subjects on the three walls without windows had evidently been done by students. There were new lighting fixtures giving adequate light without glare throughout the room. File cabinets lined one side of the room, while the wall space near a small bulletin board was shared by framed copies of the Nightingale pledge and the Nurse's Prayer. Plants, books, and current magazines created an atmosphere of informality. The general effect of the spotless room was one of efficiency without barrenness. A doorway at the side of the office was shielded from view by a screen covered with posters on nutrition.

"Before we visit the elementary schools, I'd like to have you see our rest room." Miss Wilson led the way beyond the screen. "This room is not so large and complete as in the schools where the pupils' parents are away from home working all day and therefore difficult to reach. Here we are able to take our emergency cases to the family doctor promptly, or home as the parents direct. Our rest room is used really as a first-aid station. It has only the most essential equipment."

Ruth noted the cot, the rest lounge, the small desk, sink, sterilizer, and a cabinet for supplies. Opening the cabinet for Ruth's inspection, Miss Wilson indicated the clearly printed forms posted on the inside of the door.

"These are the standing orders of the school physician; they are taught to every pupil and every teacher in school. The regulations for exclusion and quarantine approved by the health officer are also posted here."

Ruth Evans thought it looked like a miniature clinic room in the dispensary of the hospital. She wondered if the school nurse wiped it down every day! As if in answer to her thoughts she heard Jane Wilson say, "Our homemaking classes attend to the cleaning and the linen supplies as a part of their assigned practice in home nursing, on a rotation schedule. You'll see the students' names posted on the bulletin board. The senior class taking first aid and their instructor are in charge of this room, because I may be out making home visits or in another school building when something happens. That door opening directly onto the corridor permits quick use of this room without entering the health office."

As the two nurses prepared to leave the building, Ruth commented on the amount of foresighted planning that must be necessary in designing efficient administrative offices. Miss Wilson agreed and then showed her visitor another timesaving device. When they passed the desk in the admission office, Miss Wilson removed a tag marked "Nurse" from a hook in a panel near the clerk's telephone. "This tag hung in plain sight indicates that I am in the building. I take this tag with me to each school and remove it as I leave. It is a simple way of locating me, or other members of the faculty who serve more than one building."

Outside, Ruth saw that the nurse had special parking privileges indicated by a sign which held the space open for emergencies.

"We are going to visit the nearest of the two schools which houses the first to sixth grades."

"Do you visit each school every day?" Ruth asked.

"Yes, I do. The daily contact with teachers and children seems to stimulate their interest in health. I often accomplish several missions in one visit. School nurses can't always follow this schedule. Some must devote one day a week to an individual class or school. This is apt to be the case in rural areas where the distance between schools consumes much valuable nursing time. It depends on the needs of the school family."

"How does a nurse know what plan to follow?"

Ruth's question brought a smile of satisfaction to Miss Wilson's face. "The best way for a school nurse to plan her work is to ask her supervisor for help. Together they may study the needs of the community as a foundation for planning. The character of the population, their employment, the birth, death, and morbidity rates, the health facilities, indeed all the social resources need to be known in recognizing community needs. Home, school, and church are vital health centers. Every public health nurse tries to give family service; she is a health teacher as well as nurse and must reach all of the people in her community. We are placing more and more stress on the value of the home visit. She must be prepared to act as a coordinator of health services.

"Is there a supervisor of school nurses in this county?" Ruth asked.

"No; not every school nurse has an immediate nurse supervisor. Most cities and many school systems with more than one nurse designate a nurse coordinator to help the nurse in a new situation plan her program or to evaluate her service at intervals. Here, where there is only one nurse employed by the local board of education, we call upon the state department of instruction for consultation with the nurse-adviser in health education."

"Doesn't the school administrator tell you what the school wants done?"

This inquiry led to a discussion of the various forms of administrative responsibility in school health education. "There are two main types," Miss Wilson explained. "The state health department and state department of public instruction, called education in some states, both employ nurses who work in schools. Supervision is available to help the nurse utilize her opportunities. After a school health program has been outlined by a special committee composed of representatives of the board of education, board of health, school administrator, school physician, and nurse, with a representative of the parents, teachers, and students, the school nurse is responsible for coordinating and reporting on the program. Supervision of nursing service by qualified nurses is an essential part of professional growth for all school nurses."

They had now arrived at a small school building marked Springside Public School, Number 1. The nurse's parking area made it easy to leave the car and report to the principal's office promptly. Miss Wilson placed the tag marked "Nurse" on the hook near the principal's desk, as she introduced her guest.

"We are pleased to have you visit us, Miss Evans. Are you planning to specialize in school nursing?" the principal asked.

"Thank you, I'm enjoying my visit with Miss Wilson very much. But I'm not at all certain I would make a good school nurse. I think I would prefer to contribute to health education by teaching student nurses in a classroom and on the wards of the hospital."

"Hasn't Miss Wilson told you about her classroom work yet?" the principal asked with a smile at the school nurse.

"I've been saving that experience until later, because I thought Miss Evans would enjoy it most when she observes one of the classes in progress," Miss Wilson replied before Ruth could answer.

"Oh, I'm sorry to have given the surprise feature away! But it will be something to look forward to." Then, indicating a basket marked "Nurse" on a small desk near her own, the principal continued, "Here's something you will be interested in, Miss Wilson. Our teachers have completed the preliminary testing for your program of physical examinations. Their reports are here. Also, there's a call from a parent who is uncertain about her daughter's skin condition. I told her you would add her name to your list of home visits this afternoon, if it is at all possible." She gathered up some more notes.

Ruth watched while the principal and nurse continued their informal conference. She realized that similiar conferences in each school would provide work for many afternoons of the school nurse's time.

As Miss Wilson sorted the messages in her basket at the small desk on one side of the principal's office, she remarked that lack of space made it impossible to have a separate health office in each school building. A file containing the health records and several classroom files for special programs, such as the dental survey, were accessible to the principal in the absence of the nurse. Emergency report forms were used to record all first aid rendered by teachers in each school. Miss Wilson always reviewed these.

As they left the office for a visit through the building, she explained the program of teacher-nurse conferences necessary to coordinate the health service and the use of materials in the classrooms. The school nurse used the occasion of the tour for a routine sanitation inspection. Everywhere Ruth saw evidences of health education activities: in the classroom, on the bulletin boards, and in the corridors, as well as in the teachers' rest room, cafeteria, and basement lavatories. On their return to the main floor, Miss Wilson stopped at a third-grade room to call for three children scheduled to visit the dental clinic in the second school. The teacher used the few minutes while the children were getting their coats to introduce the class to the visitor.

A slightly longer drive to the second school, where the school dental clinic was located, was made lively by the children who showered the nurses with a barrage of questions and confidences. The conversation betrayed a bit of apprehension on the part of one of the young patients on this his first visit to the dental clinic. The reassuring chorus of the two old-timers, however, relieved the tension. This experience made Ruth wonder whether teaching these younger children might not have even more challenging possibilities than teaching more grown-up students.

When they entered the second elementary school, Miss Wilson directed the children to go right on to the clinic. She and Ruth went to the principal's office. After the tag marked "Nurse" had found its place, Miss Wilson examined the contents of her basket. "We tried many routines before we decided on the present policy of helping the teachers to observe and report all deviations from normal. It is eliminating class-room and office inspections by the nurse, and assisting the teachers to become more observant of their pupils' physical condition."

Ruth found the dental clinic more like a clubroom than a dentist's office. A small round table for the children was covered with books and magazines from the shelves and cabinets. A display case held materials and models on dental health. A large bulletin board was covered with comics, posters, and copies of the clinic schedules and forms. The doctor exchanged banter with the child in the chair and the two little patients who waited. The nurse's desk was covered with notes and forms awaiting her attention.

Ruth gathered that the school dentist began his work at nine each school day and worked until noon. It was part of the school nurse's work to schedule the visits and attend to the records as well as assist with the dental examinations. It sounded like a full-time job in itself to Ruth. Miss Wilson pointed out that much more could be accomplished if only a full-time clinic or a clinic room in each school were possible. Dental health problems had been seething in the minds of all health educators long before the military service examinations rejected so many young men because of bad dental conditions. She and the dentist consoled themselves with the thought that a committee was studying the problem as a community project.

Up to this time, Ruth had marveled at the smooth, quiet efficiency of the school routine. Now she was dismayed at the hum of activity and apparent lack of order. Miss Wilson explained in laughing apology that this was where most of her work, planning, and thinking originated! The phone buzzed, teachers stopped to visit on their way along the hall to recess, parents came in feeling fairly certain of finding the nurse on duty. A free exchange of ideas seemed to be stimulated by the unstudied informality. Even the supervising principal dropped in for a chat and met Ruth. The time from 10:30 to 11:30 seemed to speed by on wings, and then the three young patients were ready to return to their school and the littered desk was again clear despite all the interruptions and visitors.

On the return trip Ruth had as many questions to ask as the children! Miss Wilson felt her visitor's enthusiasm rising and the magic of their contact with the eager children infected them both.

After leaving the children at their school, the nurses returned to the high school cafeteria—a reminder of Ruth's own school days, only it seemed more noisy than she remembered! The faculty dining room was quieter, but the hum of conversation stopped only momentarily to admit the nurses. They sat with the home-economics teacher and the instructor of physical education. The conversation was lively, impersonal, and strictly nonshop! Afterward Jane told Ruth that a series of case-study conferences had shown the value of eliminating almost all meal-time gossip.

After lunch the nurse and her visitor returned to the health office. Jane began an introduction to her classroom work by showing her plan book to Ruth. "We are trying to use an old method for a new purpose here in this high school. School nurses have taught various health courses in schools for many years. Some nurses spend as much as 50 per cent of their time in classroom instruction. In other situations, circumstances favor releasing the nurse for outside-the-school contacts —meetings, home visits, and parent education. The needs of the community and the qualifications of the nurse are influencing factors. We have a required course in health problems for girls as part of education for family life. Boys, too, should consider health problems in the home, school, and community. Our vocational guidance program is correlated with physical, mental, and emotional—also social—health problems. It is a flexible course of study revised each year to include current methods and materials, the school health program, and special phases of health, such as dental, nutritional, and communicable-disease surveys. The main objective, however, is to provide an opportunity for individual contact with the school nurse so that she may learn more about the students and their needs."

During the 40-minute class that followed, Ruth sat absorbed in listening to 25 senior girls comment on their own survey of common colds among the student body and teaching staff. Miss Wilson hardly seemed to talk at all. She certainly did not "teach" as Ruth expected she would. Yet when class was over, every girl in the room had talked about the most frequent causes of the common cold and the approved methods of preventing colds, had discussed good school manners when suffering from a cold, and had agreed on when to call a doctor. Ruth admitted to herself she had learned a lot she had not known before, and also seen a demonstration of skillful group leadership in the learning process. It might be a good plan for her to study to be a school nurse after all. Teaching a group like this would be wonderful fun and a challenge to her skill.

After the bell dismissed the class, the nurse and her guest returned to the health office before leaving to make the home visits. Ruth was to join Miss Wilson for this experience another day. "There are so many things about school nursing you cannot see in a brief visit," the school nurse said regretfully. "The satisfactions of planning and working with the children, the older students, parents, teachers, administrators, and other health educators are immeasurable.

"Then, the opportunities for professional growth and for social development are particularly varied. The regularity of the school day, long holidays, and summer vacation permit time for postgraduate study, industrial or camp nursing, hospital refresher courses, or any other activity which you feel will make you a happier or better adjusted individual. Did you enjoy your day, Miss Evans?"

"Oh, yes—school nursing involves much more than I had realized! I'm glad to have had this visit with you, Miss Wilson, and grateful. I'm going to remember that the girls who enter our school of nursing from this high school will bring with them the benefit of their association with a fine school nurse. Also, I'm going to do a lot more thinking about my future teaching career before I decide where it will be carried on! I can understand now why our educational director said that school nursing is the hub of public health."

GENE V. WHITE, R.N.
School Nurse
Audubon, New Jersey

SOURCES OF EMPLOYMENT

1. Professional placement agency
2. Your local health department or board of education. whichever one is supplying nursing service to the schools. If your community is small or is already well supplied with school nurses, write to the state department of health at the state capital.
3. Private or parochial schools, colleges, or other similar institutions: directly to the principal, superintendent, or dean
4. New York State Employment Service
5. The National Organization for Public Health Nursing
6. The U.S. Office of Education, the National Education Association, and the Children's Bureau, all of which supply information and educational materials upon request
7. Any school nurse you know

CAMP NURSING

This activity, if among children, demands a lot of stamina, patience, and pep! It is not an easy job. Nurses who think, as some do, that summer camping can be used to advantage as light, out-of-door work when they are overfatigued, convalescent, or generally "run down" and in need of fresh air and sunshine, are due for a disappointment. A nurse's job in a large camp for children is not restful and cannot always be counted on to be recreational. The nurse should be in good health, able to share the camp activities, and ready for emergencies. She may have to handle an epidemic, an outbreak of food poisoning, or just a run of minor accidents, ivy poisoning, and severe sunburn, which keeps her busy 18 hours of the day. Camps for older people are not quite so strenuous.

Like other specialties, camp nursing is becoming well-defined as an offshoot of school and public health nursing. The opportunities for giving a sound foundation in good health habits and practical knowledge of how to keep well during the 6 to 8 weeks of camping, call for ability to teach, a knack of making health attractive, and skill in handling the camping group. Special workshops to help prepare nurses for effective camp service are held from time to time.[4]

Camp nursing fits in well with employment in schools and colleges, with

[4] See, for example, Institute on Camp Nursing, described in *Public Health Nursing*, p. 208, April, 1949.

university study, as a break between jobs, for private duty nurses who wish to get away from the city, or for industrial nurses employed on a seasonal basis. Knowledge of public health nursing and ability to get along with children are important assets.

Camp nursing is not recommended for nurses over fifty. Nurses from twenty to forty-five years of age are acceptable, with preference shown for those in the twenty-five to thirty-five age group.

Camps designed for patients suffering from special handicaps, such as heart disease, tuberculosis, diabetes, orthopedic, or other conditions, naturally seek nurses with advanced training and experience in the field of the specialty.

The camp nurse is responsible directly to the camp director and the camp physician whether the latter is in residence or not. She is often asked to be at the camp a week in advance of the campers and to remain a week after the date of the camp's official closing. The wise nurse will not accept a camp position if she is not assured of medical supervision and direct contact with a registered hospital in case of emergencies. Both director and nurse are responsible to the parents or relatives of the campers. The nurse works closely with the athletic, sports, or physical education director.

Some camps maintain infirmaries—temporary quarters for sick or slightly injured campers. The infirmary is, of course, the camp nurse's responsibility. She may have to use it as an isolation unit. The space may be used for teaching home nursing and first-aid procedures when not in use by patients. The camp nurse is responsible for ordering all supplies and their care, for keeping records, making reports, and winding up the service when the camp closes.

QUALIFICATIONS

Desirable qualifications include liking to be with children and enjoyment of outdoor sports and camping. Swimming is especially important. It is also desirable to have a knowledge of first aid and a thorough acquaintance with the early symptoms of communicable diseases. In addition the camp nurse needs cool judgment, quick action in emergencies, common sense, and an ability to improvise equipment. A facility for telling stories, ability to teach a handcraft or sport, and a knowledge of nature are useful assets, while an interest in child psychology is almost a "must" on this job.

Camp nurses are often asked to oversee camp sanitation—tents, lavatories, kitchens—assist in planning meals, and share responsibility as one of the camp counselors. Assistance to the doctor in pre- and postcamp examinations goes without saying.

Health inspections, "sick call," routine weighing, health teaching, and nursing care of all personnel are routine duties of the camp nurse. It can readily be understood why experience in public health nursing is especially desirable, and in many camps it is stated as a prerequisite for this job.

Working hours are irregular in camp. The nurse is always on call. Other counselors frequently give "relief hours" or alternate with her on Sunday duty.

The camp nurse need not wear her white uniform, but a distinctive washable dress is desirable and more appropriate while on duty than abbreviated shorts. A playsuit makes an adaptable uniform as the skirt can be doffed for sports and resumed for duty. However, much depends on the type of work assigned the nurse and the age and condition of the campers. It is well to have a complete white uniform on hand for formal occasions.

SALARIES

Salaries are usually paid for the season, ranging from $200 to $500, with all traveling expenses to and from camp and full maintenance in camp. This would be for a 2 months' camping period.

WHERE TO APPLY FOR A CAMP NURSING JOB

1. Local professional employment agencies (Visiting nurse associations, for example, usually know local camp needs.)
2. American Camping Association, 343 South Dearborn St., Chicago, Ill.
3. Association of Private Camps, 55 West 42d St., New York, N.Y.
4. Federation Employment Service, 67 West 47th St., New York, N.Y.
5. Directly to the camp director (See lists of summer camps in magazines and newspapers.)
6. Colleges and universities occasionally know of camp vacancies, as do settlement houses that run camps.
7. National Girl Scouts, Inc., 155 East 44th St., New York, N.Y., and similar organizations—Camp Fire Girls, Boy Scouts, Y.W. and

Y.M.C.A.'s, Y.W. and Y.M.H.A.'s; American Youth Hostels, 6 East 39th St., New York, N.Y.

8. National Jewish Welfare Board, 145 East 32d St., New York, N.Y.

9. The National Recreation Association, 315 Fourth Ave., New York, N.Y., is prepared to supply information about camping.

10. National Federation of Settlements, 214 East 53d St., New York, N.Y.

11. New York State Employment Service, Camp Unit, 1 East 19th St., New York, N.Y.

12. See list of employment agencies, p. 220.

BIBLIOGRAPHY

School Nursing

1. AYLING, WILLIAM E., and EVA F. JOHNSON: The Nurse-Teacher in a School Health Program, *Public Health Nursing*, p. 179, April, 1949.

2. CHAYER, MARY E.: "School Nursing," G. P. Putnam's Sons, New York, 1937.

3. CROMWELL, GERTRUDE: "Health of the School Child," W. B. Saunders Company, Philadelphia, 1946.

4. DEMING, DOROTHY: "Penny Marsh Finds Adventure," Dodd, Mead & Company, Inc., New York, 1940. (Rural nursing.)

5. DILWORTH, LULU P.: The Nurse in the School Health Program, *Public Health Nursing*, p. 438, August, 1949.

6. DUFFUS, R. L.: "Lillian Wald, Neighbor and Crusader," The Macmillan Company, New York, 1938.

7. GARDNER, MARY S.: "Public Health Nursing," Chap. XXV, The Macmillan Company, New York, 1936.

8. HUNTSMAN, CATHERINE: Dynamic School Health Program, *Public Health Nursing*, p. 538, October, 1949.

9. INGLIS, AGNES: What a Nursery School Can Teach You, *American Journal of Nursing*, p. 519, July, 1945.

10. OBERTEUFFER, DELBERT: "School Health Education, A Textbook for Teachers, Nurses, and Other Personnel," Harper & Brothers, New York, 1949.

11. POOLE, RAIDIE: Nursing and College Health Programs, *Public Health Nursing*, p. 192, April, 1949.

12. ROBESON, KATHRYN A.: The Part-Time Nurse in a Day Care Center, *American Journal of Nursing*, p. 104, February, 1948.

13. RUE, CLARA B.: "The Public Health Nurse in the Community," pp. 171–184, W. B. Saunders Company, Philadelphia, 1944.

14. "School Health Policies," Health Education Council, New York. See yearly index published in the December number of *Public Health Nursing* under the heading School Nursing. The April number of *Public Health Nursing* is usually devoted to the subject of school nursing.

15. SMITH, L. M.: The School System—Public Health, *Hygeia*, p. 348, May, 1945.
16. SWANSON, MARIE: School Nursing in New York State, *New York State Nurse*, p. 23, June-July, 1948.
17. WALES, MARGUERITE A.: "The Public Health Nurse in Action," Chap. III, pp. 111–155, The Macmillan Company, New York, 1941.

Camp Nursing

1. AXELSON, A. J.: The Nurse As Health Counselor in Camps, *Public Health Nursing*, p. 396, July, 1942.
2. "Camping for Crippled Children," National Society for Crippled Children and Adults, Inc., Elyria, Ohio, 1945.
3. DIMOCK, HEDLEY S.: "Administration of the Modern Camp," American Camping Association, New York, 1948.
4. FARR, MURIEL: Camp Nursing, A Summer Specialty, *R.N.*, p. 44, June, 1947.
5. FRANZ, RUTH E.: Keeping Campers Healthy, *Public Health Nursing*, p. 218, April, 1950.
6. GARNER, MADELON, Cuyamaca School Camp Health Program, *Public Health Nursing*, p. 353, June, 1949.
7. HOWETT, HARRY H.: "Camping for Crippled Children," National Society for Crippled Children and Adults, Elyria, Ohio, 1945.
8. MITCHELL, A. VIOLA, and ADA B. CRAWFORD: "Camp Counseling," W. B. Saunders Company, Philadelphia, 1950.
9. PAYNE, ELIZABETH C.: Better Camp Nursing, *American Journal of Nursing*, p. 290, May, 1947.
10. SAUNDERS, J. EDWARD: "Safety and Health in Organized Camps," Educational Series No. V and Casualty & Surety Underwriters, New York, 1931. (Still applicable.)
11. STROUP, L. B.: What Constitutes a Camp Nurse's Job, *Public Health Nursing*, p. 381, June, 1934.
12. "Suggested Standards for Camp Nursing," National Organization for Public Health Nursing, 1944.
13. THOMPSON, MARCIA A.: School Camp Nurse Counseling, *Public Health Nursing*, p. 202, April, 1948.
14. WILLIAMS, E. E.: "Keeping Campers Fit," E. P. Dutton & Co., Inc., New York, 1934.
15. WOODS, JAMES H.: Camping for Oldsters, *Recreation*, March, 1950.
16. WOODY, R. I.: Off to Camp, *Hygeia*, p. 615, July, 1937.

CHAPTER XIII

Industrial Nursing

Since the first industrial nurse started her work in 1895[1] in the Vermont Marble Company, a great variety of positions for professional nurses has developed in the industrial health field, and the character of the nurses' work is often determined by the type of industry employing them. Examples of this wide variety of jobs which are fairly typical are as follows:

1. A steel manufacturing concern in Pennsylvania, a "heavy" industry, employs 10 industrial nurses. Accidents and injuries are apt to be severe and emergent. There is a small hospital connected with the plant.

2. A textile firm in Rhode Island, a "light" industry, employs two nurses. Employees are nearly all women. There are few very serious accidents or injuries, but many medical conditions and chances for health supervision and education among the workers.

3. A large department store, state of Washington, employs one nurse and a part-time assistant. Patients include customers taken sick or hurt in the store.

4. A large hotel, Chicago, employs one nurse. Cases of all types and persons of all ages are among her patients as well as the hotel employees.

5. Service in a railroad terminal, such as in the Grand Central Station, New York, covers company employees, includes periodic examinations of food handlers, engineers, towermen, and others responsible

[1] This date is in question as it appears that the Eckly Coxe Coal Company in West Virginia engaged a nurse 7 years earlier (not verified by the author).

for running trains, seeing signals, etc., as well as offering medical and nursing care to the public taken sick or hurt on trains or within the station.

6. A gas and electric company in New York State offers both health education and sickness care to office and field staff.

7. Newspaper, printing, and editorial offices use industrial nurses.

8. A large cotton mill in the South has a nursing staff which makes home visits and includes family health supervision, as the community is made up almost entirely of the mill workers.

9. A lumber camp in the Northwest employs a nurse part of the year.

10. Itinerant labor camps, chiefly for fruit and vegetable pickers on the West Coast, are supplied with nursing service; some of these health services in camps are under the auspices of the state department of health.

11. Transportation lines, railroads, buses, airlines, and ships employ nurses (see Positions with the Transportation Lines, below).

12. A bank with 10 branches in a large city employs a nurse and a home visitor.

13. Fruit, sugar, and rubber plantations in Hawaii, Cuba, and in South America, owned by large companies in the United States, employ doctors and nurses from this country.

14. Part-time, supervised industrial nursing services are offered by visiting nurse associations to industries too small to keep a full-time nurse busy.

15. Not only do large insurance companies employ industrial nursing staffs for the care of their own employees, but a few employ and supervise salaried local staffs outside of the home office to visit policyholders whose policies entitle them to home nursing service under medical supervision. These visiting nurses are expected to be qualified public health nurses as they give care and health supervision in homes on a visit basis. Insurance companies also make contracts with visiting nurse associations for similar home nursing services. Visiting nurse associations supply nurses to make home visits to sick employees of industries carrying a form of group insurance.

16. There is a miscellaneous assortment of unique jobs for industrial nurses which are intriguing but seldom vacant. They include positions in museums, government buildings, libraries, and the United Nations headquarters in New York City.

An acceptable definition of industrial nursing is:

The practice of the art and science of nursing in industry to meet the needs of the worker for the purpose of developing and maintaining the highest potential level of health and efficiency through

1. Prompt remedial care of the ill and injured
2. Health and safety education
3. Cooperation with all health and welfare agencies[2]

The number of nurses employed by industry doubled after 1940, yet approximately 50 per cent of the industrial workers in the United States do not have the services of a nurse within the plants where they work. It is hoped that the increased appreciation of the value of nursing service will result in a continuing demand for industrial nurses. Jobs for industrial nurses increase when production rises, as in wartime, and decrease in depressions or prolonged strikes. There were 13,113 nurses in industry in 1949.[3] The states employing most industrial nurses are usually New York, Illinois, Pennsylvania, and Ohio; the lowest number are employed in the agricultural states—Idaho, Nevada, South Dakota, and Wyoming.

Industrial nursing service is one of the favorite fields among nurses and the openings in it are comparatively few. Vacancies are apt to be filled locally, by friends of the incumbents. If you know a nurse in industry, tell her of your interest. She will keep you in mind should she hear of a vacancy. Not all industrial nurses work on day shifts. It is harder to find nurses willing to work on the night shift, so that might be your opening. Once in a while, you may be lucky enough to be the first nurse employed by an industry. Your salary may be small to start with, as industry can be hard-boiled and coldly businesslike about adding your salary to the cost of production. It is up to you to give effective service and prove that health supervision, nursing care, and intelligent, fast first aid saves the plant money by keeping the worker on the job or returning him to it promptly. The nurse working alone must possess organizing ability and an appreciation of business methods. A knowledge of typing and filing is desirable.

[2] AMERICAN ASSOCIATION OF INDUSTRIAL NURSES. For addresses of organizations mentioned in this chapter, see Appendix A.
[3] *Facts about Nursing*, pp. 13 and 23, American Nurses Association, 1950.

The industrial nurse's relationship to all personnel gives her a strategic value as interpreter of health practices and promoter of good will. Her technical skill makes her the indispensable ally of the physician in the first aid, diagnostic, and treatment aspects of industrial medicine. Her close contact with workers and her knowledge of community resources aid the doctor in rounding out his health examinations and in achieving corrective measures. Her ability to evaluate the character and importance of symptoms and to record them properly, make her a valuable adjunct in the compensatory and legal aspects of industrial illness and injury.[4]

Margaret S. Hargreaves has given a very clear picture of the duties of industrial nurses. You will note that she stresses the importance of understanding the special hazards in the processes of manufacture, the necessity for keeping accurate records (inasmuch as these relate to the employees' rights under the workmen's compensation laws and the insurance regulations covering the plant), and the vital protection of securing written standing orders from the industrial physician. She has also pointed out an increasingly frequent demand made on industrial nurses: that of knowing the basic principles of rehabilitation and the adjustment of the injured worker to his job. The objective of the industrial nurse is to keep the worker well and on the job. Miss Hargreaves has shown how this goal may involve the worker's home, family, private physician, and social life. As in school nursing, we see industrial nursing merging with the community's efforts to provide adequate health service for all people whether at home, in school, at work, or at play. Its aims are, therefore, closely related to public health. This is one of the many reasons why experience in public health nursing makes a desirable background for the nurse serving industry. Employers frequently prefer a young nurse, and industrial physicians sometimes stipulate previous experience in surgical nursing. Alertness is desirable, and the industrial nurse is expected to promote employer-employee understanding, while keeping out of labor disputes. She can do much in a quiet way to interpret company policies and explain employee attitudes to management.[5] She may be called upon for a variety of skills, such as work with infrared rays, x-ray equipment, basal metabolism testing, and other laboratory procedures. She must

[4] AMERICAN ASSOCIATION OF INDUSTRIAL NURSES.
[5] See also MILLER, MYRTLE: Nurse as Industrial Health Counselor, *Public Health Nursing*, p. 119, March, 1948.

know how to find and utilize resources within the plant and in the community. She must know the Workmen's Compensation Law and how to fill out insurance records. Her records may become legal documents.

Industrial nursing is a promising field for professional men nurses.

While the industrial nurse is usually employed directly by the company, industrial nursing services are also administered by labor organizations, unions, mutual benefit associations, and under contract by insurance companies. Medical-care programs are beginning to handle contracts providing both medical and nursing care to industries.

In large plants, there is usually a full-time medical director—an industrial physician who is in charge of the health service. In small plants, the doctor may be on a part-time or "on-call" basis. The industrial nurse is then responsible to management.

There are a few pertinent questions which an applicant for an industrial position will wish to ask, in addition to the questions listed on p. 11, before accepting a job.

To whom is the nurse responsible? Is the medical director employed full time? Will there be qualified nursing supervision available to staff nurses? Exactly how are the hours of duty arranged? What deductions will be made from salary? (The nurse is subject to social security taxes in a commercial organization.) Is the nursing staff unionized? Will I be allowed to go on company time to professional meetings or annual nursing conventions? Will there be opportunity in the locality for special study on my own time? What will be my responsibilities for nonnursing duties, such as secretarial service, matron's work, care of rest rooms, etc.? What will be my own accident and sickness protection under the company's insurance?

One of the best ways to learn something about the work of the industrial nurse is to visit a large plant with a student group. (See for example, the plan of observation offered by the Simplex Wire and Cable Company of Boston, Massachusetts.)

SALARIES

In the industrial field, salaries range from $2,200 to $3,000 for staff positions, $2,500 to $4,500 for supervisors, $3,000 to $5,500 for consultant and administrative positions.

Full-time positions are nearly always on the 8-hour-day basis, with a 40- or 44-hour week, with time and a half paid for overtime. Vacations are usually 2 weeks, sometimes 3 weeks, and only rarely 4 weeks in length; sick leave and holiday time correspond to the practice among business firms in the locality. It is suggested that a copy of the approved personnel policies for industrial nurses be secured from the American Association of Industrial Nurses.

As industrial nursing positions are connected with profit-making companies, the industrial nurse is subjected to the payroll deductions of other employees. These include social security taxes, company or employee benefit and hospitalization plans of one sort or another (these may be optional), union dues (see references to Unions in the Bibliography at the end of Chap. I) and, of course, any current income taxes imposed by Uncle Sam. During the war, payroll deductions for the purchase of war bonds were expected.

Some of the positions involve night work, either the "swing shift," 3 to 11 P.M., or the "graveyard shift," 11 P.M. to 8 A.M. There are more of these during wartime.

Large industries provide cafeteria service where a meal may be purchased practically at cost. Snack bars and rest-room kitchenettes for the nurses are sometimes available.

The hospital or public health uniform is worn on duty. Laundry is sometimes furnished by the employing company.

The industrial nurse lives at home.

This is a field of work well suited to men nurses when the majority of the employed personnel is made up of men, and the work involves handling heavy machinery. There are not many men nurses employed in industry, however. Night shifts and work with construction companies and in mines suggest possible opportunities.

Miss Hargreaves' account of the work of industrial nurses follows.

Industrial Nursing—Room for All

Members of the Senior Class:

I can think of no more welcome task than this—to tell you about my own field of work, industrial nursing. This is a fast-growing field and one with a great future. There is room in this branch of nursing for older nurses, young nurses, fat nurses, thin nurses, blondes, brunettes, married or single, male or female. The essential qualities in addition to proper training and background are the ability to get along with people, the combined virtues of good judgment and resourcefulness, and the blessings of good physical health and emotional stability. An industrial nurse is a registered professional nurse specially trained in the techniques of protecting the health of the worker in industry—one who encourages the best possible care, emphasizes the preventive aspects of accidents and illness, and works with the doctor and management in planning a practical, smoothly functioning medical program. This service is most effective when a physician visits the pant and takes responsibility for diagnosis and treatment. However, not all nurses in industry have this desirable supervision.

The first duty of the nurse in industry is to care for the injured or ill employee. This is a legal and financial responsibility upon the employer, so the nurse gives the best medical and nursing care she possibly can. She keeps up to date on the newest techniques of first aid and follow-up care, and she maintains the proper facilities for carrying on this service.

Her second important function is keeping accurate records of the medical services performed. These records are useful in evaluating the work of the department, for informing management of the medical problems, and in safeguarding the interests of both employee and employer.

A third duty is the promotion of better health and safety for the worker. Through proper education of the worker and through familiarity with plant problems and processes the industrial nurse is able to assist in the control of absenteeism due to sickness and in the reduction of labor turnover for medical reasons. Often she deals with large groups, when she can apply public health principles as well as teaching preventive methods on an individual basis. She is in a good position to prevent disability by timely health counseling and education. She sees the same people again and again, when they are ill, when they are well, and in their working environment. She gains a better idea of the personality and normal behavior of the individual than does the nurse who sees only ill persons.

Is that all an industrial nurse does? Oh, no—added responsibilities are supervision of sanitary conditions, of eating facilities, of locker rooms, etc.; participation in nutrition programs, recreational activities, and other welfare plans. These added responsibilities depend on the size and nature of the industry, and the wishes of management.

This type of nursing usually carries with it Security with a big S: good pay, reasonable hours of work, added benefits in vacation pay, group insurance, social security, and retirement benefits. Management often foots

the bill when the nurse wishes to attend organization meetings and conferences, or to take special courses. Her uniforms are usually provided
and laundered. She plays an important part in the field of labor-management relations. Most of all, she gains a great many real friends and a
measure of personal satisfaction through her opportunities for improving
employee health and production. We are essentially an industrial nation
and the opportunities now for nurses in in-plant medical services are
almost unlimited.

Will you accompany me during a typical day in a busy plant?

I begin my day at the dispensary by talking with three employees who
wish to return to work after an absence due to illness. I find two apparently recovered and fit for duty, but the third I hold over for the doctor
to see later. We have a special plan for the rehabilitation of this man. Then
I see two persons suffering with headaches, then a girl who is having
difficulty with her coworkers (this will take me time to work out), another with a home problem, and still another who has an unexplainable
rash under her arm. Two workers come in for redressings on previously
injured fingers; I remove a foreign body from the eye of one of our
drivers; I cleanse and dress a simple abrasion according to the procedure
in my standing orders approved by the doctor; and I give an infrared
treatment to a man who has had it prescribed by the doctor the previous
day. Soon it is time for the doctor's visit and I call the different departments and make appointments for the employees who are scheduled to
see him. Two prospective employees are waiting to have preplacement
examinations, so I take the necessary preliminary information and prepare
the first for examination.

The doctor's 2-hour visit passes quickly but I have to be on the alert
to keep things moving swiftly and efficiently. Redressings and revisits are
cared for, then. For a short period before he leaves the doctor discusses
with me the particular phase of the health program that we are stressing
that month—it happens to be a study of known and probable diabetics.
Periodic checkups are planned on certain groups and appropriate literature and poster material selected for the drive. A short time is spent
preparing an announcement for the monthly house organ, and we both
make plans to attend a labor-management meeting the following week.

Then lunch—at last! We'll eat in the cafeteria.

After lunch there is a short lull and I have a chance to bring my records
up-to-date and to file some reference material on tuberculosis marked for
later use in the waiting room.

The afternoon is marked by one serious injury caused by a breakdown in some heavy grinding machinery. The patient is dispatched to the hospital in the company car; the doctor is notified by phone and goes at once to the hospital. A very complete record must be made of this accident for the insurance company. Late in the afternoon I attend a safety meeting and try to point out some hazards which have come up too frequently during the past few weeks. A trained first-aider replaces me while I am at the meeting. While I was gone, she cared for some simple complaints; but one employee complaining of a vague pain in his side was put to bed until I returned. After careful questioning I refer him to his family doctor. One more patient comes in just before closing time with a family problem weighing heavily on him. He suspects that his wife has cancer of the breast. He is referred to the local cancer detection clinic and goes out smiling.

I lock the files, I take off my cap, I change to street clothes, I turn off the lights and close the door. Has it been a busy and productive day?

MARGARET S. HARGREAVES, R.N.
Division Health Consultant
Liberty Mutual Insurance Co.
10 Rockefeller Plaza
New York, N.Y.

QUALIFICATIONS

Industrial nurses are realizing the need for much of the same general training, background, and experience as the public health nurse; especially is this true when the industrial nurse carries a heavy program of health teaching and home visiting. A knowledge of community resources and how to use them for the benefit of employees and their families is important. Standardized and supervised field practice is being developed for nurses in connection with some of the courses to assist the industrial nurse to prepare for these responsibilities.

The American Association of Industrial Nurses states:

Basically, courses that deal with sociology, economics, human and community relationships, public sanitation and hygiene are fundamental. These can be held in common with nurses preparing for public health nursing. The point of departure for the industrial nurse, should, we now believe, include business law and administration, personnel management, safety provisions, and related subjects. We believe too, that study of the background of industrial development, its present trends, and labor relations, should also receive attention.

Postgraduate study in industrial nursing is highly desirable, and a number of universities with accredited programs in public health nursing are offering courses in industrial hygiene for industrial nurses.[6]

It is obvious that a good surgical nurse will be sought by a heavy industry, and in all industrial positions, a practical knowledge and prompt application of first aid is an absolute essential to acceptable service. Health teaching will be stressed when the employees are women. Some employers prefer nurses who have had at least a year of experience after graduation from a school of nursing.

Supervisory positions in industry are increasing gradually. It is recommended that in staffs of two or more industrial nurses, one be appointed as supervisor. Requirements are experience in this field and special preparation through appropriate courses, including public health nursing and supervision.

There are also industrial nursing consultant positions in visiting nurse associations, in state departments of health or divisions of industrial hygiene, and in the U.S. Public Health Service. These positions are open to well-prepared nurses who have had experience and theory in both public health nursing and industrial work. Experience in supervision is desirable and usually required.

Positions with the Transportation Lines

Many of the airlines have discontinued using registered nurses as air stewardesses, preferring to train nonnursing personnel in the duties that concern the welfare of passengers. While the nurses who do apply for positions are looking for adventure, the airlines are looking for service and a fairly strict procedure is required after a training period.

Positions on airlines involving constant contact with the traveling public are usually filled by the younger nurses, though this is not the case in supervisory positions. One excellent reason for this is that there are limitations in weight and height for many of these appointments, and older nurses are apt to weigh more than those under forty! It is necessary

[6] An up-to-date list of these courses and recommended content can be secured from the American Association of Industrial Nurses.

to wear the snappy outdoor uniforms, supplied by the companies, with style; and a trig-looking, slim nurse is a definite asset to good public relations. But—make no mistake!—nurses employed on the transportation lines must be skillfully efficient and very well informed, prepared to handle all sorts of situations, including emergencies, with tact, celerity, and competency. Most of the companies give the nurse an intensive course of instruction under close supervision, and the applicant must qualify on all points before a final appointment is made. Up-to-date information on first-aid procedures and good judgment in handling difficult passengers are essential possessions for these nurses.

The usual qualifications for all applicants on the airlines are

Entering age—twenty-one to twenty-eight
Vision—20:20, *without glasses*
Height—5 feet 2 inches to 5 feet 6 inches
Weight—normal for age and height according to insurance company
   tables (a maximum of 125 is set by some companies)
Preferably unmarried
Pleasing appearance and personality
Some companies require 2 years of college education.

Only about four nurses out of 100 applicants are accepted for employment. Nurses with military service records will be given special consideration, and the air-evacuation nurses (flight nurses) have priority.

Flights have become longer and longer, farther and farther, probably faster! Round-the-world trips will not be unusual in the future. The overseas airlines prefer registered nurses as stewardesses.

Positions with transportation lines pay about as follows:

Airlines—$160 a month and up, with allowance for living accommodations
Railroads—$150 a month and up, and all expenses (not many railroads
   are using nurses on trains)
Shipping lines—$160 a month and up, with living accommodations
   (shipping lines are usually flooded with applications)

Of all the positions in industry, work on the transportation lines is most irregular, being subject to changing schedules, weather conditions, and seasonal crowds. It is usual to give the nurse a breathing space at the end of a run or flight. Trips on board ship may take her away from her home port for several weeks at a time. Turnover in these positions is not great.

The work is definitely hard. Don't apply expecting glamour, ease, and entertainment.

SOURCES OF EMPLOYMENT

In surveying the possibilities in this field, it is especially desirable to secure professional guidance before accepting a position. Therefore it is suggested that information on opportunities in general be secured from industrial nursing consultants rather than by direct application to an industry when seeking a first job.

1. Professional placement services. Your first source of guidance to a position should be a professional placement agency in preference to a newspaper advertisement or hearsay. Find out all you can about the position before you apply. Be sure that you will have adequate medical supervision and enough "tools" to work with. If you are the first nurse to be employed by the plant, you will need to proceed slowly in listing your needs until you understand just what the demands will be and what kind of service is involved. The industrial physician sometimes dictates the equipment, sometimes leaves it to the nurse.

   The American Association of Industrial Nurses will supply up-to-date outlines of recommended personnel policies and list of Duties and Responsibilities of Nurses in Industry. See especially the latter leaflet which is very clear and comprehensive.

2. Industrial nursing consultant in your state health department, the American Association of Industrial Nurses, or the nurse in this position in your local city health department or visiting nurse association[7]

3. General information regarding advanced positions may be secured from either the national association mentioned above or the industrial nursing consultants, U.S. Public Health Service. Positions in the Federal departments are under Civil Service regulations.

4. Applications for positions may be made to the medical departments of large industries.

[7] State industrial nursing sections are also being organized. These are usually known to the state health department or the national agencies.

5. New York State Employment Service, 119 West 57th Street, New York, N.Y.
6. National Manufacturers Association, 14 West 49th St., New York, N.Y.
7. Home offices of life insurance and accident companies
8. American Hotel Association, 221 West 57th St., New York, N.Y.
9. Large metropolitan hotels and stores
10. Transoceanic and coastwise steamship lines—both tourist and freight lines (usually a waiting list)
11. U.S. Maritime Commission, 45 Broadway, New York, N.Y.
12. Transportation Association of America, 40 East 40th St., New York, N.Y.; National Airlines, Inc.; Jacksonville, Fla.; United Airlines, 5959 South Cicero Ave., Chicago, Ill.; Transcontinental and Western Air, Inc., Kansas City, Mo.; Western Airlines, Inc., 6331 Hollywood Blvd., Los Angeles, Calif.
13. American Management Association, 330 West 42d St., New York, N.Y.
14. Commercial employment agencies

BIBLIOGRAPHY

1. AMERICAN ASSOCIATION OF INDUSTRIAL NURSES: Publication List.
2. AMERICAN NURSES ASSOCIATION, PROFESSIONAL COUNSELING AND PLACEMENT SERVICE: Nursing in Civilian Transportation (report), *American Journal of Nursing*, p. 234, April, 1947.
3. BOWEN, MARY: Nursing the Miners, *R.N.*, p. 41, November, 1949.
4. BROWN, DANIEL M.: Industrial Nursing at Shasta Dam, *American Journal of Nursing*, p. 268, March, 1942.
5. DEMING, DOROTHY: Serving the Traveling Public, *American Journal of Nursing*, p. 869, September, 1944.
6. DEMPSEY, CATHERINE: The American Association of Industrial Nurses, *Trained Nurse and Hospital Review*, June, 1944. (Contains brief description of industrial nurses' relationships.)
7. ELLIS, ALICE M.: An Ounce of Prevention at Sea, *Public Health Nursing*, p. 415, August, 1935.
8. HAGUE, EVA W.: Industrial Nursing in Iowa, *American Journal of Nursing*, p. 286, April, 1945. (State consultant's duties.)
9. HAMILTON, ALICE: "Exploring the Dangerous Trades," Little, Brown & Company, Boston, 1943. (Autobiography.)
10. HAMILTON, ALICE: Looking at Industrial Nursing, *Public Health Nursing*, p. 63, February, 1946.

11. HEAGLER, LOIS: Industrial Nursing in a Small Plant, *American Journal of Nursing*, p. 34, January, 1951.
12. *Industrial Medicine* (monthly magazine).
13. JAHNCKE, GLADYS A.: Industrial Nursing Today, *American Journal of Nursing*, p. 789, October, 1945.
14. KAHL, F. RUTH: Counseling and Guidance for Nurses in Industry, *American Journal of Nursing*, p. 940, October, 1944.
15. KIRALY, MARGARET: Industrial Nursing Is Human Maintenance, *New York State Nurse*, p. 16, March, 1947.
16. MACDONALD, M. G.: "Handbook of Nursing in Industry," W. B. Saunders Company, Philadelphia, 1944.
17. McGRATH, BETHEL: "Nursing in Commerce and Industry," Commonwealth Fund, Division of Publication, New York, 1946.
18. MILLER, MYRTLE: The Nurse as Industrial Health Counselor, *Public Health Nursing*, p. 119, March, 1948.
19. NATIONAL SAFETY COUNCIL: Publications List.
20. SHIRLEY, RUBY THOMPSON: Nursing Miners and Their Families, *American Journal of Nursing*, p. 347, April, 1944.
21. VINCENT, FLORENCE SMITH: Nurse in Industry Has Won Spurs, *New York State Nurse*, p. 10, June-July, 1948.
22. WILLSON, DIXIE: "Hostess of the Skyways," Dodd, Mead & Company, Inc., New York, 1944.

For descriptions of early industrial nursing jobs, see Industrial Nursing number of *Public Health Nursing*, March, 1945. Also WRIGHT, FLORENCE SWIFT: "Industrial Nursing," The Macmillan Company, New York, 1912.

All professional journals carry descriptions of industrial nursing jobs from time to time. See Index under Industrial Nursing.

CHAPTER XIV

Nursing in Doctors' Offices

As will be seen from the sketch, In Dr. Joliffe's Office, which follows, the office nurse is expected to be a Jack-of-all-trades, as well as a good manager, skillful nurse, and tactful secretary. Her duties, other than nursing, may be summarized as consisting in arranging appointments for patients and the doctor, taking messages, managing the office, ordering and caring for supplies and equipment, keeping records, taking dictation, typing, taking care of mail, keeping accounts, sending out bills, assisting in preparing reports, keeping track of tests and narcotic permits, making patients' return appointments, etc. Some of the record work is fairly complicated if the doctor carries insurance cases or is engaged in experimental work and research. A knowledge of typing is *essential*, and stenography is desirable.

Doctors differ in the amount of secretarial service they need from their office nurses. Some carry a heavy correspondence, with help in assembling reports, preparing papers, or noting references in professional journals. Most physicians expect the nurse to take care of ordering all office supplies, renewing periodical subscriptions, and keeping the accounts. There will be many details of good office housekeeping, such matters as insurance, redecorating, repairs, rent, and filing. Several handbooks are available that will give the nurse considering this sort of work a foretaste of the scope of "business duties" expected of her.[1] A very busy physician will probably ask his office nurse to be a sort of social secretary as well as office manager. She may have to keep track of his evening and week-end engagements, buy a gift for his niece, or take a grandson to the circus! One of the recent additional burdens placed on the office nurse's shoulders is

[1] See Bibliography at the end of this chapter.

the preparation of statements for the income tax. Indeed, there may come a time in office service when a nurse will need regular secretarial help if she is to keep up her nursing duties at all. A nurse, therefore, considering her prospective job, should try to find out just how heavy these non-nursing duties are. Some doctors employ both secretarial and nursing service.

The nurse is the hostess of the doctor's office and her reception room is his waiting room. She should appear in immaculate white uniform and must learn to be polite to patients on all occasions—not always an easy task. She must be accurate in recording telephone messages and be able to exercise tact and good judgment in protecting the doctor from unnecessary or time-consuming conversations. If the doctor is apt to have regular patients visit or telephone the office in his absence, the nurse must know just how far she may proceed in giving advice, medication, or treatments. She should be well informed on first-aid procedures. Occasionally she needs to act fast in emergencies. Among the visitors to the doctor's office will be representatives of insurance firms, salesmen, book publishers, lawyers, and other businessmen and women.

Nursing duties include taking patients' histories, assisting patients in preparing for the doctor's examination,[2] preparing for and assisting in treatments, tests, and any special procedures, taking the doctor's dictation, carrying out his special orders, interpreting orders to patients, following up tests, securing reports for patients' records, and conferring with patients in the doctor's absence. Much will depend on the character and size of the doctor's practice. Some physicians expect their office nurses to do practically everything, including intravenous injections and suturing. In offices where several physicians work together and more than one nurse is employed, one of the nurses may be expected to have public health nursing experience and the work may be divided into specialties. In offices where minor surgery is done, the nurse may be expected to give anesthetics. A knowledge of x-ray and the handling of special equipment for measuring basal metabolism or taking electrocardiograms, etc., may be required.

The office will receive many illustrated leaflets from pharmaceutical firms, insurance companies, magazines, and health agencies. It will be the nurse's responsibility to sort these, to file them, to give them to the doctor, or to secure his permission for use among his patients. There will be

[2] This is usually much the same routine as is expected of the nurse when assisting the doctor in examining patients on admission to a hospital.

many times when she will need to seek appropriate health education material to give to patients or to post in the office. She should try to keep up with the best in this ever-growing field.

Probably office nurses would agree that by far the most important part of their jobs concerns the doctor-patient relationships. Patients are of all types: discouraged, irritable, overanxious, unconcerned, careless, fussy, and even fakes. The office nurse must keep peace with all kinds of people, relieve the doctor of as much friction and interruption as possible, and yet know when a situation is serious enough to be placed in his hands. She must be skilled in interpreting her employer's wishes and be ready to support his orders when excited patients object to them. Professional "ethics" play a large part in handling a wide office, home, and hospital consultant practice, and the nurse must have a clear understanding from the doctor as to how he wishes her to handle some of the delicate problems that are sure to crop up. One of these is, of course, the question of the doctor's fee. One doctor is generous to a fault; the next thinks almost wholly in terms of what his practice is netting him. The nurse needs to have an insight into human difficulties and sympathy with them to settle some of these questions to the doctor's and patient's satisfaction. In short, this is a case of not only liking people but knowing how to handle them. The office nurse must be a diplomat. If you shrink from meeting new people or are easily tried by unreasonable requests, better not try office nursing!

In choosing the specialist with whom to work, consult your own preference as to patients. If you do not like children, stay away from the child specialist; if elderly people bore you, then you'd better not work for a heart specialist. There are usually enough specialists employing office nurses in large cities for you to take your choice. However, these jobs are in great demand as they fit in well with the preferences of married nurses. An office nurse is apt to hand on her job to a friend. The best office positions are rarely vacant. (See positions in group medical service offices and clinics, p. 75.)

In some offices, the doctor will have time to teach you your work; in others, he will want you to come prepared. One quality he will surely seek in you, and that is friendliness to his patients. He does not want too talkative a nurse, nor one too frigidly professional. He especially looks for a nurse who can handle telephone calls competently. Patients calling expect courtesy, warmth, and clear directions. A pleasant voice is a great asset. Patients respond to a voice over the telephone and can be cast down or cheered by the tone of the nurse. "I just called you, Miss Fritz," a patient phoned the nurse, "to tell you I slept well last night. You sounded so interested yesterday when I called, I knew you would like to hear that my ear is better!"

Furthermore, a busy doctor just can't keep on taking patients endlessly. There comes a time when patients must be refused. This takes tact, discrimination, and untiring patience. A knowledge of the other resources for care in the community is therefore valuable. Don't undertake office nursing in a totally strange city if you can help it.

Office nursing is a suitable occupation for the qualified married nurse, especially if she wants and can find part-time service, and for the older nurse, if she is alert and up to date. The doctor, however, wishes to be able to count on regular stable assistance. The nurse is expected to remain on duty as long as there are patients to be seen, and to leave things in good order. If marriage interferes with duty or if the older nurse is not able to be on her job on the days and at the hours she has agreed upon, he will prefer the young, unmarried nurse. An efficient, tactful, and technically skilled professional nurse possessing good judgment can double a doctor's practice and make the machinery of carrying on his business so unobtrusive yet productive that he will find greater satisfaction and greater success in his profession through the undisturbed attention he is able to give it.

This is one of the fields of nursing for which no advanced academic study is usually required, unless the nurse chooses to work for a specialist in a highly developed field—such as orthopedics—when she must present special training or, at least, experience.

A business course, which may be taken in the evening, covering bookkeeping, typing, and stenography is of so much use as to be practically a prerequisite.

SALARIES

Salaries paid to office nurses vary with the area of the country. The initial salary may be low, as the doctor likes to have a nurse prove her ability before making the commitment. In large cities on the East and West Coasts, they may be as high as $60 to $80 a week. In small cities, $40 to $50 may be paid. A dollar an hour is the minimum rate for part-time service. The cost of laundry for uniforms may be met by the doctor.

The nurse is usually on duty from 8:30 A.M to 4:30 P.M., or 8:00 to

4:00—sometimes from 7 A.M. to 9 P.M. Overtime is not unusual, and emergencies do occur. She may be expected to be in the office Saturday afternoons. She usually has Sundays free. She should plan to be in the office if the doctor takes his half day in the middle of the week, as is quite usual. Legal holidays and 2 or 3 weeks' vacation on pay may be expected.

In Dr. Joliffe's Office

It was a windy day in April when I walked into Dr. Joliffe's office for the first time, in answer to his request for an office nurse. It was just at noon. His waiting room was empty and he called to me from his consulting office:

"That you, Mrs. Briggs? Please come in here."

A massive man—I had to look up to his face, and I am not short—Dr. Joliffe rose to greet me from behind a cluttered desk.

"Had your lunch?" was his first abrupt inquiry.

"Yes, I stopped at . . . ."

"Good. Then you can get right to work. Do you like to fish, Mrs. Briggs?"

I smiled. This was a strange beginning to a new job! "Yes, I do. I used to go trout fish- . . . ."

"Good. Then you will understand. I want to go trout fishing and this office has been a madhouse for a month, ever since Sallie Austin left. Look at those records!" He waved toward an overflowing file box. "Not complete, not filed, no bills sent. I want you to bring order out of chaos so I can go fishing once a week. Your hours will be 8:30 to 4:00. Bring your lunch with you. Saturday till noon. I'll pay you $160 a month to start. Right?"

"Yes, I . . . ."

"Good. Now, I'll get *my* lunch. Make yourself at home. Look around. You'll find an apron in the linen cupboard that will do you for this afternoon. I'll show you the works when I get back. That's your cubbyhole."

He had risen and walked to the door of the waiting room. He waved toward its far corner where I saw a desk, files, telephone, typewriter, and a small door marked "Nurse."

"But, Dr. Joliffe, don't you want to know what experience I've had? Maybe the work here . . . ."

"Don't need to know. I called Blake. He said you were all right!" His blue eyes twinkled as he smiled down at me. "Soon find out for myself anyway! I'll be back before one. Patients begin to come then for my 1:30 office hours. You'll see." He was gone.

That first conversation was typical of Dr. Joliffe and of the work in his office. He was direct, practical, informal, and his practice moved at a fast tempo.

I found a small dressing room behind the door marked "Nurse." I shed my coat and hat, put my purse in the drawer of the desk, locked it, and started a tour of inspection, opening every door and getting a quick survey of the equipment and supplies. As I proceeded, I could feel the leisurely atmosphere of the private home where I had had my last case evaporating, and my steps quickened. There was a lot to do here.

Apparently, Dr. Joliffe handled every type of case and was prepared for any emergency, even minor surgery. He must have a heavy practice, judging by the amount of supplies.

His offices were quite new, built at the back of his private home. They consisted of the good-sized waiting room, well lighted and simply furnished, with my cubbyhole in the corner nearest the examining room. Dr. Joliffe's office opened at the left of the entrance. It connected with the examining room, and had its own small lavatory. The examining room was on a corner of the building and opened off the waiting room. It had two huge windows, was "done up" in green, and held the usual furnishings—examining table, cabinets, scales, washstand with knee-action faucets, enamel chairs, stool, dressing cart, sterilizer, and small autoclave. Two small curtained dressing rooms were on either side of a patient's lavatory. A closet contained extra supplies, including linen, and I found a white smock which fitted well enough and protected my dress. I felt fearfully unprofessional not to be in uniform but, if Dr. Joliffe did not mind, his patients probably would not. I had planned to stay off duty for a few days before starting this job, but I could see I was needed here right away.

Just as I was finishing my tour of inspecion, the telephone rang. I picked it up and uttered those three words which I have said at least a hundred times a week ever since: "Dr. Joliffe's office."

It was a Mrs. Pratt—indeed, *the* Mrs. Pratt of our town. Could she bring Junior in at three o'clock? He had skinned his knee badly in a fall from his bicycle. I didn't know what appointments Doctor had. I didn't know where he kept his appointment book. I didn't know whether he would prefer to see Junior at home. But Mrs. Pratt was Mrs. Pratt.

"Surely, bring Junior in at three, Mrs. Pratt. I'm sorry he's hurt. Is his knee bleeding badly?"

"No, and he's put a first-aid dressing on it from his Boy Scout kit. But I'd like Doctor to see it."

"Yes, indeed. We'll be ready for you."

As I cradled the telephone, the entrance door opened and a "bobby soxer" entered. (A notice on the outer door told patients to "Walk In.") She was a stout, bareheaded girl of about sixteen. She wore the regulation Sloppy Joe sweater and pleated skirt of her tribe. She flopped down in an easy chair and took up a copy of *Look*. I went over to her.

"Do you have an appointment with Dr. Joliffe? May I ask your name?"

"My name's Josie Klopec. I'm going to work for the Bruger Company. All us girls was told to come here today for 'zaminations—so we can get our papers signed."

As she spoke, the door opened again and in came another young woman. Within 10 minutes, four more had arrived. I took their names, addresses, and ages. All wanted permits to go to work for the Bruger Company, a textile firm with a batch of war orders to fill. I didn't know what records the doctor wanted made out, where they were kept, or how thorough these examinations would be.

While I was taking the names, the telephone rang twice. Dr Joliffe was wanted at the Community Hospital at 4:30 for consultation. Jennie Rose was too sick to come to the office; would Doctor please call. A search in the pile of disorderly records revealed a handwritten card for Jennie Rose—first seen a week ago. Jennie, eleven years old, had complained of aching joints.

I was just beginning to think that Dr. Joliffe's practice was largely among children, when the door admitted an old man of seventy at least, so lame he was using two canes. He sank down on the first chair he came to.

Then Dr. Joliffe returned. He beamed at the roomful, said, "Hello, girls. Are you from Bruger's? Well, Gramp! Here again. See you in a few minutes." He beckoned to me and closed his office door.

"You see? It's not one o'clock yet, yet they start crowding in for 1:30 office hours. Find where things are? That batch of girls is from Bruger's—the new employees. I examine for that company. Next Thursday, the Kay Mills will send in their crowd, and Tuesdays in May I promised to examine the boys for the Y.M.C.A. summer camp. We run off about twenty examinations in $2\frac{1}{2}$ hours. I give return appointments for more thorough examinations when it seems indicated. Here's a record. These are the points we cover. You can start getting data any time. Girls strip to the waist and put on those nightingale things in the linen closet. Use both dressing rooms—while one undresses, one is being examined and one is dressing. You'll get on to it."

"Mrs. Pratt called. She is bringing Junior in at three. Skinned knee." I was already clipping my sentences like the doctor!

"Hold everything when she comes. Private patients have priority over these contract jobs. I'll see Gramp Firkin now. His record is in that file— or should be." Doctor indicated the green steel filing cabinet at his right, marked: Current Cases. "Timothy Firkin, 80, lives on the Swamp Road. Arthritis. I'll see him in the examining room."

Dr. Joliffe went into his dressing room. Three minutes later he came into the examining room in a surgeon's spotless white coat with short sleeves. His face shone with cleanliness, his hands were immaculate.

"Here we go—Gramp first. You needn't stay. Get those girls' histories." I sent Gramp in and started my professional service for Dr. Joliffe.

Looking back, I know that afternoon was really a leisurely one. We had no emergencies, no "queer birds," as Doctor called the patients who resisted orders, treatments, and suggestions or came in on faked-up complaints. Alice Taber did not come in and have an epileptic seizure in the waiting room as she was apt to do once a month, until she finally agreed to take "that new medicine" Dr. Joliffe had been prescribing for over a year. Mrs. Pratt was very sweet and considerate and did not issue orders to me, as she has done on many subsequent occasions. The hospital did not send for Doctor to "come at once," the telephone rang only a dozen times, and I did not once have to set up for minor surgery. We did not have a single new private patient requiring a complete "admission examination." "A quiet afternoon," the doctor called it, and went off to his hospital appointment promptly at 4:15. I left a few minutes later, weary, mentally pretty much in a whirl, but thoroughly sold on my new job.

Three of the sixteen girls we examined that day for the Bruger Company were not passed for employment, but requested to return for more complete checkup. Nearly all had bad dental conditions. The doctor told two girls, under seventeen, to stop smoking. I made note of two others so much underweight that we thought the visiting nurse should visit their homes to see what could be done about better meals and more rest for them. One girl, who was overweight, was taken off candy, sodas, and cokes, and one was referred to the hospital clinic for chest x-ray. A worth-while afternoon? Why, there was enough there to keep us going a week, if we had had time to follow up those girls. I kept wondering why Bruger's did not employ an industrial nurse!

Within a week I was accustomed to my new duties and found that in an office of this sort—general practice in a small city—every kind of patient appeared. We had the rich and the poor, the young and the old, medical and surgical conditions, and within that first week a well-defined psychoneurotic case whom Doctor referred to a psychiatrist in a nearby city. I saw advanced skin cancer in an old woman who lived in the hill country and used snuff, diabetes in a child of seven, and pregnancy in an unmarried girl from "one of our best families." I went out with Dr. Joliffe on an emergency call to see old Gramp Firkin, who had a stroke and was dead on our arrival. Measles, fractured bones, and intestinal worms! I was glad I had never specialized. Even at that, the doctor floored me one day by asking me to look up yaws! Yaws! This was what the war did to us, even to a quiet Midwestern town whose boys had been all over the world.

I soon learned several things about Dr. Joliffe's office which I am passing on to you for what they are worth.

If you are in a busy office, try to get the doctor to keep his midweek half holiday—and, of course, his Sundays—free. You can be firm about this with patients and with him. He owes it to himself. Also, it is your great chance to catch up on a lot of things on that half day alone in the office.

Systematize everything that you possibly can in the way of office work, but never try to regiment the patients! Treat each one individually.

Learn to get everything ready for office hours in advance if you can, and then *work fast*. A busy doctor's general practice in a small city has no place for a lazy nurse.

Get to know the patients. The more you know about them, the better you can handle them. You will need to know what goes on in your city in a social way, as well as what resources there are to help people in different kinds of trouble. Of course, you get to know the hospitals, clinics, doctors, and other nurses, especially if you keep in touch with your professional organization.

Don't forget to be systematic about records and bookkeeping. You are the treasurer of a small business—in a way. Get help in setting up a good record, accounting, filing, and billing system if you need it. It will save time in the end.

The most important thing I have kept to the last—your professional service. You are in a doctor's office because you are a nurse. Nursing is your first responsibility. The patient is more important than any other aspect of your work. It is easy to grow careless when pressure is great, the doctor absent, and patients ignorant of what is *good* nursing. Don't let your techniques and standards slip, or you will slip out of the job. Some office nurses manage to take refresher courses.

To my way of thinking, nursing in a general practitioner's office in a small city is the most neighborly service of all and closest to the time-tested pattern of medical care for the whole family. I enjoy it very much.

ETHEL BRIGGS, R.N.[3]

SOURCES OF EMPLOYMENT

1. Professional registries
2. Commercial registries
3. Local medical societies
4. Local hospitals
5. Direct application to the physician, if he has advertised. Suggestions may usually be obtained from the local medical society, including the specialists.
6. Use of advertising pages of professional journals
7. This is one of the fields of service in which a wide circle of friends is an asset in finding employment (see also the suggestions in Chap. II).

BIBLIOGRAPHY

1. BAKKEN, HELEN D.: Clinical Courses for Office Nurses, *American Journal of Nursing*, p. 462, August, 1950.
2. BARBER, GRACE C.: Legal Problems of the Office Nurse, *American Journal of Nursing*, p. 168, March, 1941.
3. BENNETT, RUTH V.: The Nurse-Secretary, *American Journal of Nursing*, p. 360, April, 1943.
4. CAHILL, ANNE F.: Office Nurse, *R.N.*, p. 42, July, 1950.
5. CLINGER, OREL E.: Office Nurses Are Teachers Too, *American Journal of Nursing*, p. 536, September, 1950.
6. DETMOLD, MABEL: Office Nursing, *American Journal of Nursing*, p. 223, April, 1947.
7. MORSE, MINNIE G.: "The Medical Secretary," The Macmillan Company, New York, 1933.
8. PARSONS, ESTHER JANE: "In the Doctor's Office, The Art of the Medical Assistant," J. B. Lippincott Company, Philadelphia, 1945.
9. SCOTT, WILHELMINA A.: Office Nursing Today, *American Journal of Nursing*, p. 19, January, 1951.
10. WOLF, GEORGE D.: "The Physician's Business," 2d ed., J. B. Lippincott Company, Philadelphia, 1945.

[3] Mrs. Briggs prefers not to have the city in which she is working identified.

CHAPTER XV

Nursing Education

Nursing and teaching are the two most popular professions for women, and when you have prepared yourself to fill the role of both nurse and teacher you really have something to count on as a life career. "The young graduate with vision and capacity for leadership can make an important contribution to the profession by entering this field."[1] With the proper preparation through advanced courses and supervised experience, many nurses have attained a position of academic distinction in nursing education along with satisfying financial returns. Nursing education is definitely a field with a future. At the moment, its need of qualified personnel on all levels and in all specialties is greater than in most of the other fields of nursing. In schools of nursing alone, there are more than five thousand full-time instructors.

Although our aim is to consider every nurse a teacher, those who are filling positions in nursing education must prepare themselves as teachers in a formal sense. There is just as much likelihood of your being a "born teacher" as there was in your being a "born nurse." You like to nurse and you wanted to care for sick people, but that did not make you a nurse. You want to teach and you enjoy showing people how to do things, but that does not make you a teacher. However, the important first thing to decide is just that: Do you like to teach? If you do, and your scholastic standing throughout your school life has been good, talk over the question with your faculty adviser. Before the end of your course she might be able to try you out in an easy teaching assignment with students or auxiliary workers. For, after all, the way to learn to teach is to teach. There is nothing like actual experience to find out whether you can

[1] "Choose a Career in Nursing Education" (leaflet), National League of Nursing Education.

express yourself simply, explain facts clearly, and meet the unspoken questions, as well as the spoken ones, in your students' minds. It is well to have a taste of actual teaching before investing heavily in the necessary college courses. Many nurses like to "show how to do things," but when it comes to digging in and mastering a subject, organizing it in a logical way to present in successive class periods, and then patiently, skillfully, and tactfully drawing out from the students what is not clear to them and finding a new and better way of helping them learn—that is another matter. Teaching takes training and hard work. Like nursing, it has techniques of its own which you must learn to apply under varying conditions and with all kinds of students. Think of the best teacher you ever had, and you will recall that she or he had not only complete command of the subject being taught but also such skill in presenting it that your interest was roused and you learned in spite of yourself. He or she "inspired" you to learn.

The opportunities for teaching in nursing cover a range so wide that almost every taste can be satisfied. In your own school of nursing—indeed, quite possibly in high school or college—you have seen nurses teaching. You have seen them in formal classes, demonstration rooms, on the wards, at the bedside, in groups, and in individual conferences. After graduation you will see qualified nurse-teachers in the fields of specialties—public health, for example—as well as in various institutions which require nurse-educators for combined service and teaching responsibilities, as in teachers colleges, or in universities and colleges as faculty members, heads of departments, or deans of nursing education.

A fairly recent and expanding development in the teaching field is instruction in schools of practical nursing. At the present time there are about 150 of these schools, employing some 250 nurse-teachers, full or part time. This will be, many believe, a growing demand. Special preparation for professional nurses who plan to teach practical nurses is considered desirable. There are several universities offering special courses in this general area of interest. The National League of Nursing Education has information about them.[2]

The recent use of volunteers, practical nurses, and other auxiliary workers has augmented the need for supervisors—supervisors who must know how to teach as well as supervise and guide. Army and Navy nurses who have had experience in teaching corpsmen, medical technicians, and others may wish to develop their abilities and qualify for this field.

[2] For the addresses of all organizations mentioned in this chapter, see Appendix A.

It is thought that at least 25 per cent of each year's crop of graduate nurses should go into positions of responsibility as teachers, supervisors, and executives.[3] Much will depend on the skill with which student nurses are selected and encouraged to enter this field. Supervisors often ask how to find the potential teachers. Unfortunately, there is no test or criterion by which to predict the successful teacher. As Miss Stewart points out, "Many aspects of character and personality still defy objective measurement, however, and even if all the facts could be known the incalculable events of life would still conspire to upset many promising plans and careers."[4]

Certain it is that nurses should "like to teach," that they should have poise, emotional control, mature judgment, patience, and the ability to lead group thinking. They should possess that type of intellectual curiosity and integrity which keeps them seeking for the best, truest, and freshest subject matter in their special field, supported by the ability to make practical application of it to actual situations presented by the students. Nothing in nursing education is quite so tragic as the teacher who is a pure theorist and cannot demonstrate or apply her knowledge to the care of sick people or to the prevention of disease in homes and hospitals.

Teaching should not be thought of as an escape from the realities of hospital, home, and clinic situations. If that is your thought in entering this branch of nursing, it would be better for all concerned if you prepared yourself to teach an academic subject not directly concerned with sick people and forgot your nurse's preparation entirely. Student nurses and young graduates are very quick to detect failure on the part of their teachers to give practicable, possible, and simple information in answer to their questions. They expect their teachers to know the current developments and changes that affect the patients and families in their care and to suggest feasible approaches to the solution of their problems. The successful teacher never stops learning. So if you do not relish a life of reading, study, observation, and eager seeking after more knowledge from your students, your friends, and your travels, don't try to become a teacher!

Another responsibility which teaching brings to the teacher is the expenditure—sometimes in fairly sizable amounts—of personal funds to supply needed up-to-date information. Not only subscription to the pro-

[3] STEWART, ISABEL M.: "The Education of Nurses," p. 333, The Macmillan Company, New York, 1943.
[4] *Ibid.*, p. 343.

fessional journals and the purchase of books are implied in this statement, but often travel, at one's own expense, to sources of worth-while information, or pertinent activities such as annual meetings, workshops, or the like. The wise teacher does not stint herself in these essentials.

Considerable impetus has been given in the past few years to advanced preparation of instructors for the clinical specialties through Federal appropriations to nursing education. Institutes, "refresher courses," and workshops, as well as full-time academic courses, have been sponsored and the expenses of qualified instructors and students borne by government funds. How many opportunities of this sort will be available in the next few years is problematic. Most up-to-date information on these possibilities and on qualifications to be met may be secured from the Chief Nurse Officer, Office of the Surgeon General, U.S. Public Health Service. (For other scholarship opportunities, see Chap. I.)

Typical Teaching Opportunities

A few of the positions with teaching responsibilities, for which preparation as well as experience is required, are cited here just as testimony to the variety of opportunity awaiting qualified instructors. A description of teaching responsibilities as an instructor in Vanderbilt University sees them is presented on the pages following. (See Chap. V for the impressions of an instructor in obstetric nursing.)

1. Instructor in one of the clinical specialties, or in general nursing (nursing arts) in a school of nursing (example: surgical nursing)
2. Instructor in one of the nonclinical courses (example: chemistry)
3. Director (or professor), teaching a specialty in a university on the postgraduate level
4. Educational director in public health nursing agencies of all types at both state and local levels
5. Instructor of students in health, home nursing, or other related course in a teachers college or the public school system
6. Instructor of practical nurses in an approved school of practical nursing
7. Instructor of nurses preparing to teach Red Cross home nursing classes
8. Dean, director, or other chief nurse in charge of nursing departments in schools of nursing, universities, Federal or other national agencies, and her assistant

9. Special lecturer (this may be a part-time or "visiting lecturer" assignment—anywhere, and may consist in a few lectures, a "workshop,"
   an "institute," or a full series of lectures covering the academic year)
10. Educational consultant in programs of study, curriculum planning, or
    advisory service to schools in a national or state agency, such as on
    a state board of nurse examiners

The directors of the schools of nursing are well-prepared nurses who
can present academic qualifications, wide experience, and administrative
ability. This is true of the directors appointed in all schools, but especially
so of the schools connected with colleges and universities. (A list of
schools offering advanced programs to students leading to a degree in
universities or colleges may be secured from the National Nursing Accrediting Service.) Qualifications for directors should be reviewed from
time to time, as they are growing steadily stiffer.

The director of a large school of nursing has more responsibility for
administration than for teaching, but she must be equipped to secure a
satisfactory faculty and must be able to assume direction of the total
program of study or curriculum plan, unless she delegates this to her
assistant. In the smaller schools the director teaches several of the formal
courses and must sometimes substitute for other members of her staff
in times of emergency or shortages.

The nurse seeking her first experience in teaching will be wise to accept
a part-time, evening, or summer-school assignment in order to gain
confidence and be able to say that she has had some experience in the
actual handling of classes. Later, "exchange professorships," summer
courses, workshop, or special lecture requests may be accepted to add
variety, as well as experience, to a full-time teaching job.

In teaching, rather more than in other fields, the acceptance of requests to write, speak, serve on committees, or make special surveys
yields rich returns. These responsibilities serve not only to enlarge the
teacher's circle of friends—always helpful to a future job seeker—but to
widen her knowledge of the current problems in the nursing field. A
teacher tends to suffer from a narrowing horizon and the boredom of a
certain amount of inevitable repetition. Her off-duty and spare hours
should be as recreational as possible.

Something also should be said for the other less formal means of learning to teach and teach well. The university and one's field supervisor
should not have to take the full responsibility for supplying knowledge

and skills. The astute young teacher will read everything she can get her hands on relating to her field, will map out her own reading course, and will travel, visit, and observe nursing activities in her selected field whenever the chance arises. Evening lectures, attendance at national conventions, and even an occasional home study course, all have a part in "furnishing her head richly."

Nursing also stands greatly in need of trained research workers who are *nurses*. The equivalent of preparation for teaching is essential and, in most instances, a research worker must have the M.A. degree, preferably a Ph.D. Courses in statistics and statistical method as well as in the methodology of research are necessary. Nursing is fast outgrowing its adolescence, it is becoming a mature profession with enough history to make the study of its growth, changing aspects, and future possibilities a rich field for research and evaluation. Attention is called to this field because if you enjoy study, gain satisfaction from digging out facts, and like to analyze and synthesize your findings and apply them—then you may be the nurse who should head for a research job. We need this type of ability as much as any one kind of talent in nursing. Talk over your ideas with your faculty advisers. Get the best guidance you can. Research is one field in which competent workers are quite apt to find generous fellowships, study grants, and scholarships available.

The teaching field is an attractive one. The following conversation among a few students describes how a clinical instructor feels about it.

I Want to Be a Clinical Instructor

(CONVERSATION OF FIVE STUDENTS)

The students: JOAN } seniors
LOUISE

IRENE } juniors
PEG

BESS, a freshman, Joan's "little sister"

The place: Joan's room
The time: Evening

BESS (*entering*): Joan, will you help me answer this letter from a friend at home? She is a senior in high school and wants to know all about nursing.

JOAN: Sure, that's an easy one! Sit down.

BESS: The problem isn't "to be or not to be"; she has always wanted to be a nurse. She's the right type, she has brains, her father is a doctor, and since I've been writing to her from here, she is more eager than ever about the plan. The only catch is that she is anxious to hurry up and get started at once, but her father and the vocational counselor at school want her to go to a collegiate school of nursing. She is just rarin' to get into a hospital next year, and has asked me for my advice as though I were the voice of experience.

JOAN: There really isn't any doubt in your mind about what to say, is there, Bess? Tell her the college life will be fun and extra time will fly by fast. She'll actually be nursing before she knows it and be finished before she knows what happened. If she is made of good stuff and really ambitious, she won't want to sacrifice the good basic foundation of some liberal arts education to anything as common as speed. It is like comparing quality and quantity. We need more *good* nurses—people who are capable of learning and giving total nursing care. Somebody going into the hospital just doesn't have enough in back of her to learn that kind of nursing over night.

LOUISE (*entering*): 'Scuse please, but that sounded pretty good all the way over in my room! I am looking for points for the editorial in next month's *Chatter Sheet*. What prompted that remark?

JOAN: That's a newshound for you! Louise Hear-all, Tell-all!

BESS: Well, I'll explain, Louise. Joan is helping me convince a girl at home that she should have an eye to the future and plan to go to a collegiate school of nursing and not just a 3-year program.

IRENE (*entering*): Just in time for a bull session! College preparation, some say, is a matter of opinion. My sister, for instance, says it depends on what you do when you graduate.

LOUISE: There is only one answer to that! Everybody wants to get married, and if you aim to marry anybody that *is* anybody, you need to have some college background so you can at least read and talk intelligently!

JOAN: I can't argue that point—but we are just about to graduate and, if you will allow me to repeat myself, I'll say, "If you are going to be a nurse, be a good one."

IRENE: I agree.

BESS: Well, while we are on the subject, Joan, what are you going to do when you finish?

IRENE: I'm going to nominate Joan for Congress.

LOUISE: Wait, you are getting into the subject we are featuring in *Chatter Sheet* 2 months from now: "Seniors' Plans for the Future!" So, Joannie dear, prepare to make a statement for the press.

JOAN: Well, I want to be a clinical instructor. There is a terrific need for them and I rather like the idea.

LOUISE: That's not news to me. I knew you would be a teacher since the day you helped me learn anatomy. What subject are you going to teach?

JOAN: I'm not going to teach a subject, I'm going to teach girls—quoth my Latin professor in high school.

BESS: That reminds me of Miss James. She is wonderful. She makes me feel as though she really cared about me and wants me to learn. That's my idea of a real teacher.

IRENE: You know, Joan, I think you should give that idea more serious thought. You are smart enough, don't misunderstand me, but I never think of you as the studious, bookworm, absent-minded professor type. You seem interested in everything.

JOAN: Oh, Irene, your characterization of a teacher is strictly story-bookish! I'm going to be the well-adjusted, normal, human type.

LOUISE: Well, we wouldn't have elected you as president of Student Council if we hadn't thought you well-adjusted and something of an example and leader, and no fool either!

JOAN: Thanks, pal!

IRENE: But I've always imagined teaching was rather a stuffy life, and you seem so alive, Joan!

PEG (*entering*): Pardon me for knocking, but you girls should have seen Miss McDonald at the concert! She has a new hair-do and was that dress a dream! She is practically a "slick chick!" She was with that law professor.

JOAN: You see, Miss McDonald is not stuffy and she is one of our best teachers! I am sure they lead so-called normal lives. Irene, I think we get the idea that our teachers are stuffy because we see only the school side of their lives.

LOUISE: There's an idea for *Chatter Sheet!* "The Human Side of the Faculty." Maybe we could dig up a little scandal!

JOAN: It's a good thing we don't take you seriously, Louise.

PEG: But they do have lives of their own.

I suppose if you are going to guide our young students—like Bess, here—to be professional women and superior nurses, you've got to be a well-rounded person yourself and a good citizen. The students must admire you and have confidence in you, if you are going to do a really effective job of teaching.

BESS: Oh, Joan, I think that's marvelous and I know *you* will make a good teacher. But what does a clinical instructor do? What kind of teaching is it?

JOAN: She is a person who teaches us right on the ward and decides what experience we should have. She plans with the doctor when he gives us lectures and arranges the schedule. She makes out our assignments and helps plan our activities: in other words, she recognizes and capitalizes on the learning situations the patients offer.

Some schools have nurses called supervisors who teach the students and also supervise the graduates and are responsible for meeting the service needs of the hospital. I don't think education is the same as service. I think we have the best system here, where the people responsible for education are not responsible for service, because learning needs are not always the same as service needs. So I plan to be a clinical instructor giving full time to teaching.

BESS: Isn't it an awfully hard job?

JOAN: Well, it isn't particularly easy. It'll take time, but it is interesting. Of course, it's a full-time job and you have to apply yourself. But you can devote your energies to *teaching*, and that is what I want to do. Others with you have the responsibility of servicing the hospital. You are free to be with the students whenever they need your help. There's a lot of variety, you know. You teach classes, give examinations, and grade papers, and you do a lot of individual and practical teaching when you are right there to help the student take care of a patient in bed. I think that is the most important and the most fascinating kind of teaching—at the bedside—because that is where the student really learns nursing care, and that is where she needs an instructor to help her. You help the students learn how to talk with the patients and how to teach them to take care of themselves at home. And you do this both on the wards and in clinic. So you see you don't do dry, stale, "platform" teaching because you teach right where the patients are. Even though I want to teach, I don't want ever to get away from the patients. This way, you are still doing nursing and working directly with patients.

IRENE: How will you ever learn to do all of that?

JOAN: Well, naturally, I don't have it all figured out on a calendar, but I have a general plan. First, after graduation, I'm going to do general duty in a hospital. I think that is basic experience which we should all have, no matter what type of nursing we are going to do. It gives us a chance to practice what we have learned and time to grow. It is a different slant from being a student and I don't want to skip any type of experience. I want to get a complete education and, of course, I want to do some night duty. I believe I'd like to stay here for that.

IRENE: Oh, no; if I'm going to do general duty, I want to go somewhere else! Joan, don't you really want to move to new pastures?

JOAN: No, I don't think it is necessary right after graduation. It just means adjusting to a new situation and I'm not anxious to learn new techniques and routines. I want to streamline what I've already learned, and add depth and meaning to my nursing. That will be my new horizon for the present. Of course, I want some experience as a head nurse. You have to work with the people on the wards. If you haven't actually had that experience, you are likely to be too theoretical and not understand the practical problems that come up every day.

PEG: Don't you think that you could learn a lot by working as an assistant in clinical teaching?

JOAN: Definitely. If you can work with a good person, it would be excellent experience. I think also that I should have some more experience in public health or visiting nursing so I can help the students appreciate the problems in home situations and the value of preventing disease. Very few patients are well when they leave the hospital; they don't leave their sickness here, they take it home with them. I want to study the different types of patients in their home environments. Then I'll be better equipped to pass on to my students the philosophy that patients come from and go to homes and families, that they are not isolated individuals—and that their environment greatly influences them.

LOUISE: Sounds like a long road to me! We can't print all that in one issue!

JOAN: No, and it won't happen all in one year! It takes time and growing and, as Miss Robinson says, "mellowing."

BESS: Then you will have to go to school some more after you finish here?

JOAN: Yes, this is a basic education that we get here. I will need some special preparation for teaching. I plan to get a master's degree after I've had more ward experience.

BESS: Where will you go to school?

JOAN: I am not sure. I want to look around to see where I can get what I will need. But this I do know: when I go to school, I am going all out for it. I'm not going to try to do two things at one time. Working and going to school at the same time mean that you do part of each. If you are really working, it is a full-time job. And when you go to school, you need to get away from your work so you have time to think, develop your philosophy, and grow some new thoughts. You get a different perspective and see your work with new eyes.

BESS: Why don't you go right on to school next year?

JOAN: I want to work first. That gives me a chance to get on my own feet. You need to see a few of the problems to know what you want to get out of school. You can't just sit in a class expecting your teachers to pour it out, while you soak it up like a blotter. The best education is the kind you go after.

PEG: Are you going to have to save for your education as soon as you start working? You'll be a brain, but poor all your life!

JOAN: Well, I like to hope that I'll get some help. If I can start on the right foot in a place that has a good school and they think I'm worth my salt, they might help me to get better prepared, with the understanding that I'd come back to them and teach. Then, there are scholarships and loans.

IRENE: I'll have to admit you certainly have mapped out your future. But I can't decide whether I want to work all my life, or study all my life.

JOAN: That's funny! Since when did we entirely separate the two? I'm planning to combine those two activities; that is the thing about being a clinical instructor. You have to study some, but also you are in a practical situation at the same time, teaching the students right there on the ward and in the out-patient department.

IRENE: Well, I know one thing, I don't want to do the same thing over and over again.

JOAN: And I have the right answer for that one, too! I'll have contact with the patients. I'll have a chance to see them come in. They'll be sick; nobody will know what is wrong with them; tests will be run; I'll be explaining the tests to the students and helping them to do their part. Then I'll be helping the student explain procedures and tests to the patient so he won't be bewildered and his part will be easier for him. I'll help the student understand the interpretation and soon the doctor will know the diagnosis. That will be another chapter for explanations and understandings. And then there will be the treatment and I'll show the student how, and the patient will get better and we'll get him ready to go home. But it will never be a repeat performance. Every student will have a different response, some will learn fast, some slowly. I wouldn't want to teach the same old thing over and over again out of the same old books.

Working with real people will always be interesting. And there would be just enough experiments and new developments to be stimulating and challenging. Right now it is cardiac catheterization; next year it will be something else. I really think it is exciting to see new treatments giving new hope to people! And, in teaching, you get in on the ground floor of some of these things—that is, of course, provided you are in a progressive school, and who wants to be in any other kind? Yes, I think every year there would be just enough repetition to give you a chance to improve and enough new things to keep you on your toes. It would mean working along with the doctors and knowing about new drugs and treatments; and working along with the social workers, dietitians, and other nurses. You would have to know who's who in the community social and health agencies, know their policies, and keep up with changes in their programs. Oh, I think it would be thrilling!

PEG: Have you thought about the field you'd like?

JOAN: I believe it will be medicine. I think that is the field where nursing care is really important, so it is the best place to teach quality nursing. It isn't as dramatic as obstetrics and surgery or as much fun, maybe, as pediatrics. But it is difficult and a real challenge to your intellect. So many patients have chronic diseases and all the social and personality and economic problems that go along with them—all requiring expert nursing. You have a chance to study the patient himself, and work with him. Your focus is on the patient rather than on nursing techniques and procedures. I'm talking about the kind of illness where nursing is really important. Most important of all are the conditions being studied and treated now as psychosomatic disorders. The nurse is often the key person in the team—she works so closely with the patient. The nurse-patient relationship that is established is important, it can't be just incidental, and it puts real responsibility on the nurse. She can be a vital contributor in such things as observation and treatment, or if she is careless she can throw a monkey wrench in the works.

You have to have the ability to give excellent bedside care and, at the same time, recognize and deal with personality and social problems. You have to be sensitive to the patient's moods. It is relatively simple to learn mechanical duties and routine tasks, but the problems of these patients call for a truly intelligent and skillful nurse.

Sometimes your work includes diversional activities; sometimes it is health teaching; sometimes you mother a patient and let him depend on you; sometimes you have to know how to encourage his independence; and on and on—with each person it is different. Each demands real skill on the part of the nurse; that is the most stimulating and satisfying nursing. Therefore it is the best place to teach real, true, comprehensive nursing care.

BESS: Well, I want to do some work in which I can see results. I want to have the satisfaction of knowing I've done something.

JOAN: But that is just what you have in teaching! You teach a group of students just like us; you can actually see improvement and growth! I would expect to experience a sense of satisfaction with each group. I like students. I would like to work with one group after another of people like us. I can't think of anything more satisfying. It will be fun and keep me young.

PEG: One of the things I like about teaching is the idea of working with people, instead of with things, and studying people. However, I don't really think that I would care too much to grade and evaluate students. That's a very tough assignment and takes a lot of ability to size things up.

JOAN: The ability to evaluate is very important for the instructor to have and, of course, as you use it, you improve and develop better judgment of values. But you have to be really interested in students, and impersonal about it. You can't just flunk them because you don't like them, or give an "A" to everybody you like.

LOUISE: I guess the secret of success along that line is respect for the individual. You must give the student the right to be an individual and not ignore the fact that she is a person. The teacher should find the best that is in the student and work on that to develop whatever capabilities she may have.

JOAN: Yes, the instructor must be willing to listen to the student and consider her point of view. You can't teach by dictating. I want to work along with the students, show them, and explain a point so they know it for themselves and it becomes part of them. I want to convince them of the importance of what they are learning and doing, and, at the same time, give them a feeling of security and a sense of confidence in themselves. I've promised myself always to be approachable and ready to listen. I hope I'll be the kind of person the students will naturally confide in. I want them to respect me, but not be afraid of me.

IRENE: The thing I would like about teaching would be the associations. You would meet some interesting people.

JOAN: Especially when you are in a university school. Nursing is an important profession and the students should be in an educational and cultural center.

PEG: Speaking of meeting interesting people brings me back to the subject of marriage. There is Mrs. Mason. I'll have to admit she proves that you can be married and teach—that is if you are going to work at all after you are married.

LOUISE: I have another comment in support of teaching. When you teach you can branch out into writing if you have a flair for it. I think books ought to be written by people who handle the material day by day.

JOAN: Yes, and besides writing there are other things that fit with teaching. It seems that teachers do most of the research and that is what really makes progress in the profession. But as yet I am not hitching my wagon to all those stars!

One thing is sure, there is no stopping point in nursing. It is not a crowded field, you can go as high and as far as you want to. Nobody limits you or ever tells you to quit. You can improve the place where you are, or you can go on to bigger and better jobs.

PEG: That's well and good, but I want to travel. There is so much in the world that I haven't seen.

JOAN: Then you should be a clinical instructor! You don't have to stay in the same school forever, there are positions open all over the country. And besides the United States, they want experienced teachers in many foreign countries, especially if you can speak another language.

PEG: That's one of the amazing things about nursing, you can do almost any type of work and go almost any place—the world is the limit.

BESS: Do you think you have to be born to teach nursing or can anybody learn how to teach?

JOAN: I like to think of it as a happy medium. True, we say some people are born teachers, and they seem to have some of the innate qualities, but that isn't all of it. You must be able to think clearly, be able to explain, and have an abundance of patience. You'd have to enjoy studying and learning and get a kick out of mental discoveries, both in your own mind and in the minds of the students. It seems that when you teach you create, and you also encourage the students to do creative thinking. Teaching and learning are really like sharing an adventure. Of course, I think it is essential that you want to teach. No matter how brainy you are, if you don't like it, you won't be a success. You never can do your best work if you don't enjoy what you are doing.

PEG: Well, Joan, let me put my blessing upon you and wish you well, and at the same time remind you that all of us aren't brilliant and perfect. So please be tolerant, and don't forget we were all young once so we all make mistakes, and some of us are slow to catch on.

JOAN: Tolerance is a good word and I am glad you mentioned it. And now I'll tell you a secret: I am writing my memoirs. They give my feelings and views *as a student*. I plan to get them out once in a while when I am teaching and remember how it feels to be a student. I don't want ever to forget. Even though some of my ideas are wrong, nevertheless I guess they are typical of students and can't be ignored. I don't want to be a boss or a policeman, or go around catching people doing the wrong things. I want to guide and give them a chance to learn and help them apply what they learn.

BESS: To come down to earth, Joan, how do the hours of duty of an instructor compare with hours of other nurses?

JOAN: Our instructors here more or less plan their own time. As I understand it, the Dean has confidence in their ability to plan and manage their schedules, just as they do their work. They come on duty early, or when we need them in the afternoons they are there then. I think it is a matter of good planning and being on hand at the right time. In fact, their life seems very civilized to me; they don't have to punch a time clock day in and day out, year after year. They don't have a job—they have a position!

IRENE: I think I would like the vacation that teachers get because they get Thanksgiving, Christmas, and spring holidays, besides a real summer vacation.

PEG: Another thing I like about teaching is the happy combination of being a boss and being bossed at the same time. Our teachers work together on the larger problems, and they get help and advice from the higher-ups when they need it.

IRENE: How much money can you make? That seems to me an important item!

JOAN: Salaries vary in different parts of the country, but they compare favorably with those of other college instructors.

PEG: You know, the more I think of it, the more I think it is a good mixture of many types of work. You have to know human nature and be able to help the students with all sorts of problems. I think every teacher needs to be an expert in guidance.

JOAN: Absolutely. It looks like a mighty big order! It's not a job but a career.

BESS: Well, Joan, when I asked you to help me answer this letter, I didn't know we'd get into all this, but I'm glad we did. Thanks for giving me a glimpse of your future. And now I guess I'd better go answer that letter: "If you are going to be a nurse, be a good one!"

JOAN: That goes for clinical instructors, too! Good night!

BESS: Sweet dreams to you!

VIRGINIA P. CRENSHAW, R.N.
Associate Professor of Nursing
Vanderbilt University
Nashville, Tennessee

PREPARATION FOR TEACHING

In general, preparation for a full-time teaching position calls for satisfactory completion of basic nursing preparation, a bachelor's degree from a recognized university, and advanced study in the field of the specialty you plan to teach. Most authorities agree that student nurses should plan on a year of experience after graduation from the school of nursing before entering a college program or looking for a teaching position which may be accompanied by academic study. Ideally, teaching experience should start as an assistant to a well-qualified instructor. Good advice is to devote undivided time to getting some experience after graduation, followed by a year of study, and a first teaching position as an assistant instructor.

There is, however, great difference in the way in which the young graduate may approach this field, much depending on the stage of her academic accomplishment at the time of her graduation, her age, and the available resources. The best advice should be sought before signing up for either a job involving teaching or a course preparatory to it. It is highly desirable that formal academic work in preparation for teaching start within a year or two of graduation from a school of nursing. Formal teaching experience prior to entering a school of nursing places the nurse in an advantageous position if she plans to serve in the field of nursing education, as it will shorten the period of preparation necessary in many cases and give her greater confidence in the classroom.

For the advanced positions a master's degree with courses in administration (or supervision) is expected. In the future, it is quite likely that the highest academic appointments will be open only to those who have completed their work for a doctorate (Doctor of Philosophy, Ph.D.).

Public health nurses planning to prepare themselves to direct university programs of study should offer, in addition to the basic year of study in public health nursing, advanced university courses in general education, supervision, and administration in public health nursing. Also, their qualifications should include a minimum of 5 years' experience, preferably in more than one agency, 1 year of which should have been in a general public health nursing agency with direct, qualified supervision, emphasizing family health. This period should include experience as a staff nurse, supervisor, and as an executive or educational director.[5]

In summary, to become a qualified instructor of nursing in any field of nursing education requires the registered nurse to have (*a*) a college degree, (*b*) at least 6 months of supervised experience (and preferably a year of experience before advanced college work), and (*c*) advanced study in a clinical specialty, supervision, or administration. Additional experience and study (with a master's degree as a minimum) are required for appointment to the more advanced positions and those involving administrative and consultant duties.

As has been said, experience cannot be overrated. Experience as a staff nurse in a hospital, public health agency, or in private practice in a hospital of 6 months to a year is recommended before academic work is undertaken, while additional experience is a prerequisite to advanced courses. Three to five years is a minimum period of experience to offer for promotion to administrative and teaching responsibilities. The top positions in teaching, as elsewhere, are seldom available to nurses with less than 8 years between them and their school of nursing.

Duties of the directors or deans of schools of nursing have now been quite clearly defined. Because these obligations are seldom seen as a whole by students and young graduate nurses, the functions as formulated by the New York State Nurses Association may be of interest:[6]

1. Defining and interpreting the purposes and policies of the school
2. Setting up and administering the budget
3. Maintaining effective and harmonious working relationships with the personnel of the school and the staffs of the institutions and agencies with which the school is connected

[5] For faculty preparation for teaching the health and social aspects of nursing to students in schools of nursing, see the discussion in the *American Journal of Nursing*, p. 564, July, 1945, and refer to the National League of Nursing Education for the most recent statement of requirements in this rapidly developing educational field.

[6] *New York State Nurse*, pp. 24–25, October, 1947.

4. Selecting and recommending for appointment the members of the educational and administrative personnel of the school defining their respective responsibilities and relationships

5. Co-operating in the establishment of policies which will assure security of tenure, adequate remuneration, and acceptable working conditions for the school personnel and maintaining a record system which indicates the qualifications, experience, and accomplishment of each member of the staff

6. Arranging for and conducting regular staff conferenecs for policy-forming and problem-solving in areas of joint faculty responsibility

7. Arranging for and participating in programs of in-service education, including the orientation of new members of the staff; also encouraging and facilitating advanced study on the part of the personnel of the school so that they may qualify themselves for promotion and for the acceptance of increased responsibility

8. Setting up standards for admission and recruiting candidates who are eligible for enrollment

9. Setting up the curriculum, determining the general objectives and sequence of courses, planning the teaching schedule, and providing for the co-ordination of theory and practice

10. Arranging for experience in the clinical departments of the hospital and other practice fields in accordance with the plan set forth in the curriculum

11. Making provision for adequate classroom, laboratory, library and other facilities necessary for carrying out the educational program

12. Seeking and arranging for affiliation with various institutions and agencies in order to provide experience not otherwise available

13. Maintaining a comprehensive system of records showing the theoretical instruction and the experience afforded each student, personal characteristics and special aptitudes of each student, and the nature and quality of her accomplishment

14. Providing for a counseling program which will be helpful to the student in solving her problems

15. Arranging for a positive health service (including the maintenance of complete health records) and for the student care during illness

16. Securing attractive and healthful housing and living conditions for students and affording opportunities for cultural and social activities

17. Insuring reasonable hours and other conditions favorable to effective learning

18. Keeping closely in touch with the activities of the alumnae association and enlisting the co-operation of its members in promoting the interest of the school
19. Arranging for publicity concerning the school by means of announcements, bulletins and other appropriate measures
20. Maintaining cordial relationships with the community at large and especially with those groups which are directly associated with education and social welfare
21. Carrying on a continuous analysis, evaluation, and adaptation of the entire educational and administrative program

The requirements for the field of nursing education change rather constantly. The reader is advised to seek the best counsel obtainable before charting her course. Not only the adviser in the school of nursing should be consulted, but also the director of the program of study in the university of your choice. Valuable time and money may be lost by choosing the wrong institution to give you basic preparation for the specialty, or the course chosen may prove to be largely a repetition of what you may have had in your own hospital or postgraduate experience. Occasionally, exemption or credit may be granted for what you have already had. The secret to rapid and pertinent preparation for a specialty in a nursing field is consultation and planning with the best-informed advisers you can find. The National League of Nursing Education is the fountainhead of information on this subject.[7] Up-to-date information regarding scholarships may also be secured from the League, if not obtainable locally.[8]

Positions not strictly in the field of *nursing* education, but for which your teaching preparation will stand you in good stead in case a transfer from nursing becomes necessary, are

General teaching
Private tutoring
Library work[9]

[7] Besides obtaining the latest League statement on qualifications of faculty in schools of nursing, see also Qualifications of Public Health Nursing Faculty and Teaching Personnel, *Public Health Nursing*, March, 1951.

[8] The *American Journal of Nursing* carries a list of currently available courses in its advertising pages. Before selecting a course, read Chap. I of this book.

[9] Information may be secured from the American Library Association (for the address, see Appendix A).

Positions as social directors, deans of women, student personnel
    directors[10]
General personnel work
Research work
Journalism
Health education

SALARIES

Initial salaries in this field are (1950) in the neighborhood of $2,800
to $3,800; salaries paid in the advanced positions start at $3,600 and run
to $8,600 without maintenance. It may be said that in this branch of
nursing—teaching—additional academic preparation usually *does* pay.
Salaries are higher for the better prepared nurses.

This is also a field in which it is possible to do part-time work, or to
take on short, well-paid assignments in the breaks of summer vacations.
Overfatigue must be guarded against, however, as teaching is far more
demanding than the class schedule would lead one to think.

Because schools of nursing employ many of the instructors, the 1945
salaries as reported to the *American Journal of Nursing* are given here.

Salaries paid in schools of nursing in 1945, *in addition* to full maintenance:

Position	Range
Director	$4,400–$7,500
Assistant	3,200– 4,300
Supervisor	2,800– 3,500
Instructor	3,000– 4,000
Head nurse who teaches	2,500– 3,500
Ward instructor	2,500– 3,000

Salaries paid to those who receive no maintenance are $450 to $800
higher. In view of present living costs, the salary of the nurse who "lives
in" represents a better value than the one paid to the nurse who tries to
"live out" and pay her rent, food, laundry, telephone, and transportation
to and from her work. As long ago as 1928, it was pointed out that the
"living" received in the hospital was probably worth twice the allowance

[10] Refer to Council of Guidance and Personnel Associations (for the address, see
Appendix A).

to "live out" ($500 a year). The U.S. Treasury Department estimates the value of living costs provided by institutions to be from $35 to $60 a month (1945 figures).

Where to Secure Teaching Positions

This depends upon the field for which you are prepared. In general, sources of information regarding positions are the national nursing organizations, Federal services, and professional placement agencies. Direct application may be made to universities, schools of nursing, and public health agencies. Generally the nursing and hospital journals carry advertisements of teaching vacancies. The best approach is probably through the university guidance service where you have your advanced academic work. You will also find suggestions as to sources of employment at the end of the chapters in this book dealing with the specialties.

BIBLIOGRAPHY

1. Advanced Courses in Clinical Nursing, *American Journal of Nursing*, p. 579, June, 1944. (Some definitions and guiding principles.)
2. BECK, Sister M. BERENICE: Educating Nurses for the Specialties, *American Journal of Nursing*, p. 149, February, 1943.
3. BREDENBERG, VIOLA C.: Experimental Research in Nursing Service, *American Journal of Nursing*, p. 661, October, 1950.
4. BUNGE, HELEN L.: Clinical Rotations, An Aspect of Curriculum Building, *American Journal of Nursing*, p. 137, February, 1945.
5. CABOT, HUGH: Future of Nursing Education, *Modern Hospital*, pp. 47–48, February, 1943.
6. GELINAS, AGNES: "Nursing and Nursing Education," p. 36, Commonwealth Fund, Division of Publication, New York, 1946.
7. HEIDGERKEN, LORETTA A.: "Teaching in Schools of Nursing," J. B. Lippincott Company, Philadelphia, 1946.
8. KLARMAN, HERBERT E.: Prerequisites for Research in Nursing, *American Journal of Nursing*, p. 780, December, 1949.
9. McMANUS, R. LOUISE: Advanced Preparation for Nursing, *Public Health Nursing*, p. 470, September, 1949.
10. MURPHY, MARION: Do You Want to Be a Lady Professor? *Public Health Nursing*, p. 658, December, 1949.
11. NATIONAL COMMITTEE FOR THE IMPROVEMENT OF NURSING SERVICE: "Nursing Schools at the Mid-Century," New York, 1950.
12. Post Graduate Nursing Education, Some Definitions, *American Journal of Nursing*, p. 1058, December, 1945.

13. REED, ELIZABETH: Glad Return to Ivied Towers, *Public Health Nursing,* p. 432, August, 1949.
14. REITER, FRANCES: Preparation of Clinical Instructors, *American Journal of Nursing,* p. 1066, November, 1944.
15. Research in Nursing (editorial), *American Journal of Nursing,* p. 743, December, 1949.
16. SPARROW, ALMA G.: What a Public Health Coordinator Does, *American Journal of Nursing,* p. 130, February, 1951.
17. STEWART, ISABEL M.: "The Education of Nurses," Chap. VIII, The Macmillan Company, New York, 1943. See also, by the same author, A Half Century of Nursing Education, *American Journal of Nursing,* p. 617, October, 1950.
18. TAYLOR, ANNA M.: "Ward Teaching," J. B. Lippincott Company, Philadelphia, 1941.
19. Types of Clinical Courses for Graduate Nurses, *American Journal of Nursing,* p. 1162, December, 1944.
20. WAYLAND, MARY MARVIN, R. LOUISE McMANUS, and MARGENE FADDIS: "The Hospital Head Nurse," 2d ed., The Macmillan Company, New York, 1944.
21. WILLIAMS, DOROTHY ROGERS: "Administration of Schools of Nursing," The Macmillan Company, New York, 1950.

Each year the *American Journal of Nursing* and *Public Health Nursing* magazines publish, usually in their April numbers, a list of summer courses on subjects of interest to all nurses. There is something to fit almost every taste and pocketbook. Whether you are planning to study or not, read these lists. You may be able to give a fellow nurse helpful suggestions.

The reader is reminded that the National League of Nursing Education has the most recent information as to qualifications in the educational field and lists of approved postgraduate courses.

CHAPTER XVI

Nursing for the United States Government

Nurses are employed in many branches of the Federal government and in the District of Columbia. In 1950, they numbered close to 24,600.[1] Of these, civilian nurses numbered about 18,800, thus making Uncle Sam the largest employer of nurses in the world. All the positions are classified by the U.S. Civil Service Commission, with the exception of those in the armed forces, the Veterans Administration, and the commissioned personnel of the U.S. Public Health Service.

Application for Federal nursing positions may be made directly to the Commission, to one of the regional offices of the Commission,[2] or to the Federal institution of your choice. (For application procedure, see Chap. I.)

Positions are "classified" or allocated to certain grades by the Commission, which automatically determines the salary rate of the nurse applying and qualifying for the position. For example, a classification grade of P-1 or GS-5 (professional and scientific grade) for a professional nurse would currently carry a starting or "base" salary of $3,100, plus pay for overtime (1951). Higher grading means a higher salary, but also calls for higher qualifications. A grading of P-6 or GS-13, for example, calls for the completion of advanced courses of study and years of experience under supervision and in supervision, and entitles the qualifying candidate to a base salary of $7,600, plus overtime pay. The

[1] *Facts about Nursing,* p. 25, American Nurses Association, 1950.
[2] Regional offices of the Civil Service are located in Dallas, Tex.; Atlanta, Ga.; Boston, Mass.; Chicago, Ill.; Cincinnati, Ohio; Denver, Colo.; New Orleans, La.; New York, N.Y., Philadelphia, Pa.; Seattle, Wash.; St. Louis, Mo.; St. Paul, Minn.; San Francisco, Calif.; Honolulu, T.H.; Balboa, Canal Zone; San Juan, P.R.

maximum salary in the grade of GS-5 is $3,850, in GS-13, $8,600. The latest classification pay scale should be secured from the Commission, as it is revised from time to time. Also, professional nurses occasionally receive new classification, the trend being to upgrade professional nurses who, until 1945, were classified in a subprofessional grade. There is a 5 per cent increase in pay for each 3 years of service.[3]

The chief Federal agencies employing professional nurses at present are listed in this chapter, but there are others not described here that usually employ fewer than 30 nurses, or that are war-created commissions or departments that will not seek permanent nursing staffs. Information regarding new opportunities may be secured from the agencies or the Commission.[4]

Positions in these agencies are of every type, ranging from general staff nursing to some of the top administrative jobs in the profession. Federal public health departments, hospitals, clinics, and welfare agencies employ nurses of all grades. In many positions traveling is a necessary part of the job. The services are of all sizes, from small hospitals in outlying areas (as for instance the Indian Service hospitals in Alaska) to the largest institutions in the country. The positions vary in difficulty, some requiring simple generalized nursing responsibilities, others calling for highly specialized training for experimental work in pioneer fields. There is a job for almost every taste and in every place, from Alaska to Florida and over our island and territorial possessions.

The descriptions of the duties of the staff nurse and head nurse (GS-5 and GS-7) working in the Federal service will sound familiar. They are quoted from a statement from the U.S. Civil Service Commission as of October, 1950 (Series GS-610-0).

Staff Nurse: Under supervision of the head nurses renders expert nursing care to all types of patients. This care includes the following: Planning daily schedules for care of patients; preparing for and administering therapeutic treatments and medications as prescribed by the medical staff; providing for the safekeeping of drugs; recording dosages of drugs; observing and keeping accurate records of patients' conditions; meeting medical and surgical emergencies which arise in

[3] Send for the booklet, "The Nurse in the Federal Civil Service"; also for a general leaflet of information called: "Working for the U.S.A."

[4] Names of directors of individual agencies may be found in the official directory of the *American Journal of Nursing*. Professional placement agencies will assist nurses interested in Federal positions. See Appendix A for addresses.

the absence of physicians and securing their services when necessary; assisting the physicians in examining patients, in treatments and in diagnostic measures; supervising and instructing non-professional groups in their assigned duties in the care of patients; instructing patients in personal hygiene; maintaining the unit in accordance with approved sanitary standards; maintaining adequate supplies and caring for equipment in the unit and creating a pleasant and restful environment favorable to patient's recovery; performance of related duties as assigned which are of a professional nursing nature.

The nurse in the emergency room and health unit administers first-aid emergency treatment to injured employees, makes preliminary determinations as to nature of ailments for further referral to physician, furnishes health counsel for employees, maintains records of treatments administered, and as required occasionally visits homes of employees on sick leave.

Head Nurse: The head nurse is responsible for the administration of the nursing service in a single unit in a clinical department. This includes making provision for expert nursing care of the patients in the unit and maintaining good relationships with the medical attendants, relatives, and friends; arranging for the assistance required by members of the medical staff and for the carrying out of their instructions in relation to patients; providing for comprehensive and accurate records of the medical treatment and nursing care given the patients; defining the responsibilities and assigning the specific duties of the assistant head nurses, general duty nurses, student nurses, and auxiliary aides; teaching activities such as problem solving, making assignments, holding conferences, demonstrating procedures, and seeing that all opportunities are utilized for enriching the clinical experience of students and nursing staff; keeping accurate records of the nursing program and accomplishments of the students and staff; directing the housekeeping activities which insure a safe and comfortable physical environment for the patients; securing the supplies and equipment necessary for the maintenance of a high standard of nursing service; patient education and performing related duties as assigned.

The duties also involve responsibility for the supervision of the emergency room and health unit, and nurses employed therein.

American nurses are nursing all over the world under the auspices of such organizations as the United Nations, the World Health Organization, the American Red Cross,[5] the Office of Inter-American Affairs, and the Pan-American Sanitary Bureau—not to mention service with the armed forces. Occasionally, also, under special assignments from the Children's Bureau and the Division of International Health of the U.S. Public Health Service, experienced nurses are sent abroad on special missions. (See also Chap. XVII.) Facility in a foreign language is a great asset in these overseas assignments and frequently a prerequisite. Additional compensation is usually allowed for overseas service in addition to all expenses; this is known as a salary differential and is usually 25 per cent.

The sketches written by nurses in the Veterans Administration and the Indian Service (below) describe only two of the hundreds of opportunities to serve Uncle Sam, but are representative of the spirit of the services. References at the end of this chapter describe additional openings for nurses in the Federal employ. These agencies have their headquarters in Washington unless otherwise stated, and it is essential to secure descriptions of nursing requirements from the official headquarters because they change almost yearly and the information given by nurses at work today may not apply tomorrow. Furthermore, certain restrictions—such as age—may be relaxed in times of emergency or for some special assignment. It is for that reason that the qualifications for positions are not given in greater detail in this chapter.

Personnel Policies, Federal Services

HOURS OF WORK, VACATION, AND SICK LEAVE IN FEDERAL NURSING SERVICES

Personnel policies as they relate to hours of work, vacations, and sick leave in the Federal services are regulated by the rules of the U.S. Civil Service Commission and are as follows: working hours in peacetime, 40 hours a week, and an 8-hour day; the usual legal holidays; 26 working days' vacation for each year of service (or $2\frac{1}{2}$ days per month); sick leave at the rate of $1\frac{1}{4}$ days per month. Vacation days are cumulative up to 60 days, sick leave up to 90 days.

Details of these regulations, adjustment of pay, length of service entitling to leaves, etc., should be studied before a position is accepted. As these regulations are amended from time to time, it is necessary to secure the latest rulings in advance of accepting a position. The applicant con-

[5] This organization is not under Civil Service. See also The Mission Field, Chap. XVII.

sidering a job under Civil Service should read carefully the examination announcement or descriptive folder, as the personnel practices are usually outlined there.

Frequently, opportunities are offered government employees to take special training in a specialty, or in a newly developed field of service for which there is need for an entirely new type of skill or knowledge. Such courses, workshops, institutes, or periods of training, provided they are related directly to the government job, are often provided without cost and on full pay. They constitute a rare opportunity for advancement and are one of the great advantages of working for Uncle Sam.

RETIREMENT

In all the civilian services administered by Uncle Sam and subject to Civil Service regulations, one of the most attractive features is the retirement plan. Up-to-date information regarding retirement and disability benefits should be obtained when accepting a position.

The Civil Service Retirement Act, which applies to all nurses employed in the Federal government, provides a 6 per cent monthly deduction for retirement from all base salaries. Retirement is based on age and/or disability and an aggregate service of at least 5 years. No deductions are made on overtime pay. Details as to withdrawals, lump-sum payments into your fund, military-service adjustments, and methods of receiving benefits may—and should—be secured when accepting appointment. Questions may then be referred to the Retirement Division of the U.S. Civil Service Commission.[6]

Besides the benefit of one of the best retirement plans in the world, Uncle Sam is generous with the medical facilities offered to government workers.

Information regarding many of the Federal activities is given from time to time in the professional nursing journals, but one of the best and most direct ways of seeing the service in action is to observe it on the spot. Both the Veterans Administration and the U.S. Public Health Service have widely scattered regional and local representatives. If you are interested in working for Uncle Sam, try to talk with one of the nurses in charge of a regional activity. (See official directory of the *American Journal of Nursing*.)

The following are very general descriptions of the various government agencies employing nurses.

[6] "Your Retirement System" (leaflet), obtainable from the Commission in Washington, gives detailed information.

U.S. PUBLIC HEALTH SERVICE

Including commissioned nurse officers, the Public Health Service employs (1950) about 1,650 nurses.[7] The Division of Nursing, under the direction of the chief nurse officer, who holds the rank of assistant surgeon general, coordinates the work of all nursing programs in the Service. There are numerous divisions under specific bureaus. (The applicant is referred to the official list as it appears quarterly in the official directory of the *American Journal of Nursing*, giving the divisions, bureaus, and nurse officers in charge.)

The largest number of nurses is employed by the Bureau of Medical Services and the Bureau of State Services. The divisions under these bureaus include a good many specialized services and special projects—an example of the latter being the Communicable Disease Center in Atlanta, Georgia.

Quoting from a description of the work of hospital nurses in the Public Health Service[8] we learn that

Of the 26 Public Health Service hospitals, 21 care for general medical and surgical cases, two treat tuberculosis only, one specializes in Hansen's disease (leprosy) and two care for neuropsychiatric patients with emphasis on the rehabilitation of persons suffering from drug addictions.

American seamen, foreign seamen, Coast Guard officers and enlisted men, members of the Coast and Geodetic Survey, Federal employees injured at work, and veterans constitute the major segment of the patient load. The Public Health Service came into being over 150 years ago as the Marine Hospital Service to care for sick and disabled seamen.

The hospitals of the Public Health Service offer nurses manifold opportunities for a broad clinical experience. Most of these hospitals have separate departments for the medical specialties—tumor; eye, ear, nose and throat; urology; orthopedics, etc. Nurses have the advantage of rotated assignments among the services and in the normal day's work coöperate with areas of hospital activity other than their own in caring for the 'whole' patient. They may participate also in forward-looking clinical research projects. For example, the problems of drug addiction are under constant study at Fort Worth, Tex., and at Lexington, Ky.; a working relationship on the detection, diagnosis, and treatment of

[7] *Facts about Nursing*, p. 25, American Nurses Association, 1950.
[8] From a descriptive leaflet entitled: "The Nurse in the U.S. Public Health Service."

cancer exists between the hospital at Baltimore and the Service's National Institutes of Health. . . .

The hospitals of the Public Health Service need nurses, both men and women—the general staff duty nurse and the nurse who has already specialized in a clinical field or in nursing service administration.

The nurse in the Public Health Service hospital works a 40-hour 5-day week. Since most of the hospitals are in or near large cities, there are splendid opportunities for enriching leisure time—theaters, concert halls, athletic arenas, and churches. Nearby colleges and universities offer postgraduate courses and, whenever possible, individual nursing schedules are arranged so that nurses may take advantage of these ready means of professional growth.

At many of the hospitals, the nurse prefers to occupy living quarters for which a small salary deduction is made. Otherwise she may reside in the community.

Nurses may be transferred from one Public Health Service hospital to another. If the transfer is made to meet the needs of the Service, travel expenses are paid by the Government. Registration in each State to which a nurse is transferred is not required but current registration must be maintained in one State.

Under the Bureau of State Services, public health nurses serve in a wide variety of general and special public health programs. Again citing the description of the opportunities in this field, we read that

On the staff level, the general public health nurse is assigned to a local health department, where she may assist in field training for public health nurses, help to develop bedside nursing as part of the local health program or participate in demonstrations in mental health, cancer, venereal disease control, or other developing programs. In some posts, the public health nurse is a member of the Public Health Service team engaged in special field studies in heart disease, nutrition, diabetes, cancer, or one of the communicable diseases. These field studies offer opportunities for training in research methods.

As a consultant the public health nurse participates in planning and conducting in-service training programs, and in special instances, university courses for public health nurses. She consults with national, State, and local health agencies in analyzing needs and in promoting public health programs.

Public health nursing consultants may be assigned from the Division of Tuberculosis to State and city health departments to help develop the nursing phases of the tuberculosis services; they participate in community X-ray programs and they aid nursing schools in planning for teaching tuberculosis nursing to undergraduates. The public health nurse collects the data for various research projects, such as the investigation of the value of immunization in tuberculosis control and the efficacy of various therapeutic drugs. She shares in the thrill of new discoveries.

In the Division of Venereal Disease nurses are employed in institutional and public health positions. In-patient facilities for the intensive treatment of syphilis are operated by the United States Public Health Service or State departments of health to which Public Health Service nurses are assigned in staff, supervisory, or public health nursing positions. Public health nurses are assigned to State and local health departments for consultation and demonstration services. They may also be called upon to participate in research studies.

Nurses on the staff of the Cancer Control Branch of the National Cancer Institute may be assigned to universities to initiate courses in cancer nursing, to State health departments to act as nursing consultants and to conduct in-service education programs for nurses, to local health departments to assist with cancer field studies, or to cancer research centers to carry out clinical activities.

The Division of Federal Employee Health, upon request, develops and operates programs for Federal departments in the United States and abroad. . . .

In 1946 Congress passed the National Mental Health Act, recognizing mental illness as a vital problem in public health. Since then, the Public Health Service has embarked on a pioneering program in mental hygiene. In this program, both the public health nurse with special training in mental hygiene and the nurse prepared in psychiatric nursing are vitally needed. These nurses may work as members of a mental hygiene clinic team. As consultants they may participate in mental health institutes and in-service training programs, teach in universities, or consult with national, State, and local health agencies and with universities in shaping mental health programs, and in training other nurses for these programs.

Nurses assigned to the Division of Industrial Hygiene have the stimulating and satisfying challenge of developing industrial nursing programs in State and local departments of health, which are responsible for the health of 60 million workers. They assist in field studies to determine new hazards inherent in the changing technology of American industry. They also work closely with universities in developing industrial nursing curricula.

Other opportunities exist in the field of nursing education administration and research. These positions are usually on a consultant level and require both wide experience and marked executive ability.

Entrance to the U.S. Public Health Service may be by appointment to the Commissioned Corps as a regular or reserve officer or through Civil Service. A requirement for admission to the Commissioned Corps is an academic degree.

To aid in the growing work of the Public Health Service, the Reserve Corps augments the authorized strength of the Regular Corps. With few exceptions, the nurse who is a Reserve officer carries the same privileges and obligations as her colleague in the Regular Corps.

Service in the Commissioned Corps is in some ways similar to Army and Navy service. Salaries and ranks of the commissioned nurse are comparable to those of officers in the armed forces. She is expected to serve wherever the needs of the Service take her. As in the Army or Navy, her salary includes base pay plus a rental and subsistence allowance.

Although the majority of positions for nurses entering the Service are in the Civil Service grades of GS-5, 7 and 9, or in the Commissioned Corps ranks of junior assistant, assistant, or senior assistant, nurses with special qualifications may be appointed in higher grades or ranks. These grades and ranks compare with those of the armed forces as follows:

CIVIL SERVICE	COMMISSIONED CORPS, PHS	ARMY	NAVY
GS-5	Junior assistant nurse officer	Second lieutenant	Ensign
GS-7	Assistant nurse officer	First lieutenant	Lieutenant (j.g.)
GS-9	Senior assistant nurse officer	Captain	Lieutenant
GS-11	Nurse officer	Major	Lieutenant commander
GS-12	Senior nurse officer	Lieutenant colonel	Commander
GS-13	Nurse director	Colonel	Captain

"Whether she is a commissioned officer or a civil service appointee, the nurse enjoys a good salary and many benefits. These include periodic raises, opportunity for training and promotion, liberal vacations with pay, sick leave and medical care, a basic 40-hour work week, and retirement benefits."

Among the nurses now employed in the Public Health Service, about 74 per cent are in staff level positions, while among the commissioned officers, 64 per cent are above staff level.

One of the most interesting jobs for public health nurses is that of a regional nursing consultant. It is described thus by Miss McIver, Chief of the Division of Public Health Nursing in the Bureau of State Services:[9]

In addition to consultative functions common to all consultants in the regional organization of the Bureau, the nurse consultants confer with State health administrators regarding the organization and administration of nursing within State health departments. They assist State directors of public health nursing in defining standards and evaluating public health nursing practice, in establishing qualification requirements for public health nurses, in planning in-service training programs for public health nurses, and in analyzing nursing needs and determining how those needs can be met. They make surveys and studies of local nursing services, and give consultation service to State health departments on the assignment, transfer, and efficiency rating of Public Health Service nursing personnel assigned to States. They interpret public health nursing education needs of the regions to universities offering public health nursing programs, and assist these universities in arrangements for field practice facilities. They plan policies and programs of mutual concern with the Children's Bureau regional representatives, other personnel of the Service, and regional personnel of Federal agencies.

CHILDREN'S BUREAU

The Children's Bureau, now under the Social Security Administration, is another service in the Federal Security Agency. The Nursing Unit, under a nurse director, employs about fourteen nurses who serve as con-

[9] From an address presented by PEARL McIVER: "Preparing Nurses for Efficient Service within the Public Health Service," Annual Meeting, Association of Military Surgeons of the United States, New York, N.Y., November, 1950 (with permission). Functions were quoted from PHS Manual, Sec. 5-10c.

sultants to states on the care of mothers and babies, crippled children, and the handicapped. These nurses are experienced public health or orthopedic nurses; one is a nurse-midwife as well.

VETERANS ADMINISTRATION

This enormous government agency employs all types of nurses—about 13,500—in general and special hospitals caring for veterans all over the country. Many of the hospitals offer advanced clinical experience in such specialties as tuberculosis, cancer, and neuropsychiatry. There are opportunities for public health nurses in clinics in the regional offices and large metropolitan hospitals of the VA. In all, the veterans' hospitals provide about 106,450 beds.[10]

The hospitals are situated in places which will provide a healthful physical environment for veterans and, therefore, they are often located on the outskirts of town where the air is better and grounds may be more extensive.

Nurses who enjoy outdoor life will find provision for hiking, picnicking, swimming, golf, tennis, gardening, fishing, and camping. Indoor sports include bowling, Ping-pong, dancing, and card parties. Entertainments planned for the patients are often open to the nurses, and consideration is given to requests for duty hours which will make approved classwork possible. Excellent library facilities are also available for patients and personnel. Many Veterans Administration hospitals are located near colleges or universities where nurses can plan their hours to take courses if they wish.

Appointments of nurses to the VA are now directly through the agency, not the U.S. Civil Service Commission. However, the retirement benefits of Civil Service employees apply to the nursing staff. Salaries start at $3,400. The maximum salary for the top grade is $7,400. The director of nursing service receives $10,000.

The qualifications for nursing in the VA are much the same as in the other Federal services: citizenship, high school graduation, completion of a course of nursing in a school of nursing approved by the Administrator of Veterans Affairs, state registration, satisfactory physical condition, and professional experience as required in the position sought. Those applying for the administrative positions should write to the Director, Nursing Service, Veterans Administration, Washington: others may ap-

[10] *Facts about Nursing*, p. 75, American Nurses Association, 1950.

ply at the local offices of the VA. Two recent fullface photographs should accompany the application forms, which will be sent on request.[11] Appropriate white uniforms and caps are required while on duty. There is no off-duty or out-of-door uniform required.

Here is the description of the work of a nurse in a VA hospital.

With the VA

Dear Ann,

You asked in your last letter for my honest opinion about the Nursing Service in the Veterans Administration. It has been only a little more than a year since I started with the Veterans Administration and the thing that still impresses me most is the high standard of medical and nursing service. And I really can stress the cleanliness of the hospital, too. The morale is very high, principally because of the fairness and accessibility of the Chief Nurse and her Assistants. You may express your opinion openly and be respected for that opinion. That leads to a growing organization with progressive ideas from the nursing group. I'll tell you about the setup which I think leads to the friendliness and cooperativeness that is felt so soon here.

The head nurses meet every other week to discuss problems and plan for effectiveness of work. The staff nurses meet regularly and nurses from these two groups make up committees on procedures, techniques, social activities, etc. There always remains a closeness to our working group. This I think is essential, don't you? Frankly, I would have worked with the Veterans Administration long before if I had had any idea of the opportunities it offers. You know me well enough to know I'm not giving you a sales talk.

I know you are interested in all phases of our program so I will give you an idea of each service with my own ideas, of course, included.

The surgical service is a very commendable one. The Chief of Surgery respects good nurses and demands as well as commands good nursing care. Over and beyond this he is cooperative toward teaching patients. We're now beginning to do a more thorough piece of work in teaching the patients, with much more planned. It's really a challenge. With my public health background I was afraid I would not be able to do the patient

---

[11] Additional information may be secured from the Chief, Nursing Service, at the nearest hospital of the VA. Descriptions of the services appear from time to time in the professional journals. See also references at the end of this chapter.

teaching that I so enjoy. How wrong I was! On the surgical wards, for example, the nurses are teaching many patients requiring major abdominal surgery.

At one time we had six patients on one floor with colostomies. We prepared mimeographed copies of instruction for "The Care of Your Colostomy." One day during visiting hours we had a class for these six men and their wives and one sister who cared for one patient. Previously each patient had been given a demonstration and had returned the demonstration of irrigation and care of his colostomy. Each patient was well versed by the end of our class. The wives and sisters were very eager to learn about the articles needed for care and diet and asked to see the equipment and the tray we had set up for use. That was really an hour well spent. We are still hearing how much that meant to the patients and their families. But I could ramble on and on!

On the medical floors we are doing a similar job in helping the diabetic patients care for themselves. We have a tray set up for the demonstration of giving insulin. We get a return demonstration by the patient to assure safe technique. We teach the patients to test their urine for sugar. Recently several of our diabetics saw, "Diabetes, Uncomplicated," and "Diabetes, Complicated" (published by Castle Film Company and owned by Veterans Administration)—excellent films and good visual aids for diabetic teaching. We also use "Diabetic Manual," by Joslin, and "Diabetes in Pictures," by Rosenthal for references for reading for the patients, and advise the purchase of one as a guide. At present we are working on material to distribute to each patient in mimeographed form. This will be simple but sufficiently detailed to give the patient a good idea of his disease, its care and control. There are many other opportunities for teaching but I mention these only as obvious examples and ones I'm particularly interested in at the moment.

After mentioning the surgical and medical services I must give the laboratory its just due. The technologists do a terrific volume of work and competently, too. Recently they have sent out new forms to follow for all laboratory procedures which are grand and a boon to efficiency. Every week new ideas are being tried to improve our service. It's a joy to be in a growing concern.

We have many meetings offered on timely subjects for nurses and trained nurses' aides. The doctors' meetings are open to nurses. All in all, we really have a good educational plan which will become more effective as our patient-teaching program grows. Library facilities are available. In addition to a library for patients, we have a medical library containing the latest textbooks, magazines, and pamphlets—medical and nursing.

The operating room is modern, efficient, and well supervised from both the nursing and the surgical standpoint. The major surgery being done has increased tremendously over this last year and there is evidence that expansion in the way of space will occur in this department. Our blood bank is a big aid in doing major surgery. The nurses are interested in the follow-up of the patient's care after the actual operation, which demonstrates a broad viewpoint.

Our small neuropsychiatric division, in this general medical and surgical hospital, treats patients with mental illnesses. In addition to the psychotherapy given, recreational activities, occupational therapy, and hydrotherapy are prescribed for patients on an individual basis. Insulin shock therapy is used and this is often supplemented by electroshock therapy. The head nurse has prepared quite a comprehensive and complete plan for the nurse new to the ward. Acute and long-term patients are transferred to Veterans Administration neuropsychiatric hospitals.

We actually made a movie, right in another VA hospital, to show safe methods of nursing tuberculous patients. For nurses who have not had previous experience in tuberculosis nursing, planned programs of instruction give a sense of security in this interesting specialty.

This gives you an idea of our services and I'll mention a few others to give a good cross section. We have a Social Service Department so that follow-up is possible after treatment and teaching. Many problems are worked out for family adjustments as well as for adjustment of the patient.

During the war we all learned how important physical and occupational therapy were to the convalescence and speedy recovery of the patient. These departments have well-trained personnel and make daily contacts for this essential therapy.

We also have many recreational activities available through Special Services which aid in keeping patient morale high. Many vocational problems as well as training courses are also planned. All this proves that Veterans Administration and its Nursing Service are interested in the care of the whole patient and his return to take his place in his community.

I hope that you've gathered from this that there is real enthusiasm for nursing in Veterans Administration as far as I'm concerned. Drop in any time to get an idea for yourself. For that matter, choose any Veterans Administration Hospital and I'm sure you will receive a very cordial welcome.

I would be delighted to learn soon that you have joined our group. You will certainly be in a group with progressive ideas and modern facilities to keep abreast of modern medicine and nursing.

Sincerely,

Martha[12]

THE INDIAN SERVICE

Bureau of Indian Affairs. About eight hundred nurses are employed in the Indian hospitals and field stations in the United States and Alaska.[13] Those carrying on field services are public health nurses. In 1950, there were 70 public health nurses employed.

The Bureau of Indian Affairs of the Department of the Interior is charged with the responsibility of carrying out the provisions of certain treaties made by the Federal government with various Indian groups and with the development of related programs essential to the health, education, and welfare in their broadest sense for the Indians of the United States and the native peoples of Alaska which include Aleuts and Eskimos as well as Indians.

The Health Division of the Bureau of Indian Affairs administers that portion of the program which has to do with medical care, hospitalization, and public health activities. The personnel consists of a Chief Consultant in Nursing, a Consultant in Public Health Nursing, and Consultant in Hospital Nursing. In the field service there are supervisors, senior chief nurses, chief nurses, head nurses, staff nurses, junior staff nurses, field (public health) nurses, junior field (public health) nurses, and traveling nurses engaged in trachoma work. In Alaska a number of the assignments are to itinerant programs. The field organization consists of eleven areas, six of which have area consultants in nursing and area headquarters.

For the most recent salary schedule, the reader is referred to the Chief Consultant in Nursing, Bureau of Indian Affairs. (See also below.)

Most of the hospitals and field nursing stations in the Indian Service in the United States are west of the Mississippi River. A few of these are

[12] Written by MARTHA H. BROWN, a staff nurse at the VA hospital, Muskogee, Okla.

[13] *Facts about Nursing*, p. 25. American Nurses Association, 1950.

located near large cities; several are near national parks or monuments where scenic attractions provide recreation for off-duty hours. However, the majority of stations are in isolated areas where social contacts are limited and where shops and commercial amusements are not easily accessible. In these situations self-sufficiency and resourcefulness in the individual are necessary for successful personal adjustment and satisfaction. An attempt is made to transfer nurses from isolated areas to locations less isolated after tour of duty of 2 or 3 years.

To quote a "Circular of Information" from the Bureau (1950):[14]

Hospitals range in size from 18 to 335 beds with nursing staffs from 5 to 65. Except for sanatoriums and an orthopedic hospital in Alaska, all are general hospitals, admitting all age groups and both sexes. The obstetric and pediatric services are usually very active. It is customary for the nurses in hospitals, including head nurses, to rotate on all services and on all shifts. At present, due to lack of suitable quarters and the necessity for nurses to be prepared to rotate on all services, including obstetrics and pediatrics, there are no positions for male nurses. The 40-hour week is in effect, except for emergencies.

The hospital and community health programs are closely coordinated. The public health nursing service is generalized, usually developed around community clinics or hospital out-patient services. Close relationship is maintained with local and state health services to prevent overlapping of effort. . . .

The nursing service in larger hospitals is comparable to that of a well organized civilian hospital with a graduate staff.

The small hospital offers an especial challenge to the initiative and resourcefulness of the head nurse and her staff, since in these hospitals services are not segregated and the demands for all types of care, including surgery, must be met.

Nurses' aids are young Indian girls, high school graduates, who spend an academic year in class and supervised ward work under well qualified instructors at the Kiowa Nurses' Aid School at Lawton, Oklahoma. This training prepares them to render certain types of patient care under the supervision of a graduate nurse. After graduation they are employed in hospitals in the Indian Service.

[14] "Circular of Information," Bureau of Indian Affairs, Department of the Interior, Washington, D.C., 1950.

Requirements: Education. Graduation from a recognized school of nursing requires a residence of at least 2 years in a hospital having a daily average of 50 bed patients or more. The basic course must have included clinical experience in medical, surgical, pediatric, and obstetric nursing. In addition, the public health nurse (field nurse) must have successfully completed a full special course in public health nursing, extending over at least one academic year, at a college or university giving a public health course of study approved by the National Nursing Accrediting Service, or must have successfully completed a full 4- or 5-year course leading to a bachelor's degree, with major study in public health nursing, in a college or university giving a public health course of study approved by the National Nursing Accrediting Service.

Experience: Staff Nurse. At least 2 years' postgraduate experience in nursing, one year of which must have been in a hospital or sanatorium. This institutional experience must have been secured within the last 5 years.

Junior Nurse (Hospital Duty). No postgraduate experience required.

Public Health (Field) Nurse. At least 1 year of successful general public health nursing experience in a supervised rural health service or in an urban health agency which administers a general public health program. It is necessary that field nurses (public health nurses and junior public health nurses) be capable drivers, as they may drive on rural roads under all types of climatic conditions.

Junior Public Health (Field) Nurse. The above qualifications must be met with the exception that no experience is required.

It is the policy of the Indian Service to promote nurses from within the staff, thus making it possible for young nurses to build a true career service. Employees in the Indian Service receive the benefits of the Civil Service Retirement Act.

Salaries. The salary ranges in the Service (to be checked for most recent changes) are: for staff nurses, base salary, $3,100 to $3,850; for public health nurses or head nurse, $3,825 to $4,575; for chief public health nurse or director of nurses (hospital) $4,600 to $5,350.

The work that nurses perform in the Indian Service is unique. For this reason the sketch describing the duties of one nurse shows how a satisfying career may be built within the Service, starting from school-of-nursing days, and coming down to the present.

The nurse who is not happy beyond the lights of big cities and prefers pavements to grass under her feet had better not try to find a lasting career in the Indian Service. Sooner or later she will be sent into isolated areas; at least, she cannot count on remaining in the well-populated centers. The nurse, on the other hand, who craves variety, change, and something new and different from the familiar scenes around the wards of a large hospital or in the crowded slums of our great cities cannot do better than throw in her lot with the Indian Service.

A Career in the Indian Service

A very tomboy of a girl, growing up in North Dakota, used to see the Sioux Indians come to town from their nearby reservation to sell their berries and to trade in the stores. She liked to read stories telling about these people and their life. Her father also told her many stories of his pioneer experiences in Dakota Territory and his contacts with the Indians. She used to wish that she were a little Indian galloping wild and free over the prairies. That is what they were usually doing in the stories she read.

When this girl finished school in the North Dakota town and entered nurse's training at the University of Minnesota, she no longer wished to be an Indian child, wild and free; but her interest in these people continued to play a part in her plans. It was not always prominent, but remained in the background: the plan to work more closely with the Indian people.

Graduation from the school of nursing arrived. The new graduate worked in her own school hospital for graduate experience and then she made application for a Civil Service position with the United States Indian Service. The months passed, busy ones to be sure, and the Indian Service application was almost forgotten, when suddenly one morning, a telegram and the offer of a position in South Dakota in the Indian Service. Did she go? What do you think?

A ride on a bus to a little town on the banks of the Missouri River, then the next day a ride with the mailman in an old, very rattly truck and a stop at each mailbox along the 25 miles to the Indian Agency. There was also a story about the family at each mailbox from the mail carrier. The arrival at Fort Thompson, South Dakota, Agency for the Crow Creek Reservation at last; the new nurse was introduced to the superintendent at the Agency and then to the head nurse and the three other staff nurses in the two-building combination general hospital and tuberculosis sanatorium. The next morning she entered on duty in the hospital.

The patients to be cared for were mothers and new babies, sick children (mostly pneumonia or diarrhea), and grownups with numerous ailments and injuries, but all requiring the same care as any patients in any hospital, whether in a big city or a small town. These people practiced early ambulation after childbirth before it was initiated in the city hospitals. If a mother misunderstood the reason for a treatment, or a problem arose at home needing her attention, up she would get, wrap her baby in a blanket, and walk out of the hospital and home, even though the baby might be only two or three days old.

So this was how I happened to enter the Indian Service and this was my introduction to the work with the Indian people.

My entrance into the Indian Service, which I have described, took place several years ago. The methods of transportation to the Agencies have generally improved, as have the roads, and now many new arrivals come in their own cars. The hospitals have been improved greatly also. In the earlier days, I had to learn to improvise materials which I had taken for granted in the University Hospital. I learned to sterilize in a pressure cooker and in the oven of a kitchen range. Several new all-modern hospitals and sanatoria have been built, but these early experiences in improvising have helped me many times in the homes after I transferred to public health work in the Indian Service. This early hospital experience also helped me to realize the importance of a cooperative relationship between the hospital and the fieldworkers, in order to be most effective in helping the Indian people to secure better health and living conditions.

The physical surroundings may have changed since I entered the Indian Service, but the health problems have not, nor have the human relationships. The problems of infant feeding, malnutrition, and diarrhea—results of ignorance of proper feeding and also of poverty and improper sanitation, still remain. Pneumonia and tuberculosis are still found among the patients the nurses care for. Major surgery and orthopedic conditions present their problems needing skilled nursing care and later supervision when the patient goes home. The problem of helping a people who are of another race and culture and who are very proud of being Indian to understand "white man's medicine" and why the white doctors and nurses do certain things remains the same. Some of these people still rebel against the new ideas, until it is too late for help, because they don't understand;

others accept but misunderstand the instructions because of language handicaps and so fail to gain the needed help.

The nurse in her contact with the patient in the hospital and with a real desire to understand his culture and religious taboos can help him to understand much better why things are done; and he in turn will go back to his home and help his own people to understand when and if they must seek such care. The public health nurse, working in the homes and clinics, has the same opportunities, as well as being able to explain the hospital to the patient before he enters and to dispel some of the fear of the unknown. It is hard to realize, but there are in our own United States several thousand people in one Indian tribe who cannot speak or understand English. This presents a real challenge to the worker among these people and necessitates the experience of working through an interpreter. However, the satisfactions of the work are great, as the story of some of my patients shows.

Maggie Little Eagle, nine months old, in a critical condition from malnutrition was brought into the hospital in South Dakota by the public health nurse. This was a result of both ignorance and poverty. Maggie had brothers and a sister older than she, but she had had to be put on a bottle and Mrs. Little Eagle hadn't fixed the milk correctly, and sometimes there hadn't been any milk. None of Maggie's folks had ever been in the hospital and they were afraid to let Maggie go off 20 miles away with a white woman, to be cared for entirely by white people.[15] The parents finally gave in to the combined persuasion of the public health nurse—or "Blue Lady," as she was called—and the Catholic priest, and Maggie was admitted to the hospital more dead than alive. She was fed by medicine dropper every hour at first, and then by bottle at longer intervals; and after many ups and downs, Maggie finally began to look more like an Indian baby and less like a little sparrow. Maggie stayed in the hospital all winter. The nurses had a birthday party for her and the day her parents came and saw her really growing and getting better was an event. The nurses explained to them how Maggie was cared for in the hospital and started the teaching in preparation for Maggie's return home. The "Blue Lady" continued this instruction on her visits into the community and finally the great day arrived, Maggie went home a well and healthy little girl; a triumph for the combined efforts of the doctor, the nurses in the hospital, the public health nurse, and the religious worker in the field.

The public health nurse is apt to start the day feeling a little in a "what's

[15] More Indian girls are now entering nurse's training and returning to their agencies.

the use" mood. Yesterday a mother refused to allow her baby to be brought into the hospital; it was acutely ill with what appeared to be pneumonia, but the family wanted to try a "Sing" (a healing ceremony) first. The nurse fears that the next word will be that the baby has died. Last week a baby died of diphtheria on the way to the hospital because the parents stopped on their way and went home after the Trader had thought he had them on the 55 mile trip to the hospital. They had a "Sing" lasting 2 days. If the baby had only arrived sooner or had had antitoxin! What was the use? Well, on to the day's work.

The first visit is to a little four-year-old girl, Desbah Begay, who has been stricken with poliomyelitis. Her parents sought medical help and she is now at home wearing braces on both legs. The nurse is supervising the mother with the daily exercises and in crutch walking. Desbah comes to meet the nurse at the door of her home, walking alone on her crutches, very happy. She couldn't do this without help when she first came home. The visit also reveals a noticeable improvement in the muscle strength of one leg. The mother is very proud and as the nurse leaves she says that she is going to bring the nine-months-old baby Dabah in for her "shots" (diphtheria, pertussis, and tetanus) on the next conference day at the nurse's office. The mother has also been adding new foods to her diet as advised during previous visits.

The next visit is to a sixteen-year-old girl to make arrangements for her to return to a distant hospital for continued plastic work on her jaw. Mary Chischilly fell into a well when she was four years old and injured her head and jaw. She got along for eleven years without being able to open her mouth, existing by forcing soft foods and liquids through the small opening between upper and lower jaws; otherwise, her jaws were locked. Mary was very thin and unable to speak distinctly when the social worker found her. Through the combined work of the social worker and public health nurse, Mary was sent to an oral surgeon under the auspices of the State Crippled Children's Service and had her jaw operated on. She can now open her mouth and she is under the treatment of a plastic surgeon who is filling in the injuries to the jaw area. She is going to the dentist to have her teeth corrected and filled. Mary has cut and curled her hair and has found work to earn money for her clothes. She's talking about going to school next fall. The nearest thing to which the nurse can compare this transformation in Mary is a wilted bud, watered and now blooming into a flower.

The nurse travels on to her next visit. The roads don't seem nearly so rough as they were this morning. This visit is to the home of a tuberculosis patient, a father with a wife and five children. Three of the children have been enrolled in boarding school, but two are still at home. The father is anxious to go to the sanatorium, but is on a long waiting list. The family subsistence is being supplemented with a welfare grant, and the Protestant missionary helps with supplies when he can manage it. Isolation is a problem in the one-room hogan, but with the aid of an interpreter the improvisations are gone over again with the patient and his wife. The patient has his pallet on one side of the hogan, away from the others; he is burning his sputum and covering his mouth when he coughs; he has his own dishes. The members of his family have been x-rayed; his wife's condition is going to have to be watched closely. He thanks the nurse and interpreter for coming and for the cough medicine and tonic which the doctor at the clinic has sent.

The nurse leaves for her next visit—and probably her last for the day as it is 5 miles away—smiling. She is 30 miles from the Agency over a rough and winding road, but there is no more of the "what's the use" feeling. The only discouraging thought is the nagging one of the empty sanatorium bed for Chee Nakai. Will the vacancy come in time to do him any good?

A nurse who plans to enter the Indian Service should have more than average interest in people and a real desire to understand them as individuals. She should be able to be patient if results aren't forthcoming at once. The satisfaction of seeing a mother who has lost several babies because of diarrhea and improper feeding bringing her new baby for supervision and feeding instructions, and of seeing her joy and pride in the growing healthy baby, makes up for previous rejections and disappointments. The public health nurse is helped a great deal if she has an understanding of rural nursing problems. She should be able to improvise without electricity and maybe with just a homemade stove for heat. She should be able to utilize sufficient water for adequate cleanliness without being wasteful. Many of these people still have to haul their water in barrels several miles, both for drinking and for washing purposes.

The nurse should be able to create her own social relationships and amusements in small groups—she may have to depend on her own resources. Many of the stations are isolated from large centers. However, the 5-day work week and adequate annual leave allow for many opportunities to get away and renew one's friendships and interests. There are also many very picturesque places to see in the surrounding country, as the Indian people live mostly in the western part of the United States where the parks, monuments, and old historic dwellings of ancient peoples are located. There are also the ceremonials and dances of the Indian tribe with which one is working. Seeing them helps the nurse to understand the people better. There is opportunity for change and travel in the Indian Service as one has the chance of transfer to another area at periodic intervals and to learn the customs of a new group or tribe. The Indian Service also has stations in Alaska, both for hospital and public health nurses.

Doesn't it sound attractive? Why not join us!

LAURA L. CLARK
Public Health Nurse
Shiprock, New Mexico

OTHER FEDERAL SERVICES

U.S. Civil Service Commission. One nurse serves as nursing consultant in the Medical Division.

Departmental Agencies, District of Columbia. About three hundred nurses—both hospital and public health—are employed in first-aid or health rooms in Federal agencies.

Freedman's Hospital. This large Federal hospital for Negro patients employs 240 nurses. It has a school of nursing for Negro nurses.

St. Elizabeth's Hospital. There are 250 nurses at this Federal mental hospital of 7,000 beds.

Panama Canal Service. This service has about 230 nurses, mainly hospital nurses. The initial salary for service in the Panama Canal Zone is $3,875 a year. Special privileges are accorded those who work in the health department hospitals in the Zone. There is an entering peacetime age limit of thirty-five years for this service.[16]

Tennessee Valley Authority. The TVA employs 28 nurses.

---

[16] In applying for any of the positions likely to call you outside the United States, it is well to provide yourself with a set of passport photographs and a copy of your birth certificate.

THE ARMED FORCES

ARMY AND NAVY NURSE CORPS

During the Second World War, the Army and Navy Nurse Corps employed 72,978 nurses. Just how many nurses will form the permanent corps of either service cannot be stated because emergency conditions affect the monthly—one could almost say the weekly—quota needed. As these positions are not under Civil Service, inquiries should be sent directly to Washington.[17] At the present time, nurses in both corps hold commissioned rank, starting as second lieutenants in the Army and ensigns and lieutenants (j.g.) in the Navy. (For officers' ranks in the commissioned services, see classification list on p. 279.)

Currently, these two services are seeking new recruits to build up personnel available for immediate military service. It is probable that a larger reserve will be maintained in the future for defense purposes. Unless an Army nurse who served in the Second World War has applied for a reserve commission, she is not considered as in the reserve and will not be called for active duty unless she volunteers. To serve again, applicants must be under forty-five years of age, with no dependents under eighteen. Application blanks may be obtained from Washington.

It is possible at this time for Army and Navy nurses (ensigns and lieutenants [j.g.] of the Navy Nurse Corps, U.S. Naval Reserve) to apply for flight-nurse training. They must be in active service and not over thirty. Navy nurses have replaced Army nurses on board all ships.

Salaries in 1950 ranged from $2,565 to $8,379 plus subsistence and allowances (see table insert, *Facts about Nursing*, American Nurses Association, 1950). Here again, one should check with the Army or Navy for latest compensation scales.

AIR FORCE NURSE CORPS

The Air Force is offering opportunities to reserve nurse officers on active duty to become members of the regular Air Force Medical Service. (For eligibility requirements, write for "Fact Sheet" from the Air Force.) They will have commissioned rank.

A career in the armed forces thus offers opportunities for advancement and permanency; there are chances to receive postgraduate training in anesthesiology, operating-room management, nursing administration, and

[17] Names of commanding nurse officers may be found in the official directory of the *American Journal of Nursing*.

neuropsychiatric nursing; to say nothing of that familiar selling point—
"See the world." Salaries for commissioned nurse officers appear in the
section on the U.S. Public Health Service, above.

The subjects included in the training courses for flight nurses are: air
evacuation, dentistry, internal medicine, neuropsychiatry, physiology,
preventive and global medicine, surgery, flight planning, oxygen therapy,
and administration. During the last 3 weeks of the course the nurses take
part in the actual evacuation of patients within the United States.

GENERAL CONSIDERATIONS

From the personal description of nursing work in the Federal agencies
and the information regarding personnel policies, it can be seen that our
government is earnestly trying to build "a career service" for nurses as
well as for all its employees. For the young nurse who wishes to map out
a clear road ahead, running from general duty to a highly specialized
job or to administrative responsibilities, and who is willing to work and
study to qualify for each succeeding promotion, the government services
offer an enticing field with security for old age and disability benefits.

It is only fair to point out some of the possible drawbacks to Federal
employment:

1. It is quite possible that you will be transferred from place to place
   fairly frequently and required to travel a great deal. This is considered
   an asset by many nurses.
2. Personnel policies are fairly rigid—very rigid compared to the complete freedom of administration in private agencies.
3. Some of the assignments are in very large units, where you may at first
   feel lost, irked by "institutionalism," and thrown—unless you struggle—
   into a round of purely professional activities away from a normal home
   atmosphere and recreation with those who hardly know the meaning
   of the word "nurse." This situation is not nearly so unshakable, however, as it seems, and there has been great improvement in living privileges in the past few years.
4. All large administrative offices impose a certain amount of routine, red
   tape, and regimentation. Much of this can be lightened, even side-
   tracked on occasion, by the farsighted, astute administrator. The new
   employee will do well to be patient with the rules and regulations until
   she understands their purpose. Efficiency or service ratings, for example

—in other words, your supervisor's report of your work—may seem formal and highly impersonal at first. A little study and questioning will show their usefulness. If, after fair trial, you feel that the rules are unfair or unreasonable you have two alternatives: to present your complaint and resign if you feel you are up against a stone wall of indifference, or to request a transfer to another branch of the service.

5. Governmental wheels move slowly and, in agencies of long standing, changes in personnel are not rapid. Therefore, you will find nurses of the "old school" who are steeped in the disciplines and traditions of years ago. But you will also discover an ever-growing majority of highly qualified, competent, and "human" administrators and supervisors, who have the vision, the energy, and the wisdom to be true leaders. You could ask no richer experience than to be members of their staffs.

All in all, the opportunities for a satisfying, well-paid, interesting, and secure career in government service far outnumber the few possible drawbacks.

BIBLIOGRAPHY

1. ARCHARD, THERESEA: "G.I. Nightingale," W. W. Norton & Company, New York, 1945.
2. "The Army Nurse," U.S. Army Nurse Corps, Washington, D.C., 1944. (History.)
3. Army Nurse Corps Offers Unlimited Opportunities, *New York State Nurse*, p. 12 (pictures), April, 1949.
4. AYNES, EDITH A.: Army Nursing—Then and Now, *American Journal of Nursing*, P. 205, April, 1949. See also p. 232, April, 1951.
5. BURK, AUDREY RATHBURN: Forever Ugh! *R.N.*, p. 30, June, 1950.
6. CONNELLY, ELLEN H.: Shipmates in White, *American Journal of Nursing*, p. 204, April, 1949.
7. CUNNINGHAM, CLARA H.: Adventure among the Indians, *Public Health Nursing*, p. 433, July, 1941.
8. DEMING, DOROTHY: "Ginger Lee, War Nurse," Dodd, Mead & Company, Inc., New York, 1942.
9. DEMING DOROTHY: "Penny Marsh and Ginger Lee, Wartime Nurses," Dodd, Mead & Company, Inc., New York, 1943.
10. FLIKKE, JULIA O.: "Nurses in Action," J. B. Lippincott Company, Philadelphia, 1943.
11. FORBES, MARY D.: Federal Nursing Assignments outside the United States, *American Journal of Nursing*, p. 465, August, 1950.

12. FRASHER, CHARLES B.: Merit System Problems, *American Journal of Nursing*, p. 679, October, 1947.
13. HEINTZELMAN, RUTH A.: Some Points of Interest to Public Health Nurses Regarding the Federal Civil Service, *Public Health Nursing*, p. 456, September, 1947.
14. HEINTZELMAN, RUTH A., and DOROTHY DEMING: How Federal Civil Service Works, *American Journal of Nursing*, p. 319, May, 1946; p. 379, June, 1946.
15. JONES, DOROTHY E.: The Nurse Corps of the U.S. Naval Reserve, *American Journal of Nursing*, p. 287, May, 1950.
16. KEATON, MARTHA E.: My Experience in the Indian Service, *American Journal of Nursing*, p. 944, November, 1945.
17. LEIGHTON, ALEXANDER H., and DOROTHEA C. LEIGHTON: "The Navaho Door," Harvard University Press, Cambridge, Mass., 1945.
18. LUTZ, ALMA, "With Love, Jane," The John Day Company, New York, 1945.
19. MACFARLANE, JESSIE: Marine Hospitals—An Opportunity for Nurses, *American Journal of Nursing*, p. 43, January, 1946.
20. MILLER, JEAN DUPONT: "Shipmates in White," Dodd, Mead & Company, Inc., New York, 1944.
21. NEWCOMB, ELLSWORTH: "Brave Nurse," Appleton-Century-Crofts, Inc., New York, 1945.
22. PARKER, PRISCILLA: Nursing in Alaska, *American Journal of Nursing*, p. 298, May, 1949.
23. PETO, MARJORIE: "Women Were Not Expected," privately published, 1947. (Second World War. This book may be ordered from 1293 Sussex Road, West Englewood, N.J.)
24. REDMOND, JUANITA: "I Served on Bataan," J. B. Lippincott Company, Philadelphia, 1943.
25. TIBER, BERTHA M.: Nursing among the Navajo Indians, *American Journal of Nursing*, p. 552, September, 1949.
26. TIBER, BERTHA M.: The Indian Service in Alaska, *American Journal of Nursing*, p. 1114, October, 1942.
27. TRAUTMAN, J. A., and ROSALIE GIACOMO: Public Health Nursing in a Marine Hospital, *Public Health Nursing*, p. 339, June, 1949.
28. VREELAND, ELLWYNNE M.: Fifty Years of Nursing in the Federal Government Nursing Services, *American Journal of Nursing*, p. 626, October, 1950.
29. WALTERS, TRESSA: Navajos Learn by Doing, *Public Health Nursing*, p. 96, February, 1949.
30. WHITE, RUTH Y.: Army Nurses—In the Air, *American Journal of Nursing*, p. 342, April, 1943.
31. "White Task Force," Navy Nurse Corps, Navy Department, Washington, D.C. (Single copies free.)

CHAPTER XVII

Other Nursing Opportunities

POSITIONS IN NATIONAL VOLUNTARY ORGANIZATIONS

A number of national, nonprofit-making organizations, voluntarily supported (gifts, membership dues, grants from foundations, interest on endowments, etc.), employ one or more professional nurses for consultant service to their staffs or a complete staff of nurses on a national scale. Among them are the following:[1]

American Association of Industrial Nurses
American Cancer Society
American Journal of Nursing
American Red Cross
American Nurses Association
Amercian Psychiatric Association
American Public Health Association
Commonwealth Fund
The International Council of Nurses (London headquarters)
Kellogg Foundation
Maternity Center Association
National Association for Practical Nurse Education
National Foundation for Infantile Paralysis
National League of Nursing Education
National Organization for Public Health Nursing
    (*Public Health Nursing* magazine)
National Society for the Prevention of Blindness

[1] For the addresses of organizations mentioned in this chapter, see Appendix A.

National Tuberculosis Association
Planned Parenthood Federation of America
The Rockefeller Foundation

The above represent full-time positions. From time to time, other national organizations employ nurses for special studies or consultant services.[2] There are also several joint projects of the national nursing groups which are incorporated bodies, such as the National Nursing Accrediting Service, Committee on Careers in Nursing, and the National Committee for the Improvement of Nursing Services.

Most of the responsibilities of the nurses employed by national voluntary agencies call for wide experience, thorough preparation, and advanced educational qualifications. Staff members must be free to travel, able to work with and through committees, to take part in studies and surveys, to prepare reports and addresses, and to speak before audiences of all types. Considerable executive and administrative ability is essential. Knowledge of nursing and health situations on as broad a scale as possible is sought in applicants, combined with skill in handling public relations. Considerable nervous as well as physical energy is demanded in the performance of the national consultant jobs. Strenuous travel under all conditions, flexibility in judging and in making quick decisions in a wide variety of situations, and a constant demand for the tactful handling of community and individual problems call for stamina, patience, and wisdom. The nurse who does not enjoy meeting people or who likes to see a detailed piece of work perfected and completed as the reward of her effort alone, will not find satisfaction in a national agency, where results are on a long-term basis, are frequently never seen by the staff member 1,000 miles from the activity, and are nearly always the outcome of a large number of factors and persons cooperating for success.

There is very little direct contact with patients in any of the national jobs. As compensation, however, there is the excitement of being in the center of events in the nursing world, of meeting leaders who have been

[2] For lists of other voluntary national agencies see:

CAVINS, HAROLD M.: "National Health Agencies," Public Affairs Press, Washington, D.C., 1945.

GUNN, SELSKAR M., and PHILIP S. PLATT: "Voluntary Health Agencies," The Ronald Press Company, New York, 1945.

HODGES, MARGARET B. (ed.): "Social Work Year Book" (11th issue), American Association of Social Workers, New York, 1951.

Facts about Nursing, American Nurses Association (annually).

but names to you in the past, and of seeing the most progressive experiments and ideas in the making. Most of the national nursing agencies are in close touch with Washington, and there are a variety of projects cooperatively handled with the Federal nursing staffs.

If you do like travel, you will in all probability see the greater part of our vast country in the course of a national career, and extend your circle of friends and acquaintances in a most heart-warming and lasting fashion.

Salaries range (1951) from $4,000 to $8,500. All traveling expenses are met by the employer.

Applications should be made to the director of the organization.[3] A personal interview is always requested, frequently at organization expense. As these positions are for experienced nurses, those under thirty years of age can seldom qualify. There are occasional exceptions. Usually, the national organization seeks its own staff.

The American National Red Cross, in addition to employing a national advisory staff, employs local nurses for teaching home nursing, nurses' aides, and public health nurses under local Red Cross chapters. It also calls on enrolled Red Cross nurses for temporary disaster service. (About three hundred responded in 1949–1950, which included those recruited for poliomyelitis epidemics.) The positions on the headquarters staff are for experienced nurses.

The nursing services of the American Red Cross include

. . . instruction in home care of the sick and mother and baby care; disaster nursing preparedness and service; instruction and technical supervision of volunteer nurse's aides; enrollment of nurses in local Red Cross chapters; nursing in the national blood program; and educational or technical assistance to nurses in Red Cross societies of other countries.

Red Cross nursing services are planned to complement community health activities through provision of instructional and emergency nursing services, and to implement the nursing phases of disaster services, international activities, and the national blood program of the Red Cross. In a few selected situations, nursing services may engage in demonstrations or experimentations in the field of public health and health education.

A reserve of volunteer nurses is available through chapters for Red

[3] See official directory in *American Journal of Nursing.*

Cross sponsored health teaching, for emergency nursing service, and for approved community health projects.

Application should be made directly to Washington headquarters.

STATE POSITIONS

Besides the more numerous tax-supported positions for nurses on the state level, there are private agencies employing experienced nurses for promotional and administrative work. Among these, the most familiar are the state nurses associations. The responsibilities of the paid nurse-executive-secretary are quite like those of a national staff member except that they are discharged within the state's boundaries. Her qualifications are also similar. A few associations in the large cities are able to support local executive secretaries. There is a great deal of committee work involved in their duties, general and professional meetings to attend, and considerable evening work. Travel over the state is expected of the executive. A driver's license is desirable. She must be adept at handling various kinds of publicity, be able to promote happy public relations with a wide variety of groups including the press, and be able to speak easily and convincingly in public. It is essential that nurses working in state positions for the promotion of nursing interests like organization work.

In many positions, a speaking acquaintance with legislative procedure and a sound understanding of parliamentary law are important.

Positions for vocational counselors have developed at the state level in the last few years.

Salary ranges in these positions are (for full time) from $3,000 and $6,500.

THE MISSION FIELD

Opportunities as nurse-missionaries in foreign lands may be found by consulting the various missionary boards (see Bibliography at the end of this chapter) and by asking your minister. We are fortunate in having Ida Trapp's account of her work in West Africa, especially as the request reached her at a busy time. Quoting from the letter accompanying her report:

Just now I find myself virtually in charge—pro tem—of this station, with its 21 organized churches, 3 outstations, 10 elementary schools;

and then I have a weekly leper clinic 6 miles away, and the dispensers carry on 8 medical clinics twice a week out in the villages.

We have Infant Welfare Day each Wednesday and weigh 80 to 100 babies. Thursdays I have Antepartal Clinic, 16 to 30 women; besides we have 14 outstations where the evangelists have simple remedies and we dispense those. I do find such joy in the work! Here is my report:

On the Mission Field

Sudan Interior Mission
Biliri via Gombe and Jos
N. Nigeria, West Africa
May, 1951

Dear Student Nurses:

I want to tell you how wonderful it is to be a nurse on the mission field. One does not work by the clock out here. We begin early, sometimes very early, and we work until there is opportunity to stop, but our tasks are many and varied, and there is no monotony.

You won't mind if this is personal, will you? I consider nursing one of the very highest professions; more than that, it is a high calling and to be a nurse-missionary is far more than a mere occupation. Out here we nurses are few and far between, with exceedingly few doctors miles and miles away. Our district extends about 40 miles east, 50 miles north, and there are no main mission stations to the west or south of us. For some time I was the only nurse in the district. We are needed—desperately needed—and these Africans place so much confidence in us that it fairly makes us tremble. They come from miles away for help, on stretchers, on horses, on donkeys, many on foot. Is there anything that contributes more to the value of nursing than a sense of being needed? And then being trained to fill that need—it is wonderful—thrilling!

Among these pagan peoples the old grannies are the midwives. A few years ago the Government statistics reported the mortality rate of babies under one year as 80 per cent. No preparation is made for delivery. The woman in labor is in a dark hut, squatting on a rock or a small block of wood, surrounded by other pagan women. Usually one woman sits behind and one in front and from the onset of labor they make the mother bear down with every contraction. Many of the labors are reasonably short. The baby pops out head first—usually—and hits the bare, blood-and-water-soaked ground. There it lies in the cold muck until the placenta is expelled; the grannies do not cut the cord until then. If the baby cries spontaneously, all right; if not, all right too, a bit of time elapses and a grave is prepared for the little one. A tired uterus is stimulated by the grannies by rolling a cornstalk back and forth over the abdomen. A piece of cornstalk, severed with a knife and very sharp, is used to cut the cord. Then the baby is given water—clean or dirty, it makes no difference. The baby's nose is held and the water is allowed to run into the mouth until the abdomen is sufficiently distended. Prematures get the same treatment, only less care. Why waste time on them—they will die anyway! As to the mother's health, that is left out of the picture. Any laceration heals as best it can. The mother gets up immediately after delivery and goes out to bathe with hot water, washing herself with leaves.

Perhaps in a few days or weeks the baby develops a sickness. The witch doctors are consulted, appropriate "medicine" given, the little life is lost, and in an incredibly short time the pagan woman is pregnant again with no brighter prospects for health or a live baby than she had before. The Christians have separated from these terrible practices and they, as well as many of the pagan women, come to us for help.

I have been amazed at the ignorance of nurses, including myself, concerning obstetrics until we have had the privilege of taking a course in nurse-midwifery. I speak of it as a privilege, and it is all that, for I have never enjoyed any course in nursing so much as I enjoyed the 6 months at Maternity Center in New York City. [See Chap. IV.] As I look back at my cases before I had the course, I realize that my judgment and ability to make decisions were limited by my lack of theoretical training. True, many lives were saved, but I am quite sure many others might have been saved, and because I am 200 miles from the nearest railroad, telephone, doctor, or hospital, I realize more and more how often what I have to do is out of my realm as a nurse-midwife. Appreciating this I tread more softly and carefully—but there is no one else to make the decisions and carry them out!

But here comes a patient! She is carried on a cornstalk stretcher lashed together by native-woven rope. She is tied on securely and carried by four men. The stretcher is put down outside the dispensary. While the ropes are loosened, we ask for details. Then we see a live baby lying beside the mother at the end of the uncut cord. She delivered yesterday and the placenta has not been expelled. The baby is covered with dried blood and dirt. The mother is tired, dirty, unwashed, covered with blood, only leaves over her and swarms of flies follow her—altogether a terrible sight.

We tie and cut the partially dried cord, bathe and wrap the baby and give him warm, clean, boiled water. We examine the mother's abdomen, the placenta is high up and cannot be expelled by massage. Then comes the disagreeable, loathesome task of removing the filthy leaves, cleaning her body, and doing a manual extraction of a partially decomposed placenta which must be removed in small pieces. Thanks to chloroform and a competent African dispenser, the otherwise impossible task is possible and the mother is spared. What less can be done? Who else is there to do it? I find myself making decisions much more easily since taking the course in nurse-midwifery.

Another thing, we learn a simple, safe, easy, practical technique which can be used in the slum areas of New York City or 'way out in the African bush. "There is a woman in labor here," a fellow-missionary said as I approached the station; "perhaps you'd like to help us out." Right down my alley, think I, nothing suits me better; and since my stethoscope goes with me everywhere, except to church, I say: "I'll need two pieces of string, a razor blade, a bit of cotton, and some newspaper (a scarce commodity out here)." I have no gloves or finger cots, so I depend entirely on observation, instead of examination, to determine progress in labor. This is an unusually high-strung patient for an African, but she responds splendidly. In an hour and a half she is delivered of a lovely little boy—and believe me, these African babies are sweet!

While we sat there I gave the other two missionary ladies a few timely hints on obstetrics; one was a mother of two, the other had never seen a baby born. There are also several African women in our town who have learned the very simplest things about deliveries and the care of the newborn; they have saved many lives. The women in the antepartal clinic are interested in the changes during pregnancy; and when it comes to infant welfare, we realize that whatever touches the babies touches the mothers also. How happy they are when their babies gain even though they don't know an ounce from a pound! Teaching is a great challenge here.

Work in the mission field challenges the best in one. Don't forget to bring along your sense of humor! So, since you are not one to be satisfied with just the ordinary job, the extraordinary awaits you with its many and varied opportunities for service. You are needed here!

Sincerely yours in the bonds of a great and noble profession,

IDA L. TRAPP, R.N., A.B., C.N.M.

Care of the Chronically Ill, the Aged, and the Convalescent

The care of the chronically ill and the aged will offer a continuing demand for nursing service in the future as population trends indicate a growing number of persons living to "ripe old age." It is a fact that the average length of stay of patients in hospitals becomes greater with advancing age. It is also true that the disablements and diseases of old age cared for at home tend to last longer and be more incapacitating than the more acute troubles of those under fifty.[4]

One of the many lessons learned from the tragedies of war relates to that heretofore somewhat neglected period following illness that we know as convalescence. Experience with our war-wounded has proved the value of regarding convalescence as a definitely specialized field in itself, one needing much more attention and study on the part of doctors and nurses from the psychosomatic standpoint. Though much of the care in institutions for the convalescent may be carried out by nurses' aides, they should always be under professional nursing supervision, while in large institutions a regular professional nursing staff is essential. This whole field of convalescence and rehabilitation is now receiving intensive study.

The future plans of general hospitals frequently include either a division for convalescence or a country branch to which ward as well as private patients will be sent before returning to their homes.

Nursing service in convalescent homes requires a certain amount of versatility. Patients need to be kept occupied within the limits of their strength, watched carefully for untoward signs, kept from becoming homesick if possible, taught to care for themselves, and generally encouraged to want to get well. Nurses in small institutions will need to know something about dietetics, including special diets, occupational therapy, games and recreation, and, of course, first aid. As a rule, there will be nurses' aides for them to supervise. Quite a few nurses are the administrative heads of convalescent homes.

[4] "The Magnitude of the Chronic Disease Problem in the United States," The National Health Survey (USPHS), Preliminary Reports, Sickness and Medical Care Series, Bulletin 6. See also the proceedings of the National Conference on Aging, Federal Security Agency, Washington, D.C., 1950, and those of the Commission on Chronic Illness, Chicago, Ill. For general information, refer to the Division of Chronic Disease, U.S. Public Health Service, Federal Security Agency, Washington, D.C. See also, "Directory of Convalescent Homes in the United States," Burke Foundation, White Plains, N.Y.

Institutions for these three groups—the chronic, the aged, and the convalescent—abound. They may be state, county, or city tax-supported, as well as Federal facilities. A vast number of private institutions, ranging from those with sizable bed capacity to private homes for one or two patients, offer nursing service of highly varying and uncertain quality as well as quantity. All advertised homes or institutions, especially those privately owned and run for profit, should be carefully investigated by the job seeker. They should be licensed by the state or city and be able to display that license. They are supposed to be inspected regularly by state or local officials.

Professional nurses would do well to make the following inquiries before accepting a position in a privately owned or supported institution for the care of the aged, chronically ill, or convalescent.

1. Is it licensed by the state or city?
2. If supported by private gifts, is it a member of the Community Chest?
3. Is there a licensed physician in charge of all patients? Is he on call or resident?
4. Are patients accepted who are not under medical care?
5. Exactly what type of patient is admitted? (*Important*)
6. Are nurses' aides employed? How many? Who trains them? To whom are they responsible?
7. What hospital connections are there to take care of emergencies?
8. To whom will you be responsible?
9. Exactly what are the hours of duty to be?
10. Get your salary arrangement in writing.
11. Ask about tax deductions, including old age security.
12. Be sure to go over the institution or home before accepting employment. Note especially the stairs you may have to climb, the adequacy of fire escapes, and the amount of unskilled help available. Instances have occurred in which registered nurses have found themselves expected to do everything in the home, including cooking and washing dishes.[5]

Not all the chronically ill are bed patients. Many, these days, are being greatly helped by a period of hospitalization and treatment. Attention

[5] Information may be secured from the American Association of Nursing Homes, Indianapolis. (See Appendix A.)

is especially drawn to two conditions that are rapidly becoming specialties in their own right: heart disease and cancer.

HEART DISEASE AND CANCER

Heart disease and cancer, now the leading causes of death in the United States, have received more attention in the last 15 years than in all the preceding century. Both conditions, once regarded as the degenerative diseases of old age, are common among young people. The American Heart Association (for address, see Appendix A) and intensive research in the predisposing causes of heart disease have focused attention on this condition. With the establishment of the National Cancer Institute in Washington in 1937, the reorganization of the American Cancer Society (see Appendix A), grants from such sources as the Damon Runyon Cancer Fund, the inauguration of cancer-control programs in state and local health departments, and the building of several modern diagnostic hospitals for research and treatment purposes—the attack on this disease is proceeding rapidly on all fronts. Nurses are taking their part in all phases of both campaigns. They are teaching the public how to recognize these diseases assisting in early case finding, giving skilled nursing care, and promoting rehabilitation. There is a growing demand for public health nurses to work in tumor clinics and to develop the educational and preventive programs in connection with this campaign, now of national importance.

Although one in nine people die of cancer, it is growing to be a less and less hopeless disease, and any day the discoveries of the research laboratories may place it under our full control. The field is calling insistently for nurses with advanced clinical preparation. The farsighted nurse may well develop this as her specialty and expect satisfactory job opportunities.

One of the specialties within the field of cancer nursing is radiology. The growing use of radiation therapy for many deep-seated cancers makes this a likely field of the future. Training for this specialty is usually on the job.

Similarly, the study of heart disease, "rheumatic hearts," and their nursing care, offers a field of considerable future promise. There are a few institutions and children's homes and camps devoted solely to cardiac patients. Special training is usually secured on the job under the guidance of the medical staff.

Both these conditions—cancer and heart disease—warrant intensive study and practice on the part of the nurse. If you are considering entering either field as a specialty, consult the National League of Nursing Education for special courses and write or call on the two national voluntary agencies interested in securing qualified personnel: the American Cancer Society and the American Heart Association, both located in New York City. Technical manual skill and deftness, great accuracy, and close observation are expected of the nurse in many of these specialties. (For Federal positions in the specialties, see Chap. XVI.)

OTHER SPECIALTIES

There are several specialized fields in which relatively few nurses prepare themselves, such preparation being usually through experience on the job, intensive institutes, short courses, or closely supervised work with the clinical or medical director. Examples of these special fields are nursing direction of diabetic patients, special service in eye, ear, nose, and throat clinics, hospitals, and doctors' offices. The jobs may include the administration of certain highly technical tests and treatments. Assistance in office treatments and in minor operations calls for considerable judgment and skill for which nurses often develop great proficiency. This type of intensive highly developed service suits some people perfectly and frequently brings in a good income. The danger in it is that the nurse may grow away from her general knowledge of sick people and become so highly specialized that her employability as a bedside nurse after a few years is limited. It is never well to have only one string to one's bow. Refresher courses, continued reading of professional journals, and attendance at professional meetings will partly offset the danger of growing stale in specialized nursing.

One must also remember that the nurse in some of the very highly specialized jobs reaches her maximum salary in 3 or 4 years and has no future beyond that or a similar job. A review of one's situation every 3 to 5 years, a sort of stocktaking, is good practice. It will move the ambitious nurse on to a new job before she "deteriorates" in professional growth.

Other special skills for which nursing knowledge is a good foundation and which have attracted nurses who wish to "be on their own" and run their own business are cosmetology, massage, diathermy treatments, and colonic irrigations. Some of these require additional special training and a license to practice.

NURSE ANESTHETISTS

The estimated future need for nurse anesthetists is somewhat uncertain, as there is a tendency to use medical anesthesiologists in preference to nurses. There seems to be no way of knowing whether a number of nurse anesthetists will be replaced by doctors during the next 5 or 10 years. About 3,800 are employed full time, and another 1,200 part time. There are some 37 training courses available, the preferable entering age being twenty-four to thirty-five years. The courses last from 6 to 12 months.

Salaries in this field are as high as $500 a month, $250 for beginners.

Information regarding this field may be obtained from the American Association of Nurse Anesthetists (for address, see Appendix A).

X-RAY TECHNICIANS

This is a possible occupation for nurses who wish to specialize in a non-nursing activity. It is well to have a definite position in mind before going to the expense of the necessary preparation. A list of approved schools preparing x-ray technicians may be secured from the American Medical Association (for address, see Appendix A). Salaries range from $224 to $350 a month.

MEDICAL RECORD LIBRARIANS

This is usually a fairly sedentary job, adapted to a nurse with a handicap on her physical agility. A list of the approved training courses may be secured from the American Medical Association. Monthly salaries are in the neighborhood of $250.

MISCELLANEOUS OPPORTUNITIES

Nurses employed in what might be called the unclassified or miscellaneous jobs are not many—perhaps 12,000 in all[6]—but their jobs are especially interesting and frequently represent developments of a unique or highly specialized nature. These jobs may be the outcome of a lively, though practical imagination, individual initiative, unusual business acumen, or just plain chance!

Of the varied opportunities for unique, special, and part-time jobs for nurses, there is literally no end. As you were told when you entered

[6] *Facts about Nursing*, p. 13. American Nurses Association, 1950.

your school of nursing, the training for this profession, the second largest in this country for women, opens a dozen doors to jobs not usually listed or classified in the guidance books, and every year sees some new developments. Only a few of these unclassified occupations for nurses are mentioned here, only enough to illustrate how wide is the horizon for those who would look beyond the familiar demands for nursing service in hospitals and homes. Not all these are full-time jobs.

1. A nurse with a talent for drawing has become a medical artist, nearly doubling her income.
2. A nurse tied down by her family of three children has opened and equipped a nursery school, employs a trained kindergarten teacher, and also accepts little boarders over vacations and holidays. She cleared $1,000 the second year of her venture.
3. A nurse unable to do active nursing because of an injury to her spine is devoting her time to assisting in the preparation of scientific reports, studies, and speeches. She does investigation of statistical reports, laboratory findings, and discoveries as reported in medical and other journals. Magazines, newspapers, and broadcasting studios have used her services, as well as individuals.
4. The hobby of amateur photography has developed into a satisfactory business for several nurses, one of whom also plans and produces movies of medical and nursing subjects.
5. A married nurse with a teacher's background has made use of her advanced clinical preparation to conduct private classes for expectant and new mothers. Her contacts with doctors and hospitals keep her classes full. She also sells maternity and infant supplies on commission.
6. Nurses are employed full time in animal experimental laboratories. Some zoos employ nurses.
7. A good many nurses have developed their own placement services, run on a profit basis. Business experience and ability to handle and develop good public relations are essential to success in this field. There are many commercial registries run by registered nurses or employing them as managers. Workers in placement agencies should have professional backing: a professional organization or, at the least, an advisory committee of qualified professional nurses.
8. A nurse who teaches in the winter owns and runs a camp for handicapped children in the summer months.
9. A nurse has a good position as an assistant saleswoman, fitter, and

adviser in a firm taking measurements for, making, and selling surgical belts, supports, corsets, and braces of all sorts. Many of the garments are made according to prescriptions from surgeons and obstetricians.

10. Full- and part-time nurse-demonstrators are used in stores, at fairs, conventions, and other exhibitions. Occasionally, this work includes talks or informal "classes" for customers.

11. Student summer tours occasionally engage the services of nurses.

12. Positions as research assistants in laboratories or assistants in special studies, surveys, or experiments develop from time to time. The nurse who has added preparation in a second field, such as statistics, laboratory technique, or dietetics, widens her chances of employment and can frequently command a higher salary.

13. Blood banks and blood-donor centers offer both full- and part-time service to professional nurses.

14. Nurses have been able to use their own homes for the care of a few chronic or convalescent patients. Such homes must obtain a license from the state and are inspected at intervals. (See also Care of the Chronically Ill, the Aged, and the Convalescent, above.) Married nurses have also served as foster mothers, taking state wards into their homes. It is possible that mental hospitals may make use of the homes of professional nurses for the care of paroled patients (see New York State's plan).[7]

15. Teaching Red Cross home nursing classes has provided a moderate income for many nurses and part-time pay for thousands. The payment to the nurse is usually on an hourly or "course" basis and is paid by the American Red Cross, Red Cross chapter, or the sponsoring agency. Inquire of your local Red Cross chapter for requirements, opportunities, and payment rates.

16. State welfare departments occasionally employ as special consultants, or on a full-time basis, nurses for the inspection of homes for chronic, aged, or dependent persons.

17. Service on special commissions and advisory boards may bring in a small stipend or honorarium to retired but widely experienced nurses. Surveys and special studies quite frequently require the services of well-prepared and experienced nurses—full or part time.

18. Paid editorial assistance to, or direction of, professional publications occupies fewer than 50 professional nurses in this country at the

[7] CRUTCHER, HESTER B.: "Foster Home Care for Mental Patients," Commonwealth Fund, Division of Publication, New York, 1944.

present time. Free-lance writing offers a future to perhaps twice that number. Courses in journalism, experience in writing for college publications or newspapers, and unending practice form a good background for these positions. Many nurses find themselves writing textbooks as a part of their professional teaching program; a few write for recreation, for the popular magazines. *Interest* in writing is a decided asset and probably indispensable if it is to be one's main occupation. Nurses have not explored the possibilities of this field sufficiently.[8]

19. Nurses are beginning to work in the field of tests and measurements. Statistical and psychological courses on an advanced academic level are prerequisites to this field.

20. Professional nurses have been called upon as technical advisers to large moving-picture producers. (See Ref. 18.)

21. Nurses are occasionally employed by the large pharmaceutical and hospital supply agencies as saleswomen or as representatives of publishing houses interested in promoting nursing textbooks.

22. Nurses have found that running tearooms, serving as directors of cafeterias, and acting as hospital housekeepers are jobs that make good use of their knowledge of dietetics and homemaking.

23. A business of providing invalid fare, infant feeding, and special diets has been developed by a few nurses.

24. Baby-sitting, though it may sound simple, has proved a fairly steady source of income for nurses who are studying, have retired, or are in need of a few extra dollars a week.

25. Nurses are employed in migrant labor camps. These are apt to be seasonal jobs.

26. Nurses are employed in juvenile courts and domestic relations courts.

RELATED FIELDS OF SERVICE

A career book would certainly not be fulfilling its function if it did not point out the other professions for which nursing is an excellent and appropriate preparation. For each of the occupations in the following list additional study and practice are essential. Many, obviously, call for a bachelor's degree as a prerequisite. Some do not pay as well as nursing. Nurses have qualified in the following fields:

[8] For information about the Mary M. Roberts Fellowship award for the study of journalism, write to the *American Journal of Nursing*.

Anesthesia
Dental hygiene (not
  open to men)
Dentistry
Dietetics
Health education
Hospital administration
Laboratory
Medicine
Medical art

Medical library
Medical social work
Nutrition
Occupational therapy
Physical therapy
Psychiatric social work
Scientific research
Social work
Statistics
X-ray and radiology

Sources of Employment

American Cancer Society, 56 Beaver St., New York, N.Y.

American Friends Service Committee, 20 S. Twelfth St., Philadelphia, Pa.

American Heart Association, 1775 Broadway, New York, N.Y.

American Hospital Association, 22 E. Division St., Chicago, Ill.

American Missionary Association, 287 Fourth Ave., New York, N.Y.

Catholic Hospital Association of the United States and Canada, 1402 S. Grand Blvd., St. Louis, Mo.

Christian Medical Council for Overseas Work, 156 Fifth Ave., New York, N.Y.

Church World Service, 214 E. 21st St. New York, N.Y.

Council of the Congregational and Christian Churches, 287 Fourth Ave., New York, N.Y.

Council of Women for Home Missions, 297 Fourth Ave., New York, N.Y.

Federal Council of Churches of Christ in America, 297 Fourth Ave., New York, N.Y.

Home Missions, Council of North America, 297 Fourth Ave., New York, N.Y.

International Council of Nurses, 19, Queen's Gate, London, S.W. 7, England

International Grenfell Association, 256 Fifth Ave., New York, N.Y.

Lutheran Church, Board of Social Missions, 39 E. 35th St., New York, N.Y. (Also 57 Main St., Columbus, Ohio.)

Methodist Board of Hospitals and Homes, 740 Rush St., Chicago, Ill.

Methodist Church, Board of Missions, 150 Fifth Ave., New York, N.Y.

National Catholic Community Service, 1312 Massachusetts Ave., N.W., Washington, D.C.

Presbyterian Church, Board of National Missions, 156 Fifth Ave., New
York, N.Y.

Protestant Episcopal Church, National Council, 281 Fourth Ave., New
York, N.Y.

Relief Society, Women's Auxiliary of the Church of Christ of Latter
Day Saints, 28 Bishops Building, Salt Lake City, Utah

Rockefeller Foundation, 49 W. 49th St., New York, N.Y.

Rosenwald Fund, 4901 Ellis Ave., Chicago, Ill.

Salvation Army, 120 W. 14th St., New York, N.Y.

Society of Catholic Medical Missionaries, Washington, D.C.

Society of St. Vincent de Paul, 289 Fourth Ave., New York, N.Y.

Unitarian Service Committee, 9 Park St., Boston, Mass.

United Council of Church Women, 156 Fifth Ave., New York, N.Y.

United Jewish Appeal for Refugees, 165 W. 46th St., New York, N.Y

Volunteers of America, 34 W. 28th St., New York, N.Y.

World Health Organization, Palais des Nations, Geneva, Switzerland

BIBLIOGRAPHY

Nursing Abroad and Missionary Nursing

1. ASKEW, RITA L.: Nursing in the Dominican Republic, *American Journal of Nursing*, p. 814, December, 1947.
2. BYERLY, RUTH P.: Summer Nursing in Labrador, *American Journal of Nursing*, p. 302, May, 1946.
3. CANTOR, SHULAMITH L.: Nursing in Israel, *American Journal of Nursing*, p. 162, March, 1951.
4. DUNHAM, GEORGE C.: Health Makes Wealth for the Americas, *Hygeia*, p. 188, March, 1945.
5. GOFF, HAZEL A.: Preparing for Postwar Work Abroad, *American Journal of Nursing*, p. 169, February, 1943.
6. KERZE, THERESE, Nursing in a Middle East Refugee Camp, *Public Health Nursing*, p. 443, September, 1945.
7. MACKIE, JANET W.: Nursing in the Other American Republics, *American Journal of Nursing*, p. 355, May, 1945.
8. Missionary Nursing in the Postwar World, *American Journal of Nursing*, p. 297, March, 1943.
9. O'CONNOR, REV. PAUL C., S.J.: Arctic Nurses, *Public Health Nursing*, p. 508, October, 1944.
10. PETRY, LUCILE: Nursing on the World Health Front, *American Journal of Nursing*, p. 611, October, 1950.
11. WHITE, JEAN MARTIN: Modern Nursing in Old Peru, *R.N.*, p. 41, September, 1947.

See also yearly index of professional journals under the name of the country in which you are interested. Also inquire of the International Council of Nurses and the World Health Organization.

The Handicapped

1. BARTON, BETSEY: "And Now to Live Again," Appleton-Century-Crofts, Inc., New York, 1944.
2. CARLSON, EARL REINHOLD: "Born That Way," The John Day Company, New York, 1941.
3. CHERNE, LEO: "The Rest of Your Life," Doubleday & Company, Inc., New York, 1944.
4. DAHL, BORGHILD: "I Wanted to See," The Macmillan Company, New York, 1944.
5. HATHAWAY, KATHARINE BUTLER: "The Little Locksmith," Coward-McCann, Inc., New York, 1943.
6. U.S. CIVIL SERVICE COMMISSION: "A Guide for the Placement of the Physically Handicapped," Pamphlet No. 14, 4th ed., 1947.
7. WALKER, MILDRED: "Dr. Norton's Wife," Harcourt, Brace and Company, Inc., New York, 1938.

Doctors of Medicine

1. CHANDLER, CAROLINE A., M.D.: "Susie Stuart, M.D.," Dodd, Mead & Company, Inc., New York, 1943.
2. CHANDLER, CAROLINE A., M.D.: "Susie Stuart, Home Front Doctor," Dodd, Mead & Company, Inc., New York, 1944.
3. LEES, HANNAH: "Women Will Be Doctors," Random House, New York, 1940.

Miscellaneous Positions in Nursing

1. ADAMS, ELEANOR: When Spring Floods and Tornadoes Struck, *American Journal of Nursing*, p. 460, June, 1945. (Red Cross disaster service; see also p. 310, May, 1946.)
2. FREEMAN, RUTH B.: Nursing Plus—The Red Cross Nursing Service, *American Journal of Nursing*, January, 1948.
3. KRESKY, BEATRICE, and H. M. C. LUYKX: Patients Are Older and Stay Longer, *Hospitals*, p. 21, February, 1944. (Additional references to care of the aged will be found in the *American Journal of Nursing*, p. 1047, November, 1944.)
4. MEREDITH, SYLVIA R.: Nurse Plays Nurse on Television, *American Journal of Nursing*, p. 564, September, 1949.
5. Miss Merling, Registrar, *American Journal of Nursing*, p. 240, March, 1940; p. 543, June, 1940.
6. PLETCHER, KENNETH E., and FRANCES P. THORP: Aero-Medical Nursing, *American Journal of Nursing*, p. 149, March, 1950.

7. Red Cross at the Texas City Disaster, *American Journal of Nursing*, p. 400, June, 1947.

8. SCOTT, RUTH B.: Nurse to Adventurers, *R.N.*, p. 32, April, 1949.

9. STOTZ, EVELYN T.: The Red Cross Blood Program, *American Journal of Nursing*, p. 165, March, 1948.

Special Techniques

ANESTHESIA

1. Anesthesia, X-ray, Laboratory? *American Journal of Nursing*, p. 567, May, 1941.

2. "A Career for the Graduate Nurse" (leaflet), American Association of Nurse Anesthetists, Chicago.

3. COSTELLO, MARY A.: Anesthesia—A Challenge to Nurses, *American Journal of Nursing*, p. 745, August, 1944.

4. FIFE, GERTRUDE L.: The Nurse As an Anesthetist, *American Journal of Nursing*, p. 308, May, 1947.

5. HAYT, EMANUEL: Anesthesia, Legal and Illegal, *R.N.*, p. 42, February, 1948.

6. PALUMBO, LOUIS T.: Some Recent Advances in Surgery (Anesthesiology), *American Journal of Nursing*, p. 659, October, 1950.

MISCELLANEOUS

1. BAKELESS, JOHN: The Technique of Technical Writing, *American Journal of Nursing*, p. 1141, October, 1941.

2. BAKELESS, JOHN: Writing for Publication, *American Journal of Nursing*, p. 689, October, 1947.

3. COVINGTON, ETHEL: "The Efficient Dental Assistant," The C. V. Mosby Company, Medical Publishers, St. Louis, 1940.

4. HOPP, MARGARET: Roentgen Therapy and the Nurse, *American Journal of Nursing*, p. 431, April, 1941.

5. HUFFMAN, EDNA K.: "Manual for Medical Records Librarians," Physicians Record Company, Chicago, 1948.

6. HUFFMAN, EDNA K.: Training of Medical Records Librarians, *Hospitals*, p. 69, March, 1936.

7. KAKOSH, PEGGY: The Nurse as Technical Adviser in Film Production, *American Journal of Nursing*, p. 107, February, 1946.

8. LYONS, DON C.: Possibilities of Employment by the Dental Profession, *Trained Nurse and Hospital Review*, p. 33, July, 1933.

9. "Medical Laboratory Technicians, The Outlook for Women in Occupations in the Medical Services," Women's Bureau, Department of Labor, Washington, D.C., Bulletin 203, No. 4; also Bulletin 203, No. 6, "Medical Record Librarians," 1945.

10. SCOTT, RUTH B.: Medical Illustrators, *R.N.*, p. 50, April, 1947.

11. STERN, EDITH M., and META R. COBB: "Betty Blake, O.T.," Dodd, Mead & Company, Inc., New York, 1943. (Occupational therapy.)

12. TURNER, MARY ELLIS: "Karren Long, Medical Technician," Dodd, Mead & Company, Inc., New York, 1942.

CHAPTER XVIII

Practical Nursing

For the girl, woman, or man who is not qualified for professional nursing or who has passed the age when he or she may enter a professional school of nursing—usually thirty-five—practical nursing offers an interesting and satisfying occupation. Students in professional schools who find the classwork too difficult or who for family or personal reasons have had to drop out of and do not wish to resume the 3-year program, may find practical nursing the answer to their desire to nurse.[1] However, applicants must meet the standards of the approved schools of practical nursing and those who are "dropped students" from professional schools are investigated with special care. Those who have been found to have no aptitude for nursing even though they love it, those who have failed to meet the exacting demands of caring for patients or who have not met the standards of personal conduct in professional schools, will not be accepted in schools of practical nursing.

This is a possible field for older married women who need a means of support, who have always wanted to be nurses, but who have been busy raising their families or have been tied by other family obligations; and for the young women who dislike the business world. Some of the practical nursing schools will accept women in their thirties and forties who have not completed high school. This is an important point to remember because so many interesting jobs open to older women require a high school diploma or training and experience in a specialty.

At present, the general requirements for the field of practical nursing are good health, good character, a sincere interest in nursing, preferably

---

[1] Failure in classwork accounted for the withdrawal of 36 per cent of the professional nursing students in 1949–1950. *Facts about Nursing*, p. 40, American Nurses Association, 1950.

2 years of high school as a minimum (required of applicants under thirty), or completion of eighth grade for older persons. The age limits are eighteen to fifty. The schools usually administer some form of aptitude test, give a medical examination, and, of course, require evidence of the student's school grades. A personal interview is customary.

The licensed practical nurse must have completed an approved[2] course of training—usually 9 to 18 months in length—which includes theory and supervised practice in selected fields; and must meet the requirements of the state licensing body where she or he expects to practice. A list of the approved schools may be secured from the Committee on Careers in Nursing.[3]

A practical nurse has been defined as a person trained to care for sub-acute convalescent and chronic patients requiring nursing services at home or in institutions, who works under the direction of a licensed physician or a registered professional nurse, and who is prepared to give household assistance when necessary. A practical nurse may be employed by physicians, hospitals, custodial homes, public health agencies, and the lay public.

The licensed practical nurses have their own national membership organization, the National Federation of Licensed Practical Nurses, Inc., and their own state membership associations in many states.

Opportunities in Practical Nursing

Practical nurses are finding employment in an ever-increasing number and variety of positions. They have always been employed in private homes. The professional registries had over thirty thousand calls for practical nurses in 1949, and now hospitals of all types—governmental, voluntary, and proprietary—use their services. Including attendants, the total of those working in hospitals in 1949 was over 250,000, of whom probably 30,000 were licensed.[4] There are still 18 states in which practical nurses need not be licensed to practice. As might be expected, the states with the largest population employ the most practical nurses—California, Illinois, Michigan, and New York; the "rural" states, fewest—Wyoming, Utah, Idaho, and Montana.

[2] Approved by the state board of nurse examiners or other legally authorized body or by the National Association for Practical Nurse Education. Eventually, accreditation will be extended by the National Nursing Accrediting Service.

[3] For the addresses of organizations mentioned in this chapter, see Appendix A.

[4] *Facts about Nursing*, page 77, American Nursing Association, May 6, 1950.

Positions in institutions for the care of the chronically ill, the aging, the handicapped, dependent children, and convalescents are numerous. In most instances, the practical nurses work under the supervision of professional nurses.

There are a few positions in public health agencies for the well-prepared licensed practical nurse, all under professional nursing supervision. (In 1950, there were 150 practical nurses employed by 39 public health agencies.[5] These were mainly in visiting nurses associations.) It is thought that opportunities in this field will expand, however. Occasionally, the service of practical nurses—either as a part of student experience or as graduates—is used on a demonstration or experimental basis. For example, the Detroit Visiting Nurse Association is studying the function of the practical nurses (as students) in the home care of cancer patients. The cost and place of practical nursing services in the home care of the chronically ill is receiving attention in New York City. Opportunities of this sort are promising positions for well-qualified practical nurses and should be sought out.

A few licensed practical nurses are employed as assistants to industrial nurses. This function is not encouraged unless the nursing staff is large, because it is unwise to lay upon the practical nurse the responsibility of relieving the professional nurse as must often happen when the staff is a small one.

One of the largest employers of men practical nurses is the mental hospital. In many of these institutions, especially in the hospitals of the Veterans Administration, licensed practical nurses are serving in a supervisory capacity. (See also other opportunities in the Federal Services.)

Additional study and experience often make it possible for a practical nurse to advance in her chosen field or to specialize. Licensed practical nurses have become assistants in tuberculosis hospitals, in maternity divisions of hospitals, in central supply rooms, operating rooms, orthopedic wards, clinics, etc. Frequently, the acquirement of a special skill, such as massage, increases a nurse's usefulness and her salary. Nurses planning to work in doctors' offices should learn to type.

The United States Army has a school of practical nursing and will undoubtedly use its graduates in Army hospitals. The 48-week course is at the Walter Reed Hospital, Washington, D.C., and is known as the Medical Technician Procedure (Advanced) Course. If you are over thirty-five, information should be secured from the Army before planning

[5] *Facts about Nursing*, p. 79, American Nurses Association, 1950.

this course as a substitute for one of the schools which accept older men and women.

Many registries, hospitals, and homes report that they are unable to secure licensed practical nurses—in 1949, 25 per cent of the professional registry calls went unfilled—and many agencies could find a place for better qualified assistants than they now have. It appears to be a growing field for young men and women who have a genuine desire to learn to care for sick people and who are willing to devote time to the recommended training. There is less and less chance for the poorly prepared practical nurse or the misguided individual who hopes to become a "practical nurse" through a home study or correspondence course. Consult a professional nurse before wasting time and money on the latter.

Related opportunities for licensed practical nurses, some of which require additional formal training, are

> Housemother
> Doctor's office secretary
> Receptionist—clinic, hospital, otherwise
> Occupational therapy aide
> Nursery school attendant
> Masseuse
> Beauty parlor operator
> Companion or secretary to invalid
> Tearoom assistant
> Summer camp counselor

SALARIES

Salaries of licensed practical nurses vary a great deal with the area of the country, the responsibility of the position, and the attitude of the employing agencies. As a general policy, practical nurses in hospitals are paid about 75 per cent of the salaries paid professional nurses in staff positions. Pay for service in homes is apt to depend on the arrangement the nurse makes with the family, unless the nurse is employed through one of the professional registries, when the charge is usually 75 per cent of what the professional nurse is receiving in the community. For example, in 1951, licensed practical nurses were receiving $8 a day plus one meal, in cities where the professional nurses were receiving $10. However, when a family desires 24-hour service from one nurse and the patient is not in need of continuous care, the practical nurse is allowed to charge $20 with all meals and room provided.

Practical nurses, when employed on a salary basis, are usually covered by Social Security. Whether or not it is possible to work as a self-employed person when nursing in private homes—in which case the nurse pays $2\frac{1}{4}$ per cent of her earnings each month into her retirement fund under Social Security—or as a domestic, in which case the employer shares in the tax, has not been determined at the present writing. Inquiry should be made regarding the current practice when accepting a salaried position.

Personnel practices in positions for practical nurses as they relate to holidays, vacations, sick leave, and time off duty in general should be similar to those offered professional nurses. As a rule they are fair and considerate.

SOURCES OF EMPLOYMENT

1. Professional placement services
2. New York State Employment Service
3. Schools of practical nursing, especially the one from which you graduated
4. Hospitals
5. Convalescent homes and other types of institutions for the care of subacute conditions
6. National Federation of Licensed Practical Nurses, Inc.
7. National Association for Practical Nurse Education
8. U.S. Civil Service Commission
9. "Want ads" in professional journals
10. Commercial registries
11. Newspaper advertisements

BIBLIOGRAPHY

1. DEMING, DOROTHY: "The Practical Nurse," Commonwealth Fund, Division of Publication, New York, 1947.
2. DEMING, DOROTHY: Practical Nursing, Then and Now, *American Journal of Nursing*, p. 621, October, 1950.
3. DICKRAGER, HELEN, Practical Nurses Serve the Community, *American Journal of Nursing*, p. 38, January, 1950.
4. PHILLIPS, ELISABETH C.: Essentials of a Good School of Practical Nursing, *American Journal of Nursing*, p. 393, September, 1948.

5. "Practical Nursing—An Analysis of the Practical Nursing Occupation," U.S. Office of Education, Washington, D.C., 1947; also "Practical Nursing Curriculum," 1950.
6. SHARROCKS, THEODORA: Practical Nurses in a V.N.A. (letter), *Public Health Nursing*, p. 613, December, 1948.
7. STRUVE, MILDRED, and ANNE HAHN LINDBAD: Nursing Team in the Hospital, *American Journal of Nursing*, p. 5, January, 1949.
8. TUCKEY, RUTH: Practical Nurses in a Public Health Agency, *American Journal of Nursing*, p. 647, October, 1948.
9. VIGLIONE, AMY E.: Training Programs for Practical Nurses, *American Journal of Nursing*, p. 297, May, 1951.

See also publications of the American Nurses Association on the duties and functions of practical nurses; the National League of Nursing Education's "Practical Nurse Education, Manual for State and Local Leagues"; and the descriptive booklets of the Committee on Careers in Nursing, the National Association for Practical Nurse Education, and the National Federation of Licensed Practical Nurses.

Sources of Information

The organizations listed here and mentioned in the text are always glad to supply information relative to their special fields of interest. The addresses given are those of 1951 and should be checked for accuracy when used later.

Air Force Nurse Corps, Office of Surgeon General, U.S. Air Force, Washington, D.C.

American Association of Industrial Nurses, Inc., 654 Madison Ave., New York, N.Y.

American Association of Nurse Anesthetists, Inc., 18 E. Division St., Chicago, Ill.

American Association of Nursing Homes, 402 N. Holmes St., Indianapolis, Ind.

American Cancer Society, 56 Beaver St., New York, N.Y.

American Camping Association, 343 S. Dearborn St., Chicago, Ill.

American Heart Association, 1775 Broadway, New York, N.Y.

American Hospital Association, 22 E. Division St., Chicago, Ill.

American Hotel Association, 221 W. 57th St., New York, N.Y.

American Journal of Nursing, 2 Park Ave., New York, N.Y.

American Journal of Public Health, 1790 Broadway, New York, N.Y.

American Library Association, 520 N. Michigan Ave., Chicago, Ill.

American Management Association, 330 W. 42d St., New York, N.Y.

American Medical Association, 535 N. Dearborn St., Chicago, Ill.

American Medical Care Plans, 425 N. Michigan Ave., Chicago, Ill.

American Nurses Association, 2 Park Ave., New York, N.Y.

American Nurses Association Professional Counseling and Placement Service, Inc., 2 Park Ave., New York, N.Y. (Branch office, 8 S. Michigan Ave., Chicago, Ill.)

American Occupational Therapy Association, 33 W. 42d St., New York, N.Y.

American Physical Therapy Association, 1790 Broadway, New York, N.Y.

American Psychiatric Association, 9 Rockefeller Plaza, New York, N.Y.

American Public Health Association, 1790 Broadway, New York, N.Y.

American Red Cross, Washington, D.C.

American School Health Association, Kent State University, Kent, Ohio
American Social Hygiene Association, 1790 Broadway, New York, N.Y.
American Youth Hostels, 6 E. 39th St., New York, N.Y.
Army Nurse Corps, Main Navy Building, Washington, D.C.
Association of Collegiate Schools of Nursing, 2063 Adelbert Rd., Cleveland, Ohio
Association of Private Camps, 55 W. 42d St., New York, N.Y.
Bureau of Indian Affairs, Nursing Service, Department of the Interior, Washington, D.C.
Catholic Hospital Association of the United States and Canada, 1402 S. Grand Blvd., St. Louis, Mo.
Children's Bureau, Federal Security Agency, Washington, D.C.
Commission on Chronic Illness, 535 N. Dearborn St., Chicago, Ill.
Commonwealth Fund, 41 E. 57th St., New York, N.Y.
Community Service Society, 105 E. 22d St., New York, N.Y.
Division of Chronic Disease, U.S. Public Health Service, Federal Security Agency, Washington, D.C.
Family Welfare Association of America, 122 E. 22d St., New York, N.Y.
Federation Employment Service, 67 W. 47th St., New York, N.Y.
Health Education Council, 10 Downing St., New York, N.Y.
Industrial Medicine, 605 N. Michigan Ave., Chicago, Ill.
International Council of Nurses (ICN), 19, Queen's Gate, London S.W. 7, England.
Joint Orthopedic Nursing Advisory Service, 2 Park Ave., New York, N.Y.
Joint Tuberculosis Nursing Advisory Service, 2 Park Ave., New York, N.Y.
Journal of the American Medical Association, 535 N. Dearborn St., Chicago, Ill.
Kellogg Foundation, Battle Creek, Mich.
Maternity Center Association, 654 Madison Ave., New York, N.Y.
National Airlines, Inc., Jacksonville, Fla.
National Association for Mental Health, 1790 Broadway, New York, N.Y.
National Association for Practical Nurse Education, 654 Madison Ave., New York, N.Y.
National Association of Guidance Supervisors, 603 Bauch Building, Lansing, Mich.
National Committee for the Improvement of Nursing Services, 2 Park Ave., New York, N.Y.
National Committee on Careers in Nursing, 2 Park Ave., New York, N.Y.
National Conference on Aging, Federal Security Agency, Washington, D.C.
National Federation of Licensed Practical Nurses, Inc., 250 W. 57th St., New York, N.Y.
National Federation of Settlements, 214 E. 53d St., New York, N.Y.
National Foundation for Infantile Paralysis, 120 Broadway, New York, N.Y.
National Girl Scouts, Inc., 155 E. 44th St., New York, N.Y.
National Health and Welfare Retirement Association, Inc., 10 E. 40th St., New York, N.Y.

National Jewish Welfare Board, 145 E. 32d St., New York, N.Y.

National League of Nursing Education, 2 Park Ave., New York, N.Y.

National Manufacturers Association, 14 W. 49th St., New York, N.Y.

National Nursing Accrediting Service, 2 Park Ave., New York, N.Y.

National Organization for Public Health Nursing, 2 Park Ave., New York, N.Y.

National Recreation Association, 315 Fourth Ave., New York, N.Y.

National Safety Council, 425 N. Michigan Ave., Chicago, Ill.

National Society for Crippled Children and Adults, 1790 Broadway, New York, N.Y.

National Society for the Prevention of Blindness, 1790 Broadway, New York, N.Y.

National Tuberculosis Association, 1790 Broadway, New York, N.Y.

National Vocational Guidance Association, 1424 16th St., N.W., Washington, D.C.

Navy Nurse Corps, Potomac Annex, Navy Department, Washington, D.C.

New York State Employment Service, 119 W. 57th St., New York, N.Y. Camp Unit, 1 E. 19th St., New York, N.Y.

Nursing World, 468 Fourth Ave., New York, N.Y.

Planned Parenthood Federation of America, Inc., 501 Madison Ave., New York, N.Y.

Public Affairs Committee, 22 East 38th St., New York, N.Y.

Public Health Nursing, 2 Park Ave., New York, N.Y.

R.N., A Magazine for Nurses, Rutherford, N.J.

Rockefeller Foundation, 49 W. 49th St., New York, N.Y.

Rosenwald Fund, 4901 Ellis Ave., Chicago, Ill.

Social Security Administration, Federal Security Agency, Washington, D.C.

Today's Health (formerly *Hygeia*), 535 N. Dearborn St., Chicago, Ill.

Transcontinental and Western Air, Inc., Kansas City, Mo.

Transportation Association of America, 40 E. 40th St., New York, N.Y.

United Airlines, 5959 S. Cicero Ave., Chicago, Ill.

United States Civil Service Commission, Washington, D.C.

United States Maritime Commission, 45 Broadway, New York, N.Y.

United States Public Health Service, Federal Security Agency, Washington, D.C.

Veterans Administration, Washington, D.C.

Western Airlines, Inc., 6331 Hollywood Blvd., Los Angeles, Calif.

APPENDIX B

Bibliography

Guidance

(See also bibliographies in preceding chapters.)

1. ADKINS, DOROTHY C.: "Construction and Analysis of Achievement Tests," Government Printing Office, Washington, D.C., 1947.
2. ADKINS, DOROTHY C.: Construction and Analysis of Written Tests for Predicting Job Performance, *The Compass*, p. 24, January, 1946.
3. AMERICAN NURSES ASSOCIATION, PROFESSIONAL COUNSELING AND PLACEMENT SERVICE: "Manual of Counseling and Placement," New York, 1950.
4. BABCOCK, CHARLOTTE G.: Emotional Needs of Nursing Students, *American Journal of Nursing*, p. 166, March, 1949.
5. BERHARD, ROSE K., and others: A Guidance Program in a School of Nursing, *American Journal of Nursing*, p. 774, August, 1944.
6. BINGHAM, WALTER V.: "Aptitudes and Aptitude Testing," Harper & Brothers, New York, 1937.
7. BINGHAM, WALTER V., and BRUCE V. MOORE, "How to Interview," Harper & Brothers, New York, 1931.
8. CUNNINGHAM, BESS V.: "Psychology for Nurses," Chaps. XII, XIII, Appleton-Century Crofts, Inc., New York, 1941.
9. DAVIES, ELSIE, and HARRIET FROST: Health Service in a Nursing School, *American Journal of Nursing*, p. 421, June, 1940.
10. DENSFORD, KATHARINE J., and MILLARD S. EVERETT: "Ethics for Modern Nurses," W. B. Saunders Company, Philadelphia, 1946.
11. Employment Services, "Social Work Year Book," pp. 170–177 (General Background), pp. 218-225, (Guidance and Counseling), and p. 224, Bibliography, American Association of Social Workers, New York, 1951.
12. FARRELL, MARIE: The Personal Interview in Selecting Personnel, *American Journal of Nursing*, p. 303, May, 1940.
13. FELDER, ROSE: The Handicapped Nurse, *American Journal of Nursing*, p. 155, March, 1949.

14. FITZPATRICK, CHARLES P.: A Psychiatrist's View on "Guidance" of the Student Nurse, *American Journal of Nursing*, p. 588, June, 1944.
15. GARRETT, ANNETTA M.: "Interviewing—Its Principles and Methods," Family Welfare Association of America, New York, 1942.
16. GORDON, H. PHOEBE, KATHARINE J. DENSFORD, and E. G. WILLIAMSON: "Counseling in Schools of Nursing," McGraw-Hill Book Company, Inc., New York, 1947.
17. "Guidance Program for Schools of Nursing," National League of Nursing Education, New York, 1946; and "Handbook for Career Counselors," New York, 1948.
18. "Guidance—Vocational and Personal," New Jersey State Teachers College, Upper Montclair, N.J., 1945. (Lists, charts, posters, films, and publications for teaching aids in vocational guidance. See especially references under Good Manners, Good Speech and Physical Fitness, Good Grooming and Suitable Clothes. Section on Nursing is out of date.)
19. HANSEN, HELEN E.: "Professional Relationships of the Nurse," W. B. Saunders Company, Philadelphia, 1947.
20. HOPPOCK, ROBERT: "Group Guidance: Principles, Techniques and Evaluation," McGraw-Hill Book Company, Inc., New York, 1949.
21. KAUFMANN, FRITZ: "Your Job," Harper & Brothers, New York, 1950.
22. Labor standards, see *Monthly Labor Review*, U.S. Bureau of Labor Standards, Washington, D.C.; also *Facts on Women Workers*, Women's Bureau, Department of Labor, Washington, D.C.
23. LEONARD, MARGARET L.: "Health Counseling for Girls," A. S. Barnes and Company, New York, 1944.
24. LONG, LILLIAN D.: New Methods in the Selection of Public Health Personnel, *Canadian Journal of Public Health*, January, 1945.
25. McGLINCHEY, GRACE: Counseling and Placement, *American Journal of Nursing*, p. 235, April, 1947.
26. McMANUS, R. LOUISE: The Use of Tests in Professional Nursing, *Public Health Nursing*, p. 68, February, 1947.
27. MERRIAM, THORNTON W., and others: "Religious Counseling of College Students," American Council on Education, Washington, D.C., 1949.
28. MOSHER, W. E., J. DONALD KINGSLEY, and O. GLENN STAHL: "Personnel Administration," 3d ed., Parts II and IV, Harper & Brothers, New York, 1950.
29. MOSIER, CHARLES J.: Rating of Training and Experience in Public Personnel Selection, *The Compass*, p. 31, January, 1946. (Very clear and helpful explanation of methods.)
30. MYERS, GEORGE E.: "Principles and Techniques of Vocational Guidance," McGraw-Hill Book Company, Inc., New York, 1941.
31. Nursing Personnel Administration, *American Journal of Nursing*, p. 365, May, 1945.
32. *Occupations—The Vocational Guidance Magazine* (monthly), Vocational Guidance Association, Washington, D.C.

33. OED, MINNIE K.: Helping the Bewildered Adolescent, *American Journal of Nursing*, p. 296, May, 1950.

34. SHALIT, PEARL R.: Supervisor as Counselor, *Public Health Nursing*, p. 130, March, 1949.

35. SPALDING, EUGENIA K.: Orientation of the Nursing Student, *American Journal of Nursing,* p. 1047, December, 1945.

36. SPALDING, EUGENIA K.: "Professional Adjustments," rev. ed., J. B. Lippincott Company, Philadelphia, 1950.

37. SPALDING, EUGENIA K.: Your Problems—As a Nurse and a Woman, *American Journal of Nursing*, p. 945, October, 1944.

38. STRANG, RUTH M.: Appraising Family Activities Related to Student Progress, *American Journal of Nursing*, p. 44, January, 1951.

39. STRANG, RUTH M.: "Group Activities in College and Secondary School," Harper & Brothers, New York, 1941.

40. Student Personnel Work, Bibliography, *American Journal of Nursing*, p. 301, May, 1950.

41. Suggestions for Counselors of Professional Nurses, Committee on Vocational Guidance, *American Journal of Nursing*, April, 1948.

42. SUTHERLAND, JEAN E.: Counseling Professional Nurses, *Public Health Nursing*, p. 240, May, 1948.

43. TEAD, ORDWAY, and HENRY C. METCALF: "Personnel Administration, Its Principles and Practice," McGraw-Hill Book Company, Inc., New York, 1933.

44. "Training of Vocational Counselors," Superintendent of Documents, Government Printing Office, Washington, D.C. (Used by office of War Manpower Commission during the war.)

45. TRAVIS, L. E., and D. W. BARUCH: "Personnel Problems of Everyday Life," Appleton-Century Crofts, Inc., New York, 1941.

46. TRIGGS, FRANCES O.: "Personnel Work in Schools of Nursing," W. B. Saunders Company, Philadelphia, 1945.

47. U.S. PUBLIC HEALTH SERVICE: "Study of Nursing School Health Practices and a Recommended Health Program for Student Nurses," Public Health Reports, Supplement No. 189, Washington, D.C., 1945.

48. WILLIAMSON, E. G.: "How to Counsel Students," McGraw-Hill Book Company, Inc., New York, 1939.

49. WILLIAMSON, E. G. (ed.): "Trends in Student Personnel Work," University of Minnesota Press, Minneapolis, 1949.

50. ZACHRY, CAROLINE B.: "Emotion and Conduct in Adolescence," Appleton-Century-Crofts, Inc., New York, 1940.

APPENDIX C

Recruiting Nurses

Professional nurses are often asked by their younger friends, by high school teachers and vocational counselors, and by community groups to "tell about nursing" or to explain how one becomes a nurse. Young people ask: Where shall I go for my nursing course? How do I know I will like nursing as much as I think I do? Will I be able to do the work? A parent asks: Shall I let my daughter be a nurse? How many times these questions cross our paths! Recruitment is every nurse's job, but it is not always easy to know how to answer questions, how to give accurate information, or how to make an effective speech on the subject. Yet it is important to reach the 'teen-age group and their parents and advisers with reliable information about nursing as it is today. It is tragic to hear older professional nurses say: "I wouldn't advise any girl to go into nursing." Either they do not know modern nursing or they are expressing their personal frustrations in it. They are surely forgetting the strongest underlying motive for "going into nursing"—the desire to take care of sick people. If a young person wants to do that strongly enough, he or she will pursue the needed information until someone offers encouragement, but the young man or woman who is thinking about nursing as a career and weighing it against other openings, may be balked by sour comments and confusing directions as to how to go about entering a school of nursing. We need nurses. That is the reason why this appendix has been added to the book. If you can't give enthusiatic backing to the idea of a friend or relative entering nursing, at least share the following information and let the prospective student make his or her own decision.

Advice to the would-be nurse starts with the classic question: do you like to work with people? Would you prefer to work with people—rather than with things, such as books, machines, food? If this question is answered in a warm affirmative, other qualifications should be mentioned, such as the importance of steady attention to a job to be done, common sense, poise, tact, good judgment, and neatness. A person of sixteen or seventeen knows herself fairly accurately in relation to these qualities and will describe her shortcomings honestly if she sees you are trying to help her. The importance of good health need not be overstressed, and one can point out how carefully health is watched during training, but it is well to find out whether there is any history of rheumatic fever, tuberculosis, easy fatigue, or frequent respiratory infections. Do not be too optimistic with such a student. It can be said with truth that any healthy young woman or young man who is active in sports and not overtired at the end of each day will not find nursing too hard, and many will feel better than they have ever been and come out of the school better fitted for the work of the world than many of their classmates. All students are given preliminary medical examinations anyway, and no student will be accepted if there is the slightest question of physical inability to carry the work or harm to himself in so doing.

Advisers should prepare themselves to answer these questions:

1. How old must I be to enter a school of nursing?

   Most schools admit at eighteen, a few at seventeen. The upper age limit is thirty-five.

2. How long is the course?

   The diploma course is 3 years, the collegiate course 4 to 5 years. The latter combines college and nursing, conferring a B.S. degree with your R.N. Stress desirability of combined courses and experience.

3. Do I have to have finished high school?

   Indeed, yes; and you should have graduated in the upper third of your class, if possible. (For entrance requirements for the schools of practical nursing, see Chap. XVIII.)

4. How much will the course cost?

   The cost varies. It may be anywhere from a few dollars, for current expenses and books, to $1,000. A tuition fee of $200 is usual for the diploma course. However, scholarships are available. Ask about them when you apply to the school of your choice. Also, ask whether there is any government aid possible.

5. Explain what is meant by R.N.

6. Young people should be told what subjects to study in high school. If you do not have the latest suggestions, better advise the prospective nurse to write either to the school of nursing she has chosen or to the Committee on Careers in Nursing.[1]

7. How do I apply to a school?

   By letter or by a request for an interview with the director.

8. Which school should I choose?

   This is the "$64 question." Most advisers would not make the decision for a student, but friends often do on the basis of their own preference or experience. The best plan is the one recommended by the schools themselves: Give the student the following list of questions and let her seek the answers. She will learn much about what is meant by a good school, if she seeks the answers honestly. She may need help as she studies her school catalogues; but the school of *your* choice may not be the best for her.

[1] For addresses of organizations mentioned in this section, see Appendix A.

Decide first whether you wish to enter (1) a hospital school where you will spend 3 years securing a basic professional nursing education, or (2) a school of nursing connected with a college or university where you may secure both a diploma in nursing and a bachelor's degree in 4 or 5 years. Among about 1,300 schools of nursing in the United States, 140 offer undergraduate programs leading to a degree.

Then choose at least three schools which you would like to attend, and compare them carefully by asking directors of the schools, asking nurses and doctors you know, such questions as these about each school (answers should be "yes"):

1. Is it accredited under state law? (Only graduates of state approved schools are eligible to take state examinations for registration.)
2. Is it equipped to give you clinical experience in medical, surgical, maternity, and pediatric nursing? It should give you some experience, also, in psychiatric, communicable disease, and public health nursing, and in an out-patient department.
3. Is the work week, including classes, no longer than 48 hours? (Remember, you will need time for study and for recreation.)
4. Does the students' residence have single, or at most double rooms, the latter adequately equipped for two people?
5. Does the student health service include an initial and annual examination with chest x-rays, preventive inoculations, medical and nursing care in case of illness, and follow-up service throughout the entire program for correction of remediable defects?
6. Who are the school's leading graduates, and are they holding good positions?
7. Does the hospital used for practice by the school of nursing meet requirements of the American College of Surgeons?
8. Does the hospital have a daily average of at least 100 patients? If not, does it offer supplementary experience through affiliation with other hospitals?[2]
9. What salary can I expect when I graduate and have my R.N.? Beginning salaries vary with the area of the country in which you plan to work, but you can be assured that they now compare well with those of other beginning salaries for women in business. A general average would be $2,500 with yearly increases for staff work up to $3,000. However, there are higher beginning salaries in some places—$3,100, for example. If you rise to the head of your profession, you can make as much as $10,000 to $12,000 a year.

In preparing speeches on this subject, it is particularly important to stress the need for nurses; the prospect of a full, satisfying, often exciting career, which thousands of nurses combine with marriage; the desirability of the preparation for homemaking, marriage, and rearing children; and the advantages of a nursing background no matter where one goes or what the future

[2] Quoted from "*Nursing Offers You a Career, Now,*" published by the Committee on Careers in Nursing, 1951.

holds. Point out that this is a field where there is a continual demand not affected by seasons or time or place and that there are many opportunities now available for advanced study and specialization.

Since a speech full of glittering generalities does not stay with the audience, weave in specific facts, figures, and your own personal experiences. If there is time, get the facts from your state nurses association or the nearest large school of nursing. When you speak, explain why you like nursing; give a telling example of how a nurse can give effective service; and be sure to stress the new and better working conditions under which nurses serve nowadays. It will be a long time before we live down the floor-scrubbing era.

If it is possible to close a high school speech with an invitation to the seniors to visit the nearest large school of nursing and connected hospital, it makes your remarks definite and purposeful and is usually a welcome suggestion. You should make yourself available to answer questions individually. The latest career pamphlets from your state or national nursing headquarters should be distributed at the end of the meeting—not before—or arrangements may be made to show one of the new nursing recruitment films. Nursing headquarters will have information about these also.

In short, there is no excuse not to be ready to answer questions about nursing or to refuse an invitation to talk about it to any group interested. Recruitment is everybody's job.

List of Visual Aids

The following list of visual aids may be found useful as information to supplement that given in the text. The films listed are only samples of available material and should be previewed before used to make sure that the subject will fit the interests of the audience.

These films can be obtained from the distributor or producer; their full titles and addresses are given at the end of the list. In some cases the films will be available at your local film library or film distributor, or they may be borrowed from the film libraries of universities. The running time (min), and indications whether it is silent (si) or sound (sd) and motion picture (MP) or filmstrip (FS) are given with each title. The titles not listed as color (C) are black and white. All the motion pictures are 16mm, unless otherwise indicated. All filmstrips are 35mm.

Suggestions for criteria to use in selecting and handling films for educational purposes may be found in the *American Journal of Nursing*, June, 1945, p. 479, and see also, How to Find What Health Education Materials You're Looking For (reprint), *American Journal of Public Health*, January, 1948, and Adventuring with Visual Education, Winifred L. Moore, *Public Health Nursing*, March, 1949, p. 134.

Film users who wish a more complete bibliography of films dealing with nursing education, including related subjects, should obtain "Selected Motion Pictures and Slidefilms for Nursing Education," published by Indiana University, Bloomington, Indiana. Moreover, nurses and prospective nurses who wish to have information on new films should periodically examine "Educational Film Guide," a yearly catalogue with quarterly supplements published by the H. W. Wilson Co., New York, N.Y. "The Guide," a standard reference book, is available in most college and public libraries.

Occasionally a full-length dramatic film or play will offer an authentic and interesting presentation of professional nurses at work. Unfortunately, authenticity is sometimes sacrificed for sensationalism, but the vocational counselor should watch current motion picture productions and theatrical presentations for worth-while illustrations of the varying conditions and duties of different nursing jobs. Examples of such productions are *So Proudly We Hail* (Paramount), starring Claudette Colbert as an Army nurse on Bataan and Corregidor; on the stage, the play *Bataan* gave an exaggerated picture of the life of an Army nurse; *South Pacific's* heroine is a Navy nurse; and *The Hasty Heart*, which has been produced on the stage and in the movies, features British nurses.

There also appear from time to time special recruiting films for governmental or private services, such as those produced by the Army and Navy Nurse Corps. Current information regarding the latest and best in these films may be secured from the agencies themselves. (See lists at end of each chapter in this book.)

Chapter I

About Faces (MP; USPHS; 10 min). How Danny Smith took good care of his teeth and the results of inadequate dental care. Short version of a motion picture with the same title produced by the American Dental Association.

Act Your Age (MP; Coronet; 14 min). Common types of infantile reactions—temper, weeping, etc. Reasons for emotional immaturity in adolescence.

Attitudes and Health (MP; Coronet; 10 min). Simplified explanation of some of the ways in which emotional problems affect physical health.

Breast Self-examination (MP; ACS/Assn; 15 min). Importance of breast self-examination in the identification of cancer; techniques to be used.

Care of the Feet (MP; EBF; 11 min). Structural elements of the foot; how walking is accomplished; causes of structural foot ailments and remedies therefor; other kinds of foot ailments and their remedies. (Accompanying filmstrip, same title, also available.)

Care of the Skin (MP; EBF; 10 min). Good habits of skin hygiene. For juvenile audiences.

Cleanliness and Health (MP; Coronet; 10 min). Importance of cleanliness to good health.

Dale Carnegie Series (FS; Audivision; 6 filmstrips, each with accompanying record, 15 min, 16 inch, 33⅓ r.p.m.). Series based upon Carnegie's book "How To Win Friends and Influence People." Individual titles are
How To Gather Honey Instead of Stings
How To Get People To Like You
How To Make People Appreciate You
How To Make People Want To Cooperate
How To Win Your Arguments
How To Correct People's Mistakes without Making Them Sore

Dental Health—How and Why (MP; Coronet; 10 min). Research in dental health; diet and dental health; latest techniques of oral hygiene.

Ears and Hearing (MP; EBF; 11 min). Physiology of the ear; mechanics of sound wave transmission to the ear and brain; common causes of impaired hearing.

Exercise and Health (MP; Coronet; 10 min). Three instances of the value of exercise, particularly participation in athletics.

Eyes and Their Care (MP; EBF; 11 min). Physiology and hygiene of the eye; eye movements, light receptors, field of vision, night blindness, double vision, near-sightedness and far-sightedness; protection of the eyes. (Accompanying filmstrip, same title, also available.)

Eyes That Hear (MP; Lex Sch Deaf; 15 min). Program for educating the deaf at the Lexington School for the Deaf.

Hidden Hunger (MP; Swift; 30 min). A farmer conducts a one-man campaign to improve the eating habits of the nation, and prevents the kind of hunger that comes from not eating the right foods.

If It's Health You're Seeking (MP; NMPC; 30 min silent). Diet, fresh air and sunshine, exercise, sleep, posture, cleanliness, care of the teeth and eyes, vaccination and preventive inoculation.

It's Your Health (MP; So Cal Dental; 18 min). Mouth hygiene, dental care, and the importance of diet in protecting dental health.

Marriage for Moderns (MP; McGraw). Series of five films based upon the book "Marriage for Moderns," by Henry Bowman. Titles are
Choosing for Happiness (14 min)
It Takes All Kinds (20 min)
Marriage Today (22 min)
This Charming Couple (19 min)
Who's Boss (16 min)

A New Supervisor Takes a Look at His Job (MP; USOE/UWF; 13 min). A machine tool operator is made a group leader and his plant superintendent explains to him, through dramatized illustrations, the meaning of working with people instead of machines. (Problems in supervision series)

Now for Tomorrow (MP; Harmon; 45 min silent). A study of the necessity of making adequate provision for old age security, with particular application to the nursing profession.

The Nurse (MP; EBF; 11 min). Describes some of the typical activities of nurses in the pediatrics, emergency, and maternity wards of a hospital. Emphasizes the importance of nursing as a career. Educational consultant: Elizabeth S. Bixley, Yale University.

Nursing (MP; VGF; 11 min). Vocational guidance film showing various nursing opportunities and attendant responsibilities, and explaining qualifications and requirements for nursing careers.

On Your Feet (MP; USPHS; 10 min). Importance of walking correctly and comfortably; good posture; properly fitted shoes; how to walk correctly; how shoes should fit.

Placing the Right Man on the Job (MP; USOE/UWF; 13 min). Dramatized cases of five different workers, unsatisfied in particular jobs, who are reassigned to other jobs more suitable to their abilities and capacities. (Problems in supervision series)

Posture (MP; EBF; 15 min silent). Effect of posture upon the size of the chest, the position of the abdominal organs, and general personal appearance.

Posture and Personality (MP; Soc Sci Films; 12 min). Influence of posture on personal appearance and efficiency in sports and games, in making friends, and in getting a job.

Posture for Poise (MP; Iowa; 22 min silent). Natural situations in which posture is important, selected from the everyday life of a girl or young woman.

Proof of the Pudding (MP; Met Life; 10 min). Importance of good nutrition; food requirements of the body; results of good and bad diets.

Rest and Health (MP; Coronet; 10 min). Importance of rest and sleep and their beneficial effects on every daily activity.

Save Those Teeth (MP; EBF; 11 min). Importance of proper cleansing of the teeth; effect of sugar upon teeth; use of sodium fluoride in the prevention of tooth decay.

Skin (MP; EBF; 15 min silent). Structure of skin; growth of cells; secretion of sweat; structure of hair and nails.

The Supervisor As a Leader. Part 1 (MP; USOE/UWF; 14 min). Four dramatized episodes illustrating poor supervisory practices and the importance of the following rules: Always keep promises. Never take credit for someone else's work. Don't pass the buck. Don't play favorites. (Problems in supervision series)

The Supervisor As a Leader, Part 2 (MP; USOE/UWF; 13 min). Four more dramatized instances of poor supervision leading to the following generalizations: Be a leader, not an authoritarian. Show appreciation for a job well done. Do not become angry. Protect the rights and feelings of workers. (Problems in supervision series)

This Way to Nursing (MP; Yorke; 20 min). Shows theoretical and practical instruction incorporated in the student nurse course of a typical accredited school of nursing. Narrated by Milton Cross.

Working with Other Supervisors (MP; USOE/UWF; 8 min). A worker fails as a supervisor because he does not recognize the importance of working harmoniously with other people, particularly with his fellow supervisors. (Problems in supervision series)

CHAPTER VI

Family Circles (MP; CNFB/McGraw; 31 min). Interplay of home and school influences upon children.

Helping the Child To Face the Don't's (MP; EBF; 11 min). How a young child meets a world of "don't's" and how he reacts to such instructions.

Helping the Child To Accept the Do's (MP; EBF; 11 min). Child development illustrated through his acceptance of the "do's."

Life Begins (MP; EBF; 60 min). Photographic record of the Gesell studies at the Yale Clinic of Child Development.

Posture and Locomotion (MP; EBF; 11 min). Infant development from helpless immaturity to controlled locomotion; biographic series of 13 age levels based upon Gesell research studies at Yale Clinic of Child Development.

Ways to Good Habits (MP; Coronet; 10 min). Importance of habits, good and bad, and how to substitute good habits for bad ones. For juvenile audiences.

Your Child's First Visit to the Dentist (MP; ADA; 8 min). Suggestions for parents in the preparation of a child's visit to the dentist.

CHAPTER VII

A Nurse's Day with the Mentally Ill (MP; PCR; 28 min silent). Training of student nurses in a modern psychiatric department. Illustrates nursing care in excitement states (including hydrotherapy and seclusion); in tension states (including tube feeding, sedative packs, and massage); and in hypoglycemic and convulsive shock therapy.

Preface to a Life (MP; USPHS/UWF; 29 min). Parental influence on a child's developing personality illustrated through three attitudes: overly solicitous mother, overly demanding father, and both parents' acceptance of the child as an individual.

Psychiatry in Action (MP; BIS; 62 min). Treatment of war neuroses in British hospitals and results of such treatment.

Unconscious Motivation (MP; Assn; 40 min). How unconscious motives influence our everyday thoughts, feelings, and actions. Techniques used to detect troublesome, repressed ideas lying beyond conscious reach.

CHAPTER VIII

Accent on Use (MP; NFIP; 20 min). Techniques of physical therapy and their importance in the treatment of infantile paralysis.

First As a Child (MP; Va Health/IFB; 20 min). Story of a crippled child and the care he receives in a public clinic in Virginia.

How To Avoid Muscle Strains (MP; Bray; 15 min). Some of the ways that body muscles may be strained, and complications that may result.

Teaching Crutch Walking (MP; USOE/UWF; 13 min). How to teach the patient to walk in a walker; use various methods of crutch walking; sit, rise, and climb stairs; and the safety factors in crutch walking. (Supplementary filmstrip, same title, also available.)

CHAPTER IX

Cloud in the Sky (MP; NTA; 18 min). Story of a family whose mother dies of tuberculosis; the eldest daughter's symptoms of tuberculosis; and the aid of the priest in convincing the family to see the doctor.

Feeling All Right (MP; CMC; 30 min). Produced by Mississippi State Board of Health. VD case finding, detecting, treating, and educating the public in the facts about syphilis, illustrated through a story of a young man who contracts the disease. All Negro cast.

Guardians of Our Country's Health (MP; Frith; 16 min). Work of the quarantine stations of the U.S. Public Health Service.

His Fighting Chance (MP; BIS; 10 min). Treatment and rehabilitation of poliomyelitis patients in England. Produced for the British Ministry of Health.

Let My People Live (MP; NTA; 15 min). Story of a Southern Negro family whose superstitious mother dies of tuberculosis but whose son and daughter are saved, not by "cures" but by modern medical care.

Magic Bullets (MP; USPHS; 30 min). Dr. Paul Ehrlich discovers a cure for syphilis after years of experimenting with arsenic and bismuth. Short, edited version of "Dr. Ehrlich's Magic Bullets."

On the Firing Line (MP; NTA; 20 min). Visit to various sanitoriums and research laboratories to show ways in which tuberculosis was being controlled in the United States in 1939.

Striking Back against Rabies (MP; USPHS/UWF; 11 min). Typical county rabies epidemic checked by joint emergency control measures of county health department, state public health veterinarian, and federal rabies control expert.

Three Counties Against Syphilis (MP; USPHS; 17 min). Methods used in Georgia to locate cases of syphilis and to provide treatment in city and community.

With These Weapons: The Story of Syphilis (MP; ASHA; 11 min). Syphilis and its relation to personal, family, and community health.

You Can Help (MP; NTA; 10 min). Organization and activities of the National Tuberculosis Association.

Chapter XI

So Much for So Little (MP; USPHS; 11 min). Health hazards threatening a typical American family successfully controlled by a properly staffed local health department.

Your Health Department (MP; NMPC; 20 min). Functioning of a modern health department and how it affects the lives of all.

Chapter XVI

The Army Nurse (MP; USA/UWF; 13 min). Duties and work of Army nurses near battle lines, in field and evacuation hospitals, and on airplanes and vessels.

Family Life of the Navaho Indians (MP; NYU; 31 min silent). Some of the ways in which the Navaho child develops into a typical Navaho adult.

Chapter XVII

The Baby Sitter (MP; YAF; 14 min). The duties and responsibilities of a properly trained baby sitter.

Journey into Medicine (MP; **USPHS/UWF**; 39 min). One doctor's "journey into medicine"; studies in medical school, graduation, internship, further study in pediatrics, decision to specialize in public health.

SOURCES OF FILMS LISTED

ACS—American Cancer Society, 47 Beaver St., New York, N.Y.

ADA—American Dental Association, 222 East Superior St., Chicago, Ill.

ASHA—American Social Hygiene Association, Inc., 1790 Broadway, New York, N.Y.

Assn—Association Films, Inc., 35 West 45th St., New York, N.Y.; 79 East Adams St., Chicago, Ill.; 351 Turk St., San Francisco, Calif.; 1915 Live Oak St., Dallas, Texas

Audivision—Audivision, Inc., 285 Madison Ave., New York, N.Y.

BIS—British Information Services, 30 Rockefeller Plaza, New York, N.Y.

Bray—Bray Studios, Inc., 729 Seventh Ave., New York, N.Y.

CMC—Communication Materials Center, 413 West 117th St., New York, N.Y.

Coronet—Coronet Films, Coronet Bldg., Chicago, Ill.

EBF—Encyclopaedia Britannica Films, Inc., 1150 Wilmette Ave., Wilmette, Ill.

Frith—Frith Films, 1816 North Highland, Hollywood, Calif.

Harmon—Harmon Foundation, Division of Visual Experiment, 140 Nassau St., New York, N.Y.

IFB—International Film Bureau, Suite 1500, 6 North Michigan Ave., Chicago, Ill.

Iowa—State University of Iowa, Bureau of Visual Instruction, Iowa City, Iowa.

Lex Sch Deaf—Lexington School for the Deaf, 904 Lexington Ave., New York, N.Y.

McGraw—McGraw-Hill Book Co., Inc., Text-Film Dept., 330 West 42d St., New York, N.Y.

Met Life—Metropolitan Life Insurance Co., 1 Madison Ave., New York, N.Y.

NFIP—National Foundation for Infantile Paralysis, Inc., 120 Broadway, New York, N.Y.

NMPC—National Motion Picture Co., Mooresville, Ind.

NTA—National Tuberculosis Association, 1790 Broadway, New York, N.Y.

NYU—New York University Film Library, 26 Washington Pl., New York, N.Y.

PCR—Psychological Cinema Register, Pennsylvania State College, State College, Penna.

So Cal Dental—Southern California State Dental Assn., 903 Crenshaw Blvd., Los Angeles, Calif.

Soc Sci Films—Social Science Films, 4030 Chouteau Ave., St. Louis, Mo.

Swift—Swift & Co., Public Relations Dept., Chicago, Ill.

USA—U.S. Department of the Army, Washington, D.C.

USOE—U.S. Office of Education, Washington, D.C.

USPHS—U.S. Public Health Service, Public Inquiries Branch, Washington, D.C.

UWF—United World Films, Inc., 1445 Park Ave., New York, N.Y.

Va Health—Virginia State Department of Health, Richmond, Va.

VGF—Vocational Guidance Films, 215 East 3d St., Des Moines, Iowa

YAF—Young America Films, Inc., 18 East 41st St., New York, N.Y.

Yorke—Emerson Yorke Studio, 245 West 55th St., New York, N.Y.

INDEX

341